S0-CWS-934

The Challenges of Community Medicine

The Challenges of Community Medicine

Edited by

ROBERT L. KANE, M.D.

SP

Springer Publishing Company

New York

Springer Publishing Company, Inc.
200 Park Avenue South
New York, N.Y. 10003

74 75 76 77 78 / 10 9 8 7 6 5 4 3 2 1

Kane, Robert Lewis, 1940–
The challenges of community medicine.

Includes bibliographical references.
1. Community health services. 2. Medical care.
3. Hygiene, Public. 4. Epidemiology. I. Title.
II. Title: Community medicine. [DNLM: 1. Comprehensive health care. WA100 K153c]
RA427.K28 362.1'04'25 73-92198
ISBN 0-8261-1670-1

Printed in the United States of America

CONTENTS

CONTRIBUTORS

Robert H. Brook, M.D., Sc.D.
Assistant Professor, Department of Medicine
School of Medicine
University of California, Los Angeles

John Cassel, M.D., M.P.H.
Professor and Chairman, Department of Epidemiology
School of Public Health
University of North Carolina, Chapel Hill

Rodney M. Coe, Ph.D.
Professor, Department of Community Medicine
School of Medicine
St. Louis University, St. Louis, Mo.

O. Lynn Deniston
Research Associate, Department of Community Health Services
School of Public Health
University of Michigan, Ann Arbor

Hugh S. Fulmer, M.D., M.P.H.
Professor and Chairman, Department of Community Medicine
University of Massachusetts Medical School, Worcester

Ruth Henson
Department of Family and Community Medicine
College of Medicine
University of Utah, Salt Lake City

James R. Jeffers, Ph.D.
Associate Professor of Economics and Director, Health Economics Research Center
Department of Economics
College of Business Administration
University of Iowa, Iowa City

Robert L. Kane, M.D.
Associate Professor, Department of Family and Community Medicine
College of Medicine
University of Utah, Salt Lake City

Rosalie A. Kane, M.S.W.
Assistant Professor
Graduate School of Social Work
University of Utah, Salt Lake City

Thomas C. King, M.D.
Professor of Surgery
College of Physicians and Surgeons
Columbia University, New York, N.Y.

Charles E. Lewis, M.D.
Professor of Medicine and Public Health, Department of Medicine
School of Medicine, The Center for the Health Sciences
University of California, Los Angeles

Thomas M. Mack, M.D.
Assistant Professor, Department of Epidemiology
School of Public Health
Harvard University, Boston, Mass.

John M. Peters, M.D., Sc.D., M.P.H.
Associate Professor of Occupational Medicine, Department of Physiology
School of Public Health
Harvard University, Boston, Mass.

John Powles, M.B.
Research Fellow
Centre for Social Research
University of Sussex, Falmer, Brighton, England

Jesse W. Tapp, M.D., M.P.H.
Professor, Department of Family and Community Medicine
College of Medicine
University of Arizona, Tucson

Jonathan B. Weisbuch, M.D., M.P.H.
Associate Professor, Department of Community Medicine
School of Medicine
Boston University, Boston, Mass.

PREFACE

For the author or editor, the creation of an introductory text presents the task of providing enough information, without overwhelming the reader. The purpose of this book is to orient students of medicine and other health professions to the wider perspective of the community and thereby to acquaint them with the numerous factors that impinge on the health of a community. The intent is to broaden students' horizons; thus the scope of the book ought of necessity to be broad. My colleagues and I have tried to cover the major areas of community medicine and thus to provide at least a taste of each. Documentation for statements made in the text is placed at the end of each chapter, along with additional references and suggested readings where appropriate. These readings are not intended to be encyclopedic but rather to offer relevant samples of the literature available.

The appendix describes an approach to the teaching of community medicine that emphasizes the active involvement of the student in the learning process. The development of this approach by departments and teachers of community medicine is a milestone in the evolution of this branch of medical education.

One of the constant themes in this book is the multidisciplinary nature of community medicine. In fact, the development of this book is an example of the application of the team concept—a concept that currently permeates the thinking of everyone concerned with the health care system. Few teams have had to work together under such difficult circumstances. Separated by vast geographic distances, representing a variety of disciplines, beset by diverse responsibilities and time demands, our team was nonetheless able to work toward a common goal as each member carried out his assigned task. Since the authors of the various chapters represent several disciplines, the editor was faced with certain problems which required that compromises be made. In editing any multi-authored volume, one must trade off the different writing styles of the contributors against their specific competencies in their respective areas. We hope that the editing has succeeded in removing all glaring differences while permitting the individual personality of each author and the distinctive style of the discipline he represents to emerge.

All the chapters except the ones by Robert H. Brook and John Powles are original material, published here for the first time. The *Journal of Medical Education* and *Science, Medicine and Man* generously permitted us to reprint the articles by Brook and Powles, respectively. We should like to give special bouquets to three individuals whose major contributions helped make this book a reality. Ruth Henson's painstaking and meticulous technical editing brought the raw material into an integrated whole. Judy Gerlach's and Linda Twitchell's patience and diligence sustained the entire effort through times of stress.

Robert L. Kane

To Miranda, Ingrid, and Kathryn

I

The Tools of Community Medicine

For many people, community medicine is viewed as the application of epidemiologic principles to areas not traditionally covered by that discipline. In this book we shall attempt to show why it is becoming increasingly difficult to define the exclusive scope of many of the disciplines utilized by practitioners of community medicine. The boundaries between the behavioral and clinical sciences blur as we recognize the growing importance of psychological factors to physical disorders. Similarly, the distance between the disease focus of traditional epidemiology and a health focus of community medicine, or an outcome focus of health services research, is short. If we can talk about an infectious agent as the cause of a given illness, why not a therapeutic agent as a cause of recovery from that illness?

In this first section, we outline what is meant by the concept and describe some of the basic techniques used in the study and practice of community medicine. We envision community medicine as a general organizational framework which draws upon a number of disciplines for its tools. In this sense, it is an applied discipline which adopts the knowledge and skills of other areas in its efforts to solve community health problems. The tools described here include community diagnosis (which draws upon such diverse fields as sociology, political science, economics, biostatistics, and epidemiology), epidemiology itself, and health services research (the application of epidemiologic techniques to analyzing the effects of medical care on health).

Because epidemiology lies so near to the heart of community medicine, a chapter which describes ways in which these basic concepts might be effectively incorporated into medical and/or health sciences curricula appears as an appendix to this book.

1

Community Medicine: What's in a Name?

Robert L. Kane

It is ironic that a profession which began in the community should suddenly need to rediscover it. Yet several centuries of gradually institutionalized medicine, followed by a technological revolution, progressively moved medical science farther from the people to be served and closer to the artificial life support system of the medical center. Medical care providers formed communities of their own where they spoke a special language and became dependent on a complicated network of machinery. The ill entered this world of medical science for intermittent encounters—therapeutic or otherwise—without disturbing the medical milieu.

Sometime in the last fifteen years, medicine rediscovered the community at large. Along with other subdivisions of our technological society, the medical profession—more specifically academic medicine—became aware of the vast gap that exists between knowledge acquired and the implementation of that knowledge. War was declared on poverty, ignorance, and disease; in a cautious descent from the ivory tower, medical educators recognized flaws in the cult of expertise. The era of revelation gave way to the era of relevance. Amidst these rites of passage, a new discipline—community medicine—emerged.

The struggle to define this new specialty goes on. Some maintain that community medicine is not a discipline or even an area of interest, but rather a social movement. Some members of this group believe that the movement represents only a repackaging of the time-honored concepts of preventive medicine; others view it as messianic, and look forward to its success in reuniting medicine with the people. In contrast, there are those who regard community medicine as a discipline that matches other medical specialties in scientific rigor.

Community medicine is by no means limited to the activities of physicians. Community nursing, community pharmacy, community pediatrics, and community mental health are terms which illustrate the fact that the community was rediscovered simultaneously by other disciplines within the medical team. Such diverse activities have been undertaken in the name of community medicine that definition has become a real problem. In their 1962 review of the teaching of preventive medicine, Shephard and Roney listed twenty different titles for such departments (1). Perhaps the most apt was "the specialty of ?" (2).

Community medicine may be perceived as a distinct third area within medical education, producing a triad of laboratory, hospital ward, and community. Its relevance to the study of the community has been underscored by an expert committee of the World Health Organization:

> The education of every physician should . . . enable him . . . to understand how factors affecting health can be examined and measured and to discern the practical steps that can be taken to counteract hazards; he should know enough about the economics and priorities of public health programs at both the local and national levels, to recognize when the local community must make important decisions and when the national cost of health services must be balanced against those of other community services. He should understand how health services operate and are related to one another, the principles governing the delivery of medical care, what parts are played by auxiliaries and other health workers, and the effects of culture on the demands for services and of the use made of them when they are provided (3).

We prefer the definition which allows for flexibility and scope in both teaching and research: "Community medicine is the academic discipline that deals with the identification and solution of the health problems of communities or human population groups" (4). We also accept the definition of community as "a group of individuals or families living together in a defined geographic area, usually comprising a village, town or city; these may represent only a few families in a rural area or may include heavily populated cities" (5). Indeed, the concept of extending the role of the health professional beyond the curative function is by no means novel. In a seldom quoted portion of his famous report Abraham Flexner noted: ". . . the physician's function is fast becoming social and preventive, rather than individual and curative. Upon him society relies to ascertain, and through measures essentially educational to enforce, the conditions that prevent disease and make positively for physical and moral well-being" (6). The burgeoning of community medicine departments in medical schools is a formal recognition of this responsibility.

Although the roots of community medicine (and/or its cousins, preventive medicine and social medicine) can be traced to Hippocrates' observations on the winds and waters, the impetus for the academic departments began with the formulation of the germ theory of disease and its implications for possible control of infectious disease through immunization, vector control, and sanitation.* Then, as the traditional ravagers of society were subdued, new problems emerged as "diseases of medical progress"; these problems were highlighted (e.g., heart disease and cancer), aggravated (e.g., nutritional deficiency), or created (e.g., environmental toxicology) by the earlier accomplishments.

The tools of epidemiology, originally honed to carve out an understanding of the determinants of disease, were gradually turned to newer tasks. Methods for the delivery of care and containment of disease became increasingly important as prevention and cure became increasingly difficult to achieve. Studies of chronic degenerative diseases have resulted in the erosion of the concept of a single causative agent and led to an appreciation of the multifactorial determinants of disease. The behavioral sciences have assumed greater importance as tools for predicting the occurence of disease through knowledge of phenomena such as social stress (7), as well as the factors associated with compliance with prolonged medical regimens.

The black bag of community medicine is steadily expanding. Biostatistics, once the dry manipulation of complex mathematical procedures, has been freed by the computer to expand into such exciting areas as medical diagnosis, simulation models of health situations, and rapid processing of large volumes of data. Environmental health has risen out of the privy to encounter the modern worldwide ecological concern with the overabundance of people and their various waste products.

The social revolution has produced a philosophy that health care should be readily accessible and that consumers of health services

*This portion of our discussion draws upon materials prepared by the Executive Committee of the Association of Teachers of Preventive Medicine, "Guidelines for the Development of Departments of Preventive, Social and Community Medicine and Public Health in Medical Schools in the United States and Canada," 1971, mimeographed.

should participate in planning and decision making. Health administration and health education must be remodeled if they are to keep pace with developments in economics and communications. Medical care which can fulfill the three C's—continuous, coordinated, and comprehensive—is sought, but at a price society can afford. Departments of community medicine with their emphasis on developing effective delivery systems can pose the questions and help find the answers which will respond to the demands for accessibility and accountability.

While the science of medicine is forging ahead, the social setting of medicine is caught up in its own revolution. Along with the university as a whole, the medical school has been challenged to restructure its position in the community. It too is deep in the debate over the ultimate role of the university—a protected storehouse of information and pure research, or a responsive organism sensitive to the changing needs and demands of society (8).

Heedful of the changing patterns of financial support from state and federal legislatures, many medical schools have already made their commitment by accepting a major service responsibility for a segment of the adjacent community. Often they have turned to their departments of community medicine to fulfill this obligation. This is not surprising, since community medicine has frequently been associated with, if not confused with, comprehensive medical care (9) or family medicine (10). Often new departments, glad of the recognition that goes with being given a task, accept the charge without examining whether providing direct care in the community is indeed their legitimate function (11).

Medical schools across the nation have moved to establish neighborhood health centers and to increase the services available through their outpatient departments. Yet in charging medical schools with primary responsibility in their relations with the community, Surgeon General Stewart indicated that programs of teaching and research should work as partners *with*, not just *in*, the community (12). The rush to provide direct services to underprivileged segments of the community may be an overreaction on the part of medical schools to shifts in public opinion about health care. Were the nation faced with a famine, we would not turn to the schools of agriculture with demands that they grow more wheat; rather, we would expect schools of agriculture to approach the problem scientifically in search of a solution which could be utilized by farmers. Would it not be appropriate for medical schools to provide that type of consultation and leadership in this period of medical care famine?

The skills of community medicine may play a vital role in our pursuit of answers to long-standing questions rather than in reprocessing and administering the old formulae. The potential for meaningful innovation in modes of delivering and organizing health services falls clearly within community medicine's area of competence. For example, a variety of alternatives to the neighborhood health center should be developed in response to the social forces calling for increased community involvement (13). The creation of regional medical programs has provided one potential means by which a medical school can directly influence the health care delivery system without overcommitting its clinical resources. Similar opportunities for collaboration and consultation with comprehensive health planning programs exist at both the state and local levels.

The extent to which a department commits itself to a patient care project must be determined in part by its need to maintain credibility in an environment dominated by clinicians, and by its desire to develop a base for demonstration, teaching, and research. Departments of community medicine have been accused of remaining aloof from the service functions of other clinical departments, making grandiose plans for others to follow while waiting in readiness to evaluate their results and criticize their failures (14). As community medicine departments gain more confidence, perhaps they will feel less apologetic about roles which demand a necessary separation between the implementors and the evaluators.

Distinction must be made between the service and educational aspects of community medicine. Although there is merit in providing clinical training in a community environment by offering direct care to that community through such facilities as neighborhood health centers, certain drawbacks are attached to this approach. Still burdened by the traditions of charisma rather than pedagogy, the teaching of clinical medicine is scarcely able to bear the additional encumbrance implicit in working outside the medical school, especially in an impoverished setting. Medical students, as well as their tradition-oriented teachers, are apt to be overcome when the complexities of diagnosis and treatment are multiplied by the many social problems encountered in disadvantaged communities. Efforts to orient the student to the stresses of practice in the real world should not be negated; much work is needed to make medicine relevant to today's problems and issues. As yet, however, the real world has not proved to be the best laboratory for teaching clinical skills and, if clinical skills are the objective of the student's exposure, he cannot simultaneously learn about problems in health care delivery. The panacea of community involvement in a direct care project must be taken with caution and with clear purposes in mind.

The pressures to get involved are real and powerful. Communities themselves have indicated in forceful ways that they expect medical schools to respond to their demands for service. No longer will the residents of urban ghettos accept charitable crumbs of medical care; they now accuse the institutions of exploitation and demand a reckoning (15). If the school is hesitant to establish community clinics, the students may do it for them (16).

At the same time federal support, which gradually became the financial backbone of medical education after World War II, has lately shifted its emphasis. The massive spending for biomedical research that was sponsored by the postwar National Institutes of Health has been leveling off, or decreasing. Priorities are being transferred to the delivery of health care and to the application of knowledge already acquired from research. Like the proverbial donkey chasing the carrot on the end of the long stick, the university is being enticed, cajoled, and coerced into offering more direct services. Such a transition may well require a new set of ethics and philosophy (17).

Some educators now believe that if a student is to appreciate the community, its social systems and their interactions with the medical care system, he must become a part of that community. While moving from the fortress of the hospital to the outpost of the clinic will provide a more realistic spectrum of medicine than will the one out of a thousand persons seen at the university medical center (18), it still does not offer a total perception of the health problems and their potential solutions. But depending on the time the student spends in the community, the degree of his immersion, and the amount of help he has to reflect on the experience, the exposure can introduce valuable information, skills, and attitudes:

> In a community the physician may develop concern for the medical care of all the people. He may more effectively contribute to prevention and early recognition of illness. He can influence social and psychological adaptation of patients to illness and health. He can affect the accessibility of medical care to the population. He can become involved in the development of educational programs on health and health care. He develops a deeper appreciation for the economic and personal needs for improving the present health-care system (19).

No single formula has been developed for teaching community medicine. Some departments have established programs wherein the student visits and perhaps works in a variety of settings in which several types of community health problems are present (20). Others have established more permanent operational units in one or more communities in which medical students and house staff can work with and become involved in community health problems (21). Another alternative is the placement of students in a specific community for the express purpose of studying the community as one would study a patient. Students are encouraged to view the community as an ecological system with multiple subsystems, but while so doing to utilize the basic approaches and language with which they are most comfortable, those of clinical medicine (22).

Regardless of the precise name they go by or the specific learning experiences they structure, the several departments of community medicine have a common area of concern; that is, the problems of health among groups of people—*health* being defined in the sense of the World Health Organization definition of maximal physical, mental, and social well-being. Such a concern with the health problems of populations leads inevitably to a broad range of interests —from the cause, prevention, and control of disease to the organization, financing, and effectiveness of health care delivery.

Perhaps community medicine represents a bridge between medicine and society. It may even loom as the conscience of medicine, for it constantly questions what difference medical treatment makes, raises issues about the potential "mirage of health" (23), seeks to measure the impact of new developments, and challenges the efficiency and effectiveness of care, if not also the efficacy (24). Some force—community medicine, perhaps—is probably necessary to maintain medicine's relevance to real world problems, to help keep medicine in context.

The ultimate test of community medicine lies not in its ability to consolidate a multiplicity of theoretical frameworks but in its application to actual problem-solving situations. Community medicine is not merely a subject to be studied and debated; it is a method for accomplishing social ends (25)—a means by which rational action can take the place of rhetoric. Case studies in community medicine include such efforts as neighborhood health centers but are by no means limited to these thrusts. Community medicine is not the practice of medicine in the community. It is a discipline which requires a precise definition of health problems and a specific commitment to examine them and treat them in the full scope of their implications. When it fails to do this, when it becomes a tool of public pacification, confusion and discouragement follow.

The various chapters in this book deal with several areas which exist under the umbrella of community medicine. They start with community analysis and the basic skills of epidemiology as a tool for applying the scientific method to medical problem-solving, and build to encompass a variety of different but often overlapping disciplines, including medical economics, behavioral science, environmental health and ecology, health services research, and demography. The synthesis of these multiple techniques and concerns represents the methodology and body of knowledge that we recognize today as community medicine.

REFERENCES

1. Shephard, W. P., and Roney, J. G., Jr. The teaching of preventive medicine in the United States. *Milbank Memorial Fund Quarterly*, 1964, *42*, Part II.
2. Wolf, G. A., Jr. The speciality of ? *The Journal of Medical Education*, 1965, *40*, Part 2, 13-19.
3. *World Health Organization Technical Report Series*, 1967, *355*. The use of health service facilities in medical education.
4. Tapp, J., and Deuschle, K. The community medicine clerkship—a guide for teachers and students of community medicine. *Milbank Memorial Fund Quarterly*, 1969, *47*, 411-447.
5. Deuschle, K. W. Organizing preventive health programs to meet health needs. *Annals of the American Academy of Political and Social Science*, 1961, *337*, 36-45.
6. Flexner, A. *Medical education in the United States and Canada. A report to the Carnegie Foundation for the advancement of teaching.* Bulletin No. 4. Boston: Merrymount Press, 1910. P. 26.
7. Scotch, N., and Levine, S., eds. *Social stress*. Chicago: Aldine, 1970.
8. The two sides of this controversy are perhaps best illustrated by Clark Kerr's *Uses of the university* (Cambridge, Mass.: Harvard University Press, 1963) and Jacques Barzun's *The American university: How it runs and where it is going* (New York: Harper and Row, 1968).
9. For an example of this confusion see Reeder, G. Teaching community medicine. *Annals of the New York Academy of Sciences*, 1965, *128*, 582-588; Popper, H. New objectives in medical education. *Annals of the New York Academy of Science*, 1965, *128*, 473-479; and Stewart, W. Community medicine—An American concept of comprehensive care. *Public Health Reports*, 1963, *78*, 93-100.
10. For example see Walker, J. H., and Barnes, H. G. Teaching of family and community medicine. *British Medical Journal*, 1966, *2*, 1129-1130.
11. Seldin, D. W. Some reflections on the role of basic research and service in clinical departments. *Journal of Clinical Investigation*, 1966, *45*, 976-979.
12. Stewart, W. H. The relationship of the medical school to its surrounding community. *Journal of the American Medical Association*, 1967, *202*, 401-403.
13. Sheps, C., and Seipp, C. The medical school, its products and its problems. *Annals of the American Academy of Political and Social Science*, 1972, *399*, 38-49.
14. Kaplan, N. Community medicine as an academic discipline. *Archives of Internal Medicine*, 1972, *129*, 124-128.
15. See Ehrenreich, B., and Ehrenreich, J. *The American health empire: Power, profits and politics* (New York: Vintage Books, 1970), particularly Chapters XVI and XIX for examples of struggles between aroused communities and the health establishment.

16. For example see McGarvey, M. R., Mullan, F., and Sharfstein, S. S. A study in medical action—The student health organization. *New England Journal of Medicine,* 1968, *279,* 74-79, and Freidin, R., Levy, R., and Harmon, R. A student-community plan project for the poor. *New England Journal of Medicine,* 1970, *283,* 1140-1147.
17. See Ramsey, P. The ethics of a cottage industry in an age of community and research medicine. *New England Journal of Medicine,* 1971, *284,* 700-706, and Stallones, R. Community health (editorial). *Science,* 1972, *175.*
18. For the complete calculation of this surprising figure see White, K., Williams, T. F., and Greenberg, B. The ecology of medical care. *New England Journal of Medicine,* 1961, *265,* 885-892.
19. Reynolds, R., and Cluff, L. The medical school and the health of the community: Programs developing at the University of Florida. *American Journal of Public Health,* 1971, *61,* 1196-1207.
20. A number of courses on issues in medical care have been developed in departments of community medicine; see, for example, the March 1972 issue of the *Journal of Medical Education.*
21. Reynolds, R., and Cluff, L. The medical school and the health of the community: Programs developing at the University of Florida. *American Journal of Public Health,* 1971, *61,* 1196-1207.
22. This approach is more fully described in several articles from the Department of Community Medicine at the University of Kentucky. See for example Tapp, J. W., Fulmer, H. S., Deuschle, K. W., and McNamara, M. J. The Kentucky experiment in community medicine. *Milbank Memorial Fund Quarterly,* 1966, *44,* 9-22, and Fulmer, H. The community medicine program in Kentucky. *Canadian Medical Association Journal,* 1967, *99,* 725-730.
23. The biologic philosopher, René Dubos, has questioned the effectiveness of medical care in actually changing the health of the world. He sees these changes as generally antedating medical developments and attributes them more to social and environmental changes than to medical changes. For a more complete discussion see his book, *Mirage of health* (New York: Harper and Brothers, 1959).
24. The concept of cost benefit analysis has been increasingly applied to health care delivery, for example: Klarman, H. E., O'Francis, J., and Rosenthal, G. S. Cost effectiveness applied to the treatment of chronic renal disease. *Medical Care,* 1968, *6,* 48-54; Levin, A. Cost effectiveness in maternal and child health. *New England Journal of Medicine,* 1968, *278,* 1041-1047; May, P. R. A. Cost efficiency of mental health care, III. Treatment method as a parameter of cost in the treatment of schizophrenia. *American Journal of Public Health,* 1971, *61,* 127-129; Klarman, H. Present status of cost benefit analysis in the health field. *American Journal of Public Health,* 1967, *57,* 1948-1953.
25. Kane, R. Community medicine on the Navajo reservation. *HSMHA Health Reports,* 1971, *86,* 733-740, and Kane, R., and Kane, R. *Federal health care (with reservations!).* (New York: Springer Publishing Company, 1972).

2
Community Diagnosis

Jesse W. Tapp

Community diagnosis is a process for identifying and solving community problems, in this case, health problems. It is presented here by one who has used it as an educational tool with medical students. Because comprehensive community analysis is rarely reported in the medical literature, it is difficult to determine to what extent it is actually done. Analyses that are reported have usually been done for a specific applied purpose. You may be familiar with communities that have conducted self-studies for special purposes, such as obtaining information when planning for a new neighborhood health center or other form of health service. These studies rarely reach formal publication for they have only local application.

If one defines community medicine as the identification and solution of the health problems of human communities, then it covers all health services and the total status of the population and community served. Community medicine views whole phenomenon rather than just one piece of it. Community diagnosis is the attempt to identify as fully as possible what the health problems and the health care resources are; it enables the practitioner of community medicine to implement solutions.

Community diagnosis has a long history which extends back to the time of Lemuel Shattuck's epidemiological studies in Massachusetts in the mid-nineteenth century (1) and of John Snow in England (2). These early epidemiologists made tremendous contributions, but they focused their attention mainly on disease. Haven Emerson, in 1927, described well the importance of community diagnosis. Labeling it public health diagnosis in an address which still has a contemporary ring, he called for periodic diagnosis of the community just as one would recommend the regular health assessment of an individual patient (3).

Another aspect of community diagnosis arose with the increase in popularity of medical care studies, in contrast to disease studies. One of the forerunners in this field was John Grant who, in the 1950s, wrote about the importance of community diagnosis and what he referred to as social diagnosis. He lamented that there was no laboratory for social diagnosis such as medical schools have for physical diagnosis, and suggested that we should work toward the time when community or social diagnosis would be just as important to medical students as physical diagnosis in individuals (4).

McGavran was not alone in suggesting that the scientific diagnosis of the community be likened to the diagnosis of a patient's illness, but in recent years he has been one of the more articulate formulators of the analogy that the community is a patient and should be studied in a similar fashion (5). At least those who have a background in patient care or patient diagnosis ought to be able to understand this concept. And now the advent of comprehensive health planning legislation focuses on the importance of looking at the total community.

Community diagnosis need not be comprehensive. It may include a study of a part of a community, whether an epidemiologic study, a medical care study, or an immunization survey to see how well-covered the community is. The term community diagnosis may be used rather loosely in this regard. It has been said that the definition of the pattern of disease in a community constitutes a community diagnosis, and that if health data about a country have been collected and analyzed, a community diagnosis has been done (6). But in this discussion community diagnosis is used mainly in terms of a locality, a specifically defined local community. It may be a town or a county, or perhaps a whole state; however, on a national level, at least in a large country, such a diagnosis becomes too broad to be useful.

A partial community diagnosis might look at a piece of the community picture and link several parts, without attempting to make all possible connections. In contrast, a comprehensive community diagnosis represents an attempt to study all aspects of the community and to relate them to each other, and tries to arrive at some basis for establishing priorities. The actual process of establishing priorities goes beyond diagnosis and enters into the area of treatment. Data are necessary for cost-benefit and cost-effectiveness analyses on which priorities depend. In order to do such analyses a body of information must be established—a data base.

A comprehensive diagnosis begins with a description of the community—its background, its history, and its geographic determinants. What kinds of natural resources are there on which to draw when trying to solve problems? The people must be characterized—not just their demography, but their culture—what it is that makes them tick. Why do they behave the way they do? Are some of their health problems rooted in religion, or in genetics? This sociocultural context would include the basic governmental and social constitution; that is, how do the people generally approach living together? Is it a democratically based society, or is it a culture in which groups have a more authoritarian approach to community organizations?

Next, the more familiar area of health indicators may be considered. What is known about the community from its health records, from its vital statistics, morbidity, and mortality records? What kinds of information sources are available about this community, including health services, the number of professionals, number of facilities, and so forth? These data are usually recorded in existing documents. Particularly today we must also give special consideration to the environmental conditions. Even in the most modest community, the environment is not just something that is simply inherent in the place, but is the resultant of what has been done in an ongoing series of interactions.

Once the data base has been developed on the basis of a review of the history and an actual examination of the community, it is possible to formulate a problem list and consider a plan for problem management. This plan would include a possible prognosis for the community. Given various possible alternative treatments, what results can be expected? What would happen if no treatment took place? At this point, it would become the task of the therapeutic community medicine men to undertake management of the defined problems.

Several examples of a limited community study may be cited as examples. Koos's classic, *Health of Regionville,* was an intensive interview study of a sample of households, about 25 percent of the homes in an unnamed community (7). It is a collection of data from respondents who were not aware that they were participating in a health study. (This approach was used in an attempt to eliminate bias.) The interview cycle continued over a period of four years. This is not the type of study one would cite as an efficient or practical means of making a community diagnosis, but it is one way to obtain health behavior information with a high degree of validity. Nevertheless, even with such information, Koos stated that his formulation of problems in the community was based largely on professional judgment and personal values.

Martin County, Kentucky, is a typical mountain community in eastern Kentucky where approximately ten thousand people participated in an intensive project to eradicate tuberculosis (8). Over 99 percent of the households were interviewed and over 95 percent of the people were skin-tested. Yet, this still falls far short of a comprehensive community diagnosis since the same degree of scrutiny was not given to the environment, to the health services, and to other aspects of the community.

Another example of limited community diagnosis is the sample survey in which, for a number of years, the Washington Heights health district in New York City has been a sampling frame for various kinds of epidemiological and sociological studies (9). But there too, no attempt has been made to look at all aspects of the community, even though the population itself has been thoroughly sampled.

The health survey constitutes still another type of partial diagnosis. For example, the United States National Health Survey provides us with good data on a nationwide sample (10). However, such data are not generally applicable to a particular locality other than to make predictions as if that community were typical of the total national sample. A series of studies on chronic disease in the U.S. in both rural and urban areas was published in the late 1950s. The extensive studies in Hunterdon, New Jersey, and Baltimore are also excellent sources of very useful data-gathering instruments, with standardized interview and physical examination schedules, but they made no attempt to look at the entire community; rather they were concerned only with the extent of chronic disease in those particular sample areas (11,12).

The need for limited studies is evident in the purposes they serve. To deal with tuberculosis, it is necessary to find everyone who has it. If the goal is to have the population better immunized, it is helpful to find out how well immunized the population already is. These are ad hoc community studies. In contrast, a comprehensive study is based on the premise that many major health problems cannot be isolated and examined individually in test-tube fashion. Health problems today are increasingly a part of the whole fabric of society. The only way one can begin to think about solving behavioral problems, whether drug abuse or the decline in family life, is first to acquire a thorough understanding of all aspects of community life. For example, an attack on cardiovascular disease, at the level of better coronary care, may have a definite clinical benefit, but it is certainly not going to solve the basic etiologic problems of coronary artery disease. For that, it will be necessary to look at all pieces of a community that contribute to the disease, i.e., nutrition, recreation, transportation, employment, tobacco use, and so on.

The complexity of health problems and their solutions is what lies behind the new impetus for community studies (13). This approach is equally valid for looking at an established community or for that relatively rare occasion when a new town is being planned and one wants to project what will be needed to plan for prevention of problems in the future. Public demand and expectation that community medicine can perform such analyses is increasing and the public is being told that it should turn to universities and medical schools for help in this endeavor. There will always be new health problems but, unless they are explored in a comprehensive context, it will not be possible to define the full extent of their effects.

Furthermore, studies of medical care quality, efficacy, and quantity must have at least population denominators to have any meaning (14,15,16). When a medical care study is done as part of a larger view of the community, it is possible to say whether the medical care in question is appropriate in terms of the total overall needs of the community. On the other hand, pure research continues to be the reason for some major community studies, such as the study of the population of Tecumseh, Michigan (17). For several years the population has been under careful surveillance for a variety of disease conditions. Many specific studies on the natural history of cardiovascular disease and arthritis have been underway, as they have also been in Framingham, Massachusetts. However, it would appear that Tecumseh is not being used as a laboratory for health planning, nor are there any local attempts to solve the problems being analyzed.

Given the need for community diagnosis, the next question is who ought to be involved in the process. One popular answer to this is the self-study—community members looking at their own problems. However, such studies must have some guidance by experienced investigators. Consumers of health care are usually not very well informed about how to study their own communities. They require leadership to avoid wasted time and motion. On the other hand, the people who intend to use the information for health action certainly should be involved in community studies even though this may be difficult to accomplish. If public health nurses and sanitarians can be persuaded to become involved in collecting useful data, they should have some interest in the study outcome and in using the results in their future activities in the community. Nevertheless, it is difficult to get personnel at some levels of public health administration to realize that this would be a valid use of limited time, in lieu of traditional duties.

There are relatively few practitioners of comprehensive community study, judging from the dearth of published reports, although there are many reported studies of selected areas. The literature on interviewing techniques and on standardized research methods is extensive (18,19,20). Indeed, epidemiologists are highly trained specialists accustomed to looking at pieces of a community, but few of them appear to see that their job includes getting a comprehensive view. There is a need to develop more interest in this area.

Now let us look at some of the methods and sources for getting information about the whole community. Data are available from the United States census and from vital statistics (21,22) with rates standardized for factors such as age, sex, and socioeconomic status. In dealing with rates for small communities, however, apparent differences may be misleading. It would not be unusual to find the infant mortality rate for a county at 45 one year and 12 the next. The explanation usually lies not in changes in the health care system, but in the small number of births per year which cause the rate to be severely influenced by one or two deaths. When dealing with such small numbers it is generally necessary to work with five-year averages when making comparisons over time or between locations.

Hospitals have become better sources of data because of the increased use of automated reporting systems, such as the Professional Activity Survey-Medical Audit Program (PAS-MAP), which makes information on hospital activities and diagnoses readily available. However, one must recognize that this is numerator information; it reflects only that portion of the community which enters the hospital.

A mortality rate which shows an unusually high peak of mortality in one period, compared to the expected rate for that period, may be a means of identifying an epidemic and possibly correlating it with other factors. For example, there may be a marked increase in urban deaths in times of temperature inversion and subsequent massive air pollution.

It is important to emphasize the usefulness of nonmedical

sources that may not be immediately obvious as sources of health information. Police records are a valuable source of data about accidents, emergencies, problems with alcoholism and drug addiction, and other types of behavior that take place in a community. Welfare departments have a large amount of information, but they are justifiably reticent about its use because of the need to protect the confidence of their clients. With assurance that individual records are not of specific interest, but that concern is only in how many people are receiving aid, or how many people are in the aged or disabled group, this kind of information is more readily available.

Schools have information about the health of the community which may be derived from absenteeism, dropout rates, availability of sex education or driver education. Public works offices can often provide environmental information about the availability of community services, what projections there are for future water supply and sewage disposal, or where new roads are going to be built. A community that is isolated today may be within easy access of health care services within the next year or two, and a planned elaborate rural health center may be unnecessary. It would be hard to justify building a hospital or health care facility in a particular location if the same amount of money invested in a road would make it unnecessary.

Ambulance services should maintain records which would reflect the emergency and acute problems of the community. Moreover, the emergency care provided by the service itself could be a valuable part of a community study.

These items are all important in the history taking of a community—the looking at information that is already in existence. Making such a community survey is much like taking the history of a patient, i.e., finding out from the patient what he can tell and then studying him by physical examination. This analogy bears emphasis. The traditional way of taking the history of a community is to do a community survey—actually to go to the people in the community and to the practitioners to obtain information—to examine them, as it were. Generally, a total population survey is not justified unless one intends to deliver some specific kind of service at the same time—for example, immunize everybody or skin-test everybody. Then everyone must be included. But if only information is needed, then a sample will do.

There are numerous sources of useful information on sampling methods. Suffice it to say that it is relatively easy to plan a reliable sample of households in either a rural or urban community. In some communities the use of a city directory, or the tax rolls, or the utility company list of addresses will provide the base from which a sample can be drawn (23). Or one may start from scratch to establish a sampling frame by conducting a quick household census.

Often a community study is conducted by knocking on doors, but mail and telephone surveys have been reasonably well standardized and validated (24,25). There are times when these are useful expediencies. For some kinds of information, better responses are obtained over the telephone as one can minimize the respondent bias: that is, the individual may be more willing to reveal some socially unacceptable response over the telephone than face to face. In this context, the health diary is another standardized technique for gaining information about the health of a respondent—not relying on what he can recall at any moment, but having him keep a record of his health status over a period of weeks or months.

The actual physical examination of individuals in a sample, whether done in the home or at some examination center, is the next step in gathering information about a population. There is currently quite a controversy about whether responses on the doorstep are valid. Those who advocate the use of medical records as the primary source of information consider doorstep information hardly worth the effort. Those who have tried to validate this information by studying the medical records have found that there may be a 60 percent correlation between recall of what the patient says is wrong with him and what the doctor's record shows (11). They have also found that there are items in a doctor's record which the patient did not mention. It is important, therefore, to decide how much error or how much lack of information is acceptable before deciding what kind of method should be used. Of course, environmental inspection can be undertaken at the same time as a household interview.

A number of other important problems involving methodology should be mentioned. One must not underestimate the difficulty and importance of attempting to standardize techniques to eliminate bias. Investigators have gone to great lengths to develop special kinds of survey machines to measure blood pressure, for instance, and other kinds of objective measurements to eliminate observer bias. One of the major objectives of the National Health Survey, in addition to trying to collect information about the population of the United States, has been to test various methodologies (26). The report of this survey contains much valuable information on which approaches might be most suitable for obtaining particular kinds of information.

As to community study guides or forms, few have been published. The American Public Health Association (APHA) has put out several editions of its Community Study-Health Study form, but this still leaves much to be desired when used in an attempt to interrelate various kinds of information about the community (27). The western branch of the APHA has published a comprehensive health planning book, which includes a rapid self-study outline (28).

The modern technology of automatic data processing should provide solutions to many of these problems. Acheson's record-linkage system has the potential of giving an automated view of the community from the standpoint of the health experiences of the population—their utilization of care in doctors' offices, hospitals, and mortuaries (29). In this country with its uncoordinated medical care system, there does not appear to be a possibility for record-linkage systems to work at this point in time. Perhaps with national health insurance and all bills paid through the same system, it will sometime be possible to get some idea of the health experience of a population by pushing a button. The Indian Health Service, with its Health Program System Center at Tucson, has devised a patient record-summary system for the 6000 people on the Papago reservation which can provide a continuous daily profile of the health care and disease pattern on the reservation.

The Michigan State College of Human Medicine and the Michigan State Health Department are engaged in a collaborative program to formulate a self-study which will be made available to municipalities in Michigan. For the past three or four years they have offered a package plan whereby communities, first of all, make a comprehensive environmental survey. This establishes a frame of reference and enables them to know who is living where—not by name, but according to which dwelling units are occupied, what the environmental conditions surrounding the units are, what degree of dilapidation the neighborhood is in, and what appears to be happening in terms of decay or rehabilitation. From this perspective, a simple probability sample of the households in the community can be drawn and then interviewed. The sanitarian and the public health nurse do the initial interviewing. Sometimes public health staff need to be reminded that there are a lot of normal people in a community who have service needs; it is not just the pathological households about which they need to be concerned.

This regular and continuous random sampling of households is fed into a data processing system; it receives the data generated routinely from other health activities in the community and from welfare activities. This makes possible comparison of data about the environment and data about households with what is happening in regard to arrests for alcoholism, for instance, and other antisocial behavior. The system also receives data about the location of families in which illegitimate pregnancies have occurred, as shown on birth certificates. As an embellishment, the program includes computer mapping of data so one can see at a glance where the pathology is occurring. The sampling system is arranged in such a way that every household is returned to the sample pool after a year. If the sampling is continued year in and year out, one can have a constant assessment of the whole community. One can generate a very good profile of a neighborhood yet not be able to go back and "break the code," or locate information about a particular individual; this is a legitimate concern in our haste to get everybody on tape.

Returning to the community as patient, how is the problem list for a community formulated? The quickest way is to list disease problems. It is easy to talk about the prevalence of tuberculosis or the incidence of VD, but more difficult to characterize the chronic disease situation. We often accept the fact that an epidemic of chronic diseases exists; but is the epidemic worse in a particular community than is to be expected? And if it is worse, is there any way to explain it, or do something about it? Certainly the occupational and other environmental problems in a community can be portrayed in the same disease-oriented manner. What are the probable disease outcomes from the conditions found? What are the observed disease outcomes?

Another way of organizing these problems is in terms of the structure or function of the community. Similarly, it might be oriented toward the problems observed in the economy—poverty, economic potential, and so forth, or in terms of the problems in health service organizations, or the problems of changing demography—aging, crowding, and the population explosion. When 14 to 15 percent of the population is over 65, for instance, one can anticipate added demands for health services.

If one differentiates between specific diagnoses, and functional, physiologic, and anatomic abnormalities, one may still be left with symptoms which cannot be explained. The findings of a community study may reveal that people report symptoms of illness, but the causes may still be hidden. Or, the findings may reveal that people aren't eating well, that nutritionally the population is in bad shape as a result of cultural patterns or lack of money or of food. It may require considerably more study to move from recognition of the symptoms to definition of the more specific and potentially treatable problem.

Comprehensive community analysis is unlikely to come up with a single diagnosis. Medical schools may still teach that one ought to try to find a single cause to explain a patient's problem, but that is certainly not true in terms of a community. If one looks, he will most likely find many things wrong in terms of health problems.

The approach to priorities for solving problems is largely a matter of political realities (30). Many priorities are established essentially on the basis of what is politically expedient, what will appear to pay off quickly, or what will give a result that appears beneficial for the least amount of money. But there are more rational ways to weigh priorities, such as the cost-benefit and cost-effectiveness approach. If funds are spent for A, they will not be be available to spend on B; if spent on C, the result will benefit a certain age group, but it will mean that there will not be enough money to pay for heart transplants, for instance. Also, traditional and ethical demands in a community may be overbearing in the value they place on prolongation of life, or the obligation to keep the fetus alive in all circumstances. However, the recent drastic change in priorities on abortion suggests the possibility of a similar change in priorities in other areas.

In conclusion, it appears that community diagnosis may be rising in popularity. At the same time it is unfortunate that the quality of the art and the potential for improving it are limited. The crises faced in health care and in so many other parts of life today may overwhelm any possibility for actually doing comprehensive community studies. The demands to do something "right now" can keep us from looking at all the problems and cause us to fail to develop the necessary long-term solutions.

Priorities have suddenly become a fashionable topic. Organ transplantation rises and falls in popularity; now almost everyone has discovered that he lives in an unhealthy environment. How is a medical student to know what faction will prevail—whether he should devote himself to molecular biology or to the economics of health care distribution? One hopes that intelligent people will continue to sort themselves into productive pathways but without the limitations of the past. Some critical priorities will always be decided on the basis of politics; physicians must become more involved and effective in guiding such policy decisions. They need to be more informed in making their personal decisions, too. The student must have accurate information about what society needs before he commits himself to far-reaching career decisions.

The community is the most realistic place for the student to get the information and experience which he needs to guide his decisions and future professional performance. The community promises to play a meaningful role in medical education regardless of whose values or priorities may be championed. Career choices will be influenced by study in and about the community, but the effectiveness of teaching community medicine should not be judged completely by students' career choices. The surgical student can be influenced in his future professional behavior as much as one who chooses medicine. Just as the community needs the molecular biologist who pursues relevant research, it needs the family physician who will be ruthlessly critical of the value and outcome of his practice.

The student activists' plea for relevance may have become monotonous, but our failure to respond meaningfully suggests that we have ignored the community in community medicine. Everyone in the community—consumers, practitioners, health care agencies, populators, and polluters—needs to become involved with medical teachers and students in identifying the problems and prioritizing them; all must participate in the application of the available social and medical information to the task. The diagnosing and solving of community problems should be pursued with the same diligence and care that individual patients with rare and exotic conditions have regularly experienced in the teaching hospital. Work with real community problems should be as respected a pursuit as traditional clinical practice. However, while developing better models and solutions to health care, it is all too easy to become isolated from those already working in the community and to forfeit the potential contribution of their experience. It is essential to find ways to build mutual respect and collaboration, rather than simply to exist side by side.

The community can become a primary unit for concern. The doctor should know when and how to deal with it. Individuals and groups constitute the community; their health results from their relationships with and in the community. Hospital medicine represents only a limited fragment of the community panorama. Priorities in medical education should emphasize the problems and opportunities of using the community wherever possible to achieve this perspective.

REFERENCES

1. Shattuck, L., et al. *Report of the sanitary commissioners of Massachusetts, 1850*. Cambridge, Mass.: Harvard University Press, 1948.
2. Snow, J. *Snow on cholera*. London: Oxford University Press, 1936.
3. Emerson, H. *Public health diagnosis*. Chicago: Fifth Sedgewick Memorial Lecture, 1927.
4. Seipp, C., ed. *Health care for the community: Selected papers of Dr. John B. Grant*. American Journal of Hygiene Monograph Series Number 21. Baltimore: The Johns Hopkins Press, 1963.
5. McGavran, E. G. Scientific diagnosis and treatment of the community as a patient. *Journal of American Medical Association*, 1956, *162*, 723-727.
6. Morris, J. N. *Uses of epidemiology*, 2nd ed. Baltimore: Williams & Wilkins Company, 1967.
7. Koos, E. L. *The health of Regionville, what the people thought and did about it*. New York: Columbia University Press, 1954.
8. Hochstrasser, D. L., Nickerson, G. S., and Deuschle, K. W. Sociomedical approaches to community health programs. *Milbank Memorial Fund Quarterly*, 1966, *44*, Part 1, 345-359.
9. Gill, C., and Elinson, J., eds. The Washington Heights master sample survey. *Milbank Memorial Fund Quarterly*, 1969, *47*, Part 2.
10. Origin, program, and operation of the U.S. National Health Survey. *Vital and Health Statistics*, PHS Publication 1000. Washington, D. C.: National Center for Health Statistics, August 1963, Series 1, No. 1.
11. Trussel, R. E., and Elinson, J., eds. *Chronic illness in a rural area: The Hunterdon study*. Volume 3 of *Chronic illness in the United States*, by the Commission on Chronic Illness. Cambridge: Harvard University Press, 1956.
12. *Chronic illness in a large city, the Baltimore study*. Volume 4 of *Chronic illness in the United States*, by the Commission on Chronic Illness. Cambridge, Mass.: Harvard University Press, 1957.
13. National Commission on Community Health Services. Action-planning for community health services. In *Report of the Community Action Studies Project*. Washington, D. C.: Public Affairs Press, 1967.
14. Sullivan, D. F. Conceptual problems in developing an index of health. In *Vital and Health Statistics*, PHS Publication 1000. Washington, D.C.: National Center for Health Statistics, May 1966, Series 2, No. 17.
15. Shackelford, M. F., Dyal, W. W., and Waldrop, R. H. *Collection and use of mortality data in community evaluation by social strata*. PHS Publication. Atlanta: National Center for Disease Control, July 1968.
16. Shapiro, S. End result measurements of quality medical care. *Milbank Memorial Fund Quarterly*, 1967, *45*, Part 1, 7-30.
17. Epstein, F. H., et al. The Tecumseh study, design, progress, and perspectives. *Archives of Environmental Health*, 1970, *21*, 402–407.

18. *Premises and home environmental health survey.* Public Health Service, Indian Health Service, Health Program System Center, Tucson, 1968.
19. *10th Report of World Health Organization Expert Committee on Health Statistics.* Sampling methods in morbidity surveys and public health investigations. World Health Organization Technical Report Series #336, Geneva, 1966.
20. Serfling, R. E., and Sherman, E. L. *Attribute sampling methods for local health departments.* PHS Publication #1230. Atlanta: National Center for Disease Control, Epidemiology Branch, March 1965.
21. *12th Report of the World Health Organization Expert Committee on Health Statistics. Morbidity statistics.* World Health Organization Technical Report Series #389, Geneva, 1968.
22. *13th Report of the World Health Organization Expert Committee on Health Statistics.* Statistics of health services and of their activities. World Health Organization Technical Report Series #429, Geneva, 1969.
23. Wilson, E. A., and Kane, R. L. Health knowledge among residents of a rural Kentucky county. *Journal of Kentucky Medical Association,* 1969, *67,* 113-114.
24. Mooney, H. W., Pollack, B. R., and Corsa, L., Jr. Use of telephone interviewing to study human reproduction. *Public Health Reports,* 1968, *83,* 1049-1060.
25. Colombotos, J. Personal versus telephone interviews: Effect on responses. *Public Health Reports,* 1969, *84,* 773-782.
26. Plan and initial program of the health examination survey. *Vital and Health Statistics.* PHS Publication 1000. Washington, D. C.: National Center for Health Statistics, July 1965, Series 1, No. 4.
27. *Guide to a community health study,* 2nd ed. American Public Health Association, 1961.
28. Blum, H. L., et al. *Health Planning, 1969.* San Francisco: Western Regional Office American Public Health Association, 1969.
29. Acheson, E. D. *Medical record linkage.* London: Oxford University Press, 1967.
30. Butterfield, W. J. H. *Priorities in medicine.* The Nuffield Provincial Hospital Trust, 1968.

3

General Epidemiology: A Guide to Understanding Biologic Information

Thomas M. Mack

The scope of epidemiology is confusing; at least some attempt should be made to explain the confusion. Most professional biologists can easily tell whether or not a given topic is within their discipline. Some, like ophthalmologists or geneticists, define their fields on the basis of an anatomic or a functional system. Others, such as parasitologists, veterinarians, botanists, and pediatricians, specify a special set of organisms. Marine biologists and tropical health specialists phrase their definitions in terms of the physical environment. Other biologists emphasize particular environmental influences; that is, the adverse influences which interest the toxicologists, medical microbiologists, and radiobiologists, or the favorable influences which are manipulated by agronomists, sanitary engineers, and pharmacologists.

Epidemiologists, however, may be interested in any anatomic or functional system and concerned with any environmental or genetic influence, whether adverse or favorable. And, although the roots of the word "epidemiology" indicate a concern with humanity, individuals who accept that label may find themselves studying leukemia in cats, encephalitis in horses or birds, or even the behavioral peculiarities of mosquitoes.

Because the subject boundaries of epidemiology cannot be neatly described, epidemiologists who are asked to describe their work tend to provide one of a number of succinct but misleading definitions. For example, epidemiology is sometimes said to be the science of preventing ill health. Since a knowledge of cause must precede action to prevent, almost all research could be so defined.

Moreover, ill health is not easily definable. If too strict criteria are used, minor conditions which are very common and thus economically important may not be included. If asymptomatic conditions, however serious, are excluded, the health problems of inarticulate or uncomplaining people are neglected. If ill health is considered present only when accompanied by a measurable physiologic malfunction, our interests are limited by our understanding of and our ability to measure function. Any of these limitations in scope would preclude a rational examination of public problems, as opposed to an individual's private problems.

Because of such limitations, ill health is frequently defined as "the sum of those conditions other than complete physical, mental, and social well-being." Such a definition permits concern not only with disease in its usual sense, and with diseases in populations, but also with the broader intrinsic and extrinsic origins of man's illnesses. But because this definition encompasses the many wide areas that are of interest to epidemiologists, it fails to distinguish these scientists from the other biologists who attempt to prevent human suffering.

Another conventional definition of epidemiology is "that body of knowledge used to explain and prevent epidemics." While historically this may be defensible because it emphasizes the biology of populations as opposed to individuals, it no longer fully describes current practice. Modern epidemiologists turn their skills toward the achievement of many goals in addition to that of curbing outbreaks of disease—elucidation of cause, measurement of therapeutic efficacy, planning and evaluation of programs and services. They are interested in variations in disease frequency other than those that occur with the passage of time—variations such as are manifest in the changing endemicity of disease or in the differences in the risk of disease with increasing age.

Many view epidemiology as an analytic method, but few agree on specifics. Phrases such as "in the field" and "disease ecology" call attention to the direct observation of natural causes. Needless to say, indirect evidence is often found to be important. Furthermore, epidemiologists are also interested in the genetic, nosocomial, behavioral, and iatrogenic determinants of disease.

Others specify that epidemiologists are those with a concern for disease "in populations." However, they share such a concern with demographers, actuaries, sociologists, and medical economists, not to mention ordinary diagnosticians, whose efforts are meaningless in the absence of knowledge about the distribution of diseases in populations.

Some definers of epidemiology emphasize the implicit or explicit mathematical processes by which disease frequencies are compared. True, a common contribution of the epidemiologist is the demand for an explicit mathematical comparison, whether in the form of controls or of denominators; but clinicians, laboratory researchers, and policy makers must also make the same demand.

In the end, one need not hotly defend any exclusive conceptual niche for the epidemiologist. One can easily imagine a world in which clinicians, basic scientists, administrators, and environmentalists may all function optimally without the services of epidemiologists. However, such a world would be replete with epidemiology, if not epidemiologists. In society today, decisions that depend on the distribution and determinants of the conditions, qualities, and experiences which detract from well-being are often made by persons whose skills and vantage points are imperfect. The clinician too frequently ignores the daily setting of his patients and too frequently neglects the many healthy persons from whose ranks the sick emerge. The basic scientist often has difficulty assessing the generalizability, the impact, and the usefulness of his findings because he rarely needs to consider human environments, populations, or programs. The administrator often has no feeling for the validity of the evidence upon which he bases his decisions, or for the complexity of the relationships affected by them.

In short, the epidemiologist provides the service of advising both the producer of information, the scientist, and the consumer of information, the decisionmaker, on the quality of information —particularly that information which deals with the determinants and the distribution of human disease. In current practice he is more actively interested in the classic epidemic diseases and in important diseases of obscure etiology such as cancer. In addition, he frequently indulges in certain methodologic activities; for example, designing disease control programs, testing hypotheses of environmental causation of disease, and counseling others on the methodologic problems of study design and of program evaluation. Therefore, rather than asking the epidemiologist to define his niche, it would be better to ask what useful skills can be learned from him. In that spirit, the discussion of epidemiology which follows seeks to acquaint the reader with an empirical bag of tricks. Such is the scope of the field that most readers will find some familiar ground; hopefully, they will also find bridges to unfamiliar territory.

The text of this chapter is organized into three sections: the uses of information, the qualities of information, and the production of information. Terms are sometimes introduced without definition and, if they cannot be found in the glossary, it must be understood that noncontroversial definitions are easily available. Idiomatic terms that refer to fine, cloudy, or controversial distinctions; terms that refer to subjects for which references are not readily available; and those that provide convenient tags for purposes of outside reference, are defined.

Before reading any farther at this point, please turn to page 61 and read the summary of the objectives which it is anticipated the reader of this chapter will achieve.

USES OF INFORMATION

Before considering information per se, the consumers of information and the process of consumption of information (that is, decision making) should be considered.

The first step in decision making consists of setting problem priorities and then choosing a problem that will be pursued as a goal. Such a choice must be based on several considerations. The first and most familiar consideration is the simple value judgment, the quantitative equivalent of a definition of disease. In deciding whether or not the world would be better off without disease A or without disease B, both the frequency and the severity of each are considered, and they are ranked. The next consideration is less straightforward. The decision maker estimates the relative likelihood that any action will be instrumental in actually ridding the world of disease A or disease B. Not only is the ranking of priorities in practice affected by these considerations, but priorities must be assigned to each recognized disease and, in addition, to each suspected but unsubstantiated threat of disease. In the list along with leukemia and acne, then, must go the as yet unfamiliar but preventable conditions which might result from lunar contamination or from cumulative exposure to birth-control pills.

Epidemiologic information is itself useful for setting priorities. The sudden appearance of a high frequency of diphtheria or of an unusual cancer in a sharply circumscribed area or group implies a novel cause, and thus a high likelihood of preventability and a high priority.

The various users of data may not set the same priorities as those who compile the data, nor as those who ultimately pay for and receive the services derived from the data. The citizen consumer is wholly responsible for listing his own concerns. The clinician is obligated to deal with the patient's concerns (his symptoms) but at the same time is free to superimpose his own version of priorities. The recent trend toward problem-oriented records minimizes this tendency but cannot eliminate it. Public servants, such as administrators of mass screening or Medicaid programs, must ultimately answer to the priorities of their constituents; but in the meantime they can proceed with their personal priorities. Only occasionally are researchers asked to explain an incongruity between the goals of the research and of the sponsoring philanthropy. Decision makers in the private sector, such as pharmaceutical company managers, are perfectly free to ignore all other priorities (and even to conceal their own) as long as they meet their contractual obligations. Congruity between the priorities of any two of these priority setters is rarely complete.

Once the goal has been specified, a decision as to how the goal is to be reached is made in steps. Each step utilizes qualitative and quantitative information about the host, his exposures, the natural history of disease, and the available modes of intervention.

1. Alternative outcomes to the desired goal are specified.
2. Alternative courses of action are reviewed.
3. Alternative hypotheses are proposed, each of which specifies both the course of past events (diagnosis) and of probable future events (prognosis).
4. Under each complete hypothesis a probabilistic prediction of goal achievement is specified under each alternative course of action.
5. Each complete hypothesis is assigned a probability, such that the sum of all the alternatives is unity.
6. On that basis, the probability of achieving the goal is calculated under each set of contingencies (hypothesized course of events, course of action).
7. That single course of action which maximizes the probability of the desired goal is chosen.

This process is easy to see in a clinical setting. The goal is usually complete recovery; the alternatives are death, residual impairment, or continued acute discomfort. Therapeutic modalities are listed. All observations are reviewed. The alternative diagnostic possibilities are listed, assigned probabilities, then quantitatively revised after new observations. The various probabilities of recovery are calculated using the probability of each hypothesis together with the probability of recovery after treatment with each alternative therapy. A therapeutic mode is chosen.

When the jump is made from the problem of the individual patient to that of the population, each step becomes more complex, but the steps follow in the same order, whether the decisions affect long-term policy matters or short-term tactical procedures.

The research scientist goes through the same process as other decision makers. He must set priorities based on the likelihood of a useful outcome, keeping in mind all the while his constituent population. Each investigation is considered in the context of specific goals. Alternative hypotheses about truth—the course of etiologic events—are assigned probabilities; mutually exclusive and collectively exhaustive study designs are outlined; conditional probabilities are assigned; and a decision is made, just as in the clinical model.

What, then, does any decision maker require for raw materials? Only one kind of information is directly useful—predictive information. For example, it is useful to know that smoking will be associated with a high probability of cough; that a person with cancer is likely to experience premature death; that if a dog has a cold nose, it will probably be healthy.

Of course, such predictive information derives from general information (theories) and specific observations through a process of deductive reasoning. Thus, as healthy dogs generally have cold noses, and as four-legged hairy beasts that bark tend to be dogs, and as the concern is with a four-legged hairy barking beast with a cold nose, one predicts that such a beast will be healthy. In addition, the general information has itself been derived from specific observations through a process of inductive reasoning. In a large number of dogs, under a wide variety of conditions, coldness of the nose was observed more often than chance might dictate, in conjunction with a state of health.

The usefulness of items of information, whether predictions, specific descriptive observations, or theoretical generalities, can be evaluated by certain features which may be only implied or may be expressly detailed. The set of organisms to which the information applies and the conditions under which it applies must be clear. The two or more qualities, variables, or conditions being related must be specified. The relationship between them should be qualitatively and quantitatively described. Finally, there should be some feeling for the truthfulness or dependability of the statement.

The decision maker consumes information when specifying goals and alternative outcomes, when proposing hypotheses, when assigning probabilities to the various outcomes, when listing alternative courses of action, and when estimating the probable course of events under each contingency. The more confident the decision maker is in his ability to predict outcome, the less arbitrary and thus the less difficult the decision. It follows that if the difficult choices (those made under conditions of uncertainty) are to be made rationally, the decision maker must not only be familiar with the qualitative and quantitative logic of decision making, but he must be a connoisseur of information. He must therefore ask at least four rhetorical questions before he can judge the usefulness of a piece of information:

1. Can it be considered to have sufficient scope for application to the setting, period, and population of the proposed decision without making untenable assumptions?
2. Can the definitions (classifications) of the two variables (conditions, events, characteristics, experiences) be considered appropriate to the proposed usage without making untenable assumptions?
3. Can the nature and strength of the relationship described be considered appropriate to the proposed usage without making untenable assumptions?
4. Can the information be considered dependable without making untenable assumptions?

Each of these criteria, indispensable guides for the information shopper, must be discussed at greater length.

THE QUALITIES OF INFORMATION

Scope

The first criterion of usefulness is scope, or generalizability; i.e., the conditions of time and space under which the statement holds true. If such conditions cannot be specified, a prediction is not possible, and the information is useless. Because the units being studied are usually persons, the spatial dimensions are usually expressed in terms of populations.

To evaluate scope, the words available must actually define the population studied in space and time, rather than simply describe their characteristics. If information was gathered in the Massachusetts State Correctional Institute for Women, it may be true but misleading to state that it pertains to young New England women. Because no two populations live under precisely the same conditions, the aim is to permit one to identify relevant differences between the population to which the statement pertains and the population of interest if differences exist; because relevance can be judged only by the consumer, he should be provided with a relatively complete definition of the study population.

On the other hand, the more detailed the definition of the study population, the less likely that the scope of the information will appear to include the population of interest to a given decision maker. It always falls to the decision maker to make assumptions about the similarity between the population studied and the one with which he is concerned. An obvious and relevant discrepancy may permit the decision maker to recognize quickly that the information is not appropriate for his purposes; the absence of any discrepancy may only indicate the paucity of detailed definition and description.

Sometimes scope is difficult to define because the reference population is difficult to define. Studies which compare one group of cases to a second group of cases of a different disease, or one group of exposed people to persons with a different exposure, provide special problems because the reference population includes many groups that were never sampled. In these instances, the conclusions represent a statement of the difference between two partially defined groups, rather than information about a specific population inferred from the difference between an expected and observed value in samples of the same population.

Some common errors made by decision makers who judge the usefulness of information without properly evaluating its scope often include unwarranted jumps: 1) from observations in animals to decisions affecting people; 2) from observations about hospital patients to decisions for healthy people; and 3) from observations in the United States or Western Europe to decisions for the residents of Africa or Asia.

Classification

The second important criterion in judging the usefulness of information is the appropriateness of the various definitions (classifications) of the variables. Just as the words used to describe the conditions of the study must permit an evaluation of the scope of the resultant information, so the words used to describe the subject matter variables must precisely specify the qualities, events, conditions or exposures measured, and the alternative qualities, events, conditions or exposures. Words are not always efficient for this purpose because, for example, the alternative to *symptomatic* may be either *asymptomatic*, or *normal*, or *dead*, or, for that matter, any combination of the three.

Substantive errors in the interpretation of subject matter definitions are also common. Frequently, investigators who purport to explain the etiology of an infectious disease have studied the infection but not the disease. Statements about the efficacy of drugs usually describe the effect upon a laboratory test or a physical sign, rather than the short- or long-term effect upon overall morbidity or mortality.

In addition, classification is closely related to measurement. Any classification of a subject variable, that is, any list of mutually exclusive and collectively exhaustive conditions, qualities, or experiences can be thought of as a scale of measurement. There are different kinds of scales, and familiarity with the differences between them is important because the amount of information presented depends upon the type of scale chosen.[1]

Nominal scale: An unordered list of mutually exclusive and collectively exhaustive categories.

Examples: Race: black, white, oriental, other.
Name: Melvin, George, Gertrude, other.
State of health: diseased, not diseased.

Ordinal scale: A similar list of categories amenable to and arranged in some logical order but without any systematically assigned divisions between categories.

Examples: Pigmentation: very dark, dark, medium, light, very light.
State of health: died, recovered with residua, symptomatic without residua, asymptomatic carrier, uninfected.

Interval scale: A similar ordered list with systematic assignment of intervals but without a meaningful absolute reference point.

Examples: Prothrombin time in seconds.
White blood cells/cubic millimeter.
Wavelength of light at which the optical density of a solution (by colorimetry) is maximum.
State of health: days of work lost through illness.

[1]Note in relation to scales: 1) Any scale other than a nominal one can be divided into discrete divisions for purposes of classification or, alternatively, can be left continuous so that an infinite number of categories is possible. 2) Any set of measurements recorded on one scale can be degraded into a scale providing less information. For example, IQ can be presented as it usually is on a ratio scale, or as raw scores on an interval scale. It can also be presented on an ordinal scale with the observations divided between categories of high, average, and low; or it can be degraded to a nominal scale by dichotomization into categories of average and other. 3)The more complex the scale, the more information provided by each observation. 4) The more complex are each of the two or more scales being related, the more complex are the biostatistical manipulations necessary to quantitate the association and assess its reliability.

Ratio scale: As above, but including a meaningful absolute reference point.

Examples: IQ (ratio of individual score/standard score).
Percent aneuploidic cells among white cells in sample.
Schistosoma eggs found/gram feces.
State of health: percent of previous year spent in sickbed.

Probability scale: As above, but with scale altered to reflect not only the relationship of each value to a reference point, but of the distribution of all values to a standard theoretical distribution.

Examples: Examination score in percentile units.
State of health: probability by chance of observed weight for age in standard deviation from normal growth curve.

Scales must often be adjusted to insure a standard time of measurement. One common problem is the duration of an attribute. A measurement of the frequency of events over time (for example, incidence of cases diagnosed annually) must not be compared with a measurement of the frequency of a condition at a given point in time (for example, prevalence of active cases on January 1). For comparison, one of these scales must be converted to the other, a simple procedure if assumptions or predictions can be made about the pattern of incidence and duration of the condition over time. Standard time units (week, month, year) are specified when using incidence. Of course, when comparing two prevalences or two incidences, it still must be valid to assume that the measurements occurred over a comparable period or at a comparable point in time or in life.

Sometimes the nature of the problem will permit the assumption that, whatever the calendar time involved, the net risk to the group has been the same in each circumstance. Thus all persons diagnosed or attacked (during the entire risk period) are counted and the sum reported with a definition of the nonstandard time period (pregnancies experienced before menopause, smallpox cases within 21 days of exposure to the first case). In these latter circumstances, then, any comparison is between numbers of units attacked, not between true incidences.

Measurements may be more useful when transformed into some mathematical function, such as the logarithm or the square of the original observation.

The most common and necessary adjustment is for the number of units at risk in the population observed. This is accomplished by calculating and using frequency rates rather than the raw numbers as shown in the following examples: a cancer incidence rate of 15 per 100,000 persons per year; a cancer prevalence rate of 1 per 1000 population on January 1, 1972; a smallpox attack rate of 90 percent among household contacts within 21 days of exposure; or a congenital anomaly rate of 10 cases diagnosed per 1000 babies delivered and followed through their third year. Note that attack rates such as the latter two can be thought of as incidence rates (persons who experienced the event, per unit population, per time interval of exposure) or, alternatively, as prevalence rates (persons having experienced an event as of the termination of the time interval of exposure, per unit population).

Adjustment of scale can be simultaneous for both time and the number of units observed, when combined time-unit segments such as person-years (5 persons for 1 year each equals 1 person for 5 years) are used. This method is usually employed when small numbers of individuals are followed (measured) for varying periods of time. Note that it can be validly used only when it is reasonable to assume that the likelihood of an event in a given segment, such as a person-year, is not affected by the number of previous time-segments of risk in the same person. When the latter assumption is not valid, life-table adjustments may be necessary.

Rates which have not been adjusted for anything other than time or unit factors are referred to as crude rates. The term adjustment is reserved for manipulations which are less commonplace than those for time or number of units at risk, but which still are routine corrections for well-understood confounding variables such as age and sex. Age adjustment, then, describes the process of manipulating overall rate measurements by breaking them down into their age-category parts and recombining them into a standardized form based on a common age standard. A rate which applies only a single, presumably homogeneous category, is called an age-specific rate.

Lastly, there are the extremes of manipulation represented by mathematical models. Models may be constructed in order to predict, for purposes of decision making, the future course of some important and complex variable under most likely or under alternative contingencies. Models which emphasize the probabilistic nature of the various outcomes are called stochastic, and those which provide the single most probable estimate in a given circumstance are called deterministic.

Measurements of the state of health can be classified on any scale, and can be adjusted for any number of complex factors. The selection of a scale or of any classification is always an arbitrary judgment. A conventional wisdom among clinicians is that "each patient is unique," but for practical purposes clinicians must still classify patients and their diseases. While diseases were originally classified according to their untoward manifestations (scrofula, phthisis, pox, cholera, dropsy, lupus), such schemes were amended to facilitate predictions of outcome (cholera morbus, smallpox). As therapeutic and preventive modalities developed, classifications based on management implications appeared (failure to thrive, fever of unknown origin). Similarly, as knowledge of etiology advanced, causal factors, partly by virtue of the preventive and therapeutic implications, formed the basis of new classifications (tuberculosis, Gram-negative sepsis, honeymoon cystitis, farmer's lung). The current disease nomenclature is the composite result of all of these processes. It is important to realize that because our familiarity with pathophysiology and manifestations, our understanding of etiology, and our capacity to prevent or cure are incomplete at any one point in time, systems of disease classification are all arbitrary and dynamic. As soon as a subclassification proves useful, it appears ("splitting"); and as soon as a division becomes irrelevant it is ignored ("lumping"). Furthermore, even at a given point in time, no single scheme of classification will serve equally well the purposes of the clinician, the hospital administrator, and the researcher. All schemes are artificial.

Therefore, the first step in evaluating a classification is to examine its purpose and to identify the variables that are actually operative. Exposure classes, risk classes, and outcome classes should be so constituted as to separate those who would be regarded differently in the decision process. If the ultimate goal is to minimize work output lost, then morbidity should be more useful than mortality. If the aim is to prevent the spread of infection, then virus excretion is a better criterion of disease than is fever. If the need for hospital beds is anticipated, prevalence is a better measure than is incidence. If new case onsets are being explained, incidence is a wiser choice than prevalence.

However, the most appropriate classification may not be feasible in practice and must be replaced by the alternative which is most specific (that is, minimizes the proportion of false positives) and also most sensitive (that is, minimizes the proportion of false negatives). For example, if one is interested in studying in retrospect a possible association between the use of a certain drug and the occurrence of hepatitis, neither a precise history of drug ingestion nor a uniform evaluation of liver function is apt to be available. It might ultimately prove necessary to classify people by 1) whether or not they actually purchased the drug by prescription (pharmacy records) within a specified 30-day period, and 2) whether or not their hospital or outpatient record mentions jaundice, abnormal serum bilirubin, elevated SGOT or SGPT, or, if none of the above, three from a series of six symptoms which are most indicative of hepatitis.

Nature of Relationship

The third criterion of usefulness is the qualitative and quantitative nature of the relationship proposed. The qualitative alternatives are only three in number. The two or more variables described may be related by 1) definition, 2) noncausal association, or 3) a causal connection.

The statement, "Preeclampsia is associated with pregnancy," seems to convey information; but in fact it does not because, by definition, preeclampsia cannot exist in the absence of pregnancy. Such absurd propositions are encountered more frequently than one might expect. Consider "A history of hallucination (or a family history of schizophrenia) is common in schizophrenia." Only after reviewing the criteria for diagnosis (classification) does one realize that this statement is in part tautologic.

Distinctions between cause and association, and between various subcategories of cause, are less easily clarified. Philosophically, cause is not easy to define but, in the context of medicine, one can feel operationally comfortable with the following proposition: A cause is something which, if prevented, removed, or eliminated, will prevent the occurrence of the event in question, and/or if permitted, introduced or maintained, will be followed by the event in question.

Causes are spoken of as necessary and sufficient. In the case of a true sufficient cause for any disorder, the disease would inevitably follow in everyone exposed. But if such a danger really existed, then any means by which only some people were exposed would constitute a second cause and belie true sufficiency. Sufficient can only mean sufficient in a specific contingency, like the straw that broke the camel's back.

Empirically, it is easier to think of a candidate for a necessary cause. The lepra bacillus causes a truly distinctive set of clinical and pathological syndromes, as do the rabies and smallpox viruses. On the other hand, if we were sufficiently adroit, we could surely produce an identical clinical syndrome with some other carefully directed form of danger; because there are only a finite number of susceptible end-organs, the various permutations of end-organ response must also be finite. There have been many instances of a symptom complex having been thought to be a discrete and homogeneous disease, but which has been later divided into several etiologic entities on the basis of further knowledge. A good example of this process is the attrition of the rubric "acute yellow atrophy" of the liver, which has over the past decades been divided into various infectious, toxic, and residual unknown etiology categories.

In some infectious diseases (tuberculosis and tetanus, for example), a clear clinical and/or pathologic heterogeneity seems to result from a common single agent. In such cases, the empiric basis of invoking the agent as a necessary cause of any specific clinical syndrome, such as scrofula, pulmonary cavitary disease, or pleurisy, is not firm; there is clear evidence that other causes determine the form the disease will take. If all clinical forms of such an infection are considered to be one disease, defined etiologically (tuberculosis), then the causal agent (M. tuberculosis) is a necessary cause by definition.

Examples at the other extreme are those ubiquitous infectious agents such as Proteus vulgaris, which are responsible for urinary tract infections, bacteremia, and Gram-negative sepsis. Unless it is done by definition, to invoke such an agent as either a necessary or sufficient cause is ridiculous, for such organisms are ubiquitous and pervasive, and a wide variety of other Gram-negative bacilli can promote a similar syndrome in a given patient. In addition, we recognize that the most useful determinants of the symptom complex, such as the antibiotic resistance pattern or the endotoxin released, frequently have nothing to do with the taxonomy of the bacterial agent. Thus, when considering the notion of multiple causation in the context of infectious disease, it is easy to picture several different varieties of determinants acting simultaneously. Certainly, a vector or vehicle which transmits the agent to the host and a toxin which alters cell function are both indisputably causes; they differ only in their degree of proximity to the clinical effect. Moreover, on each link in the causal chain, there are recognizable side chains, each also composed of individual causal links; for example, stagnant water causes the mosquito vector, or pH causes the toxin to function.

For every syndrome, there is, then, a web of infinite causes. We choose to regard some causes as more important than others. The criterion is not one which divides necessary from sufficient, or direct from indirect, or primary from contributory, although all of these criteria are often cited. The criterion is therapeutic or prophylactic usefulness. If one can identify a cause that explains a disease distribution or a cause that will permit the development of a prophylactic measure, that cause is of interest. Hence, there is no reason to presume that among diseases of unknown etiology, single useful causes predominate.

Presuming agreement on what constitutes a cause, the next issue is the differentiation of causal and noncausal associations. That problem can never be conceptually solved. Two phenomena can be inseparably associated without a causal relationship, either because both result from the same cause or because (which is the same thing) one is closely associated with a cause, or an effect, of the other.

On a practical level, however, it is sometimes possible to say when two factors are *not* causally related. First, if they are not in a consistent sequence, one cannot be consistently causing the other. Second, if the statistical association between variables is very weak, it implies that either the presence of other simultaneously operative causes is also necessary, or that only a small proportion of cases is really being caused by the factor in question. Although causality cannot be truly ruled out in such a circumstance, the cause being considered will ultimately prove to be of limited usefulness, because too few cases would be prevented if the exposure were eliminated. Third, causality may be judged less likely in light of current biologic theory, that is, on the basis of the inconsistency of data derived from different study conditions or from different approaches and disciplines.

Frequently, a causal association cannot be excluded on the basis of sequence or theory and the association is sufficiently strong to be of interest, yet there is reason to believe that the association may be wholly explained on a spurious basis. Such potential errors may result from bias or from confounding. These are usually described as sources of invalidity—that is, of invalid inferences of causality. First, let me explain bias.

Several different kinds of problems may originate during the processes of selection and classification of study subjects. If the population from which the subjects are chosen is an unusual or special one, then the scope of the study may be unusual. If the control subjects are not randomly chosen from the population of origin there must be some assurance that the measure of expectation taken from them is appropriate. In neither of these circumstances is the validity of the study necessarily endangered—knowledge of a true and valid association may be produced under either condition.

Picture the simplest of studies, in which a group of subjects is first divided into exposed and nonexposed, and then each of these two classes is further divided into diseased and nondiseased subgroups (neither the order of the two classifications nor the complexity of the scale affects the point). If errors are made in either or both of the two classification steps, whether predominantly in one direction (e.g., true disease unrecognized) or in both directions (e.g., true disease and true nondisease unrecognized), they are errors of misclassification. Because they usually result in inefficiency (tend to obscure the perception of a true association), such errors do not themselves endanger validity. Validity is only threatened by a misclassification when it is biased, that is, when it is not independent of the other classification process in the study. For example, if ulcer patients and controls are both asked about their exposure to spicy foods, bias occurs when the patients preferentially recall spiciness, even when the two diets have been identical.

An analogous problem exists when the selection or sampling process identifies and either includes or excludes preferentially those persons who would fall into one of the four cells defined by the interaction of the two classification scales—for example, those cases who had been exposed. This bias also might result in the demonstration of a nonexistent association. For example, a study of maternal measles and malformation in infants could be ruined if the reporting process is more efficient for malformed children because their doctors recognize and wish to report preferentially the combination of infection and malformation. Bias, then, is any error in selection and classification which tends to produce the invalid appearance of an association. Notice that an error might be committed by the investigator, by a technician, by a subject, or by some intermediary agent.

The second category of reasons for suspecting that an inference of causality might be invalid is referred to as confounding and is exemplified by the statement "Nicotine-stained fingers can be shown to cause lung cancer." Any association between two variables which occurs because there exists a third variable which itself determines one of the two, and is associated with the other, is described as confounded. The third variable is referred to as a confounding variable, factor, or cause. Thus, in the example given, cigarette smoking is the confounding factor, and the causal association between stained fingers and lung cancer is a confounded association and is not a valid one.

The same confounded noncausal association can be used to advantage when the noncausal condition or experience is useful as a risk factor or predictor. Thus knowledge of an association, even when it is recognized not to be causal, may be a valuable commodity. Imagine that there is an identified cause of a disease and a specific prophylactic measure is developed. However, the application of this prophylactic measure is expensive, either in terms of dollars or in terms of complications, and the nature of the disease is such that the cost is too great to warrant application of the measure to the population at large. An example of such a situation is rabies, an uncommon disease in the United States. Rabies may be prevented by live rabies vaccine, but this can produce a considerable number of complications. Because individuals who will be exposed cannot be identified in advance, it is worthwhile to utilize the risk factors, known to be noncausal, in order to predict those at greatest potential risk. Predictors, such as place of residence, age, sex and/or occupation, can thus be used as criteria for the establishment of rabies vaccine priorities.

Because bias and confounding are very similar and closely related concepts, they seem to apply to different facets of the same problem. Bias usually implies a human error in design and a source of error in the final measurement; but confounding usually refers to subject complexities rather than to study design and to problems which can frequently be measured and controlled in the analysis.

More specifically, bias can be minimized in several ways. Misclassification can be minimized by choosing the most specific and sensitive instruments available and by incorporating procedures to identify systematic human errors and to rectify random and mechanical errors. Bias can be minimized by ensuring that selections and classifications are made blindly, that is, without knowledge of status with respect to the other scale.

Confounding may be minimized by ensuring that, insofar as possible, a comparison is always made between groups which differ in only one respect—the variable under study. This can be accomplished in several ways:

1. One can gather a large amount of data, record for each individual all possible sources of confounding, and hope that after the study is complete, the data can be rearranged so that the measurements in both study and comparison groups can be presented within categories or strata comprised of persons identical with respect to the confounding factors.
2. One can identify persons to be studied so as to assure that only such homogeneous categories or strata will be present after the data are collected. This may be done by:

   a) Identifying or systematically arranging two heterogeneous populations that are so similarly distributed in all relevant respects that one can reasonably assume that no confounding exists (comparing city A with city B).

b) Stratifying the subjects into categories defined by confounding factors (studying individual age, sex, and racial groups).

c) Eliminating all subjects except those identical with respect to the confounding factors (studying only white males between six months and one year of age).

d) Matching each exposed individual with an unexposed individual who is identical with respect to all confounding factors (a study of identical twins, for example, cannot be confounded by genetic factors).

3. Lastly, one can divide a set of subjects into two subsets by means of chance, and chance alone, by randomization. This method has the advantage that, within the limits of chance, the two groups will be composed identically with respect to all confounding factors, whether recognized or not. It has the disadvantage that chance can dictate an unequal distribution of subjects with respect to some confounding factor. This latter disadvantage can be abrogated in several ways. The randomization can take place within strata defined by known identifiable confounding factors, or information about each subject can be collected to enable an estimate of the importance of chance confounding, or the numbers can be increased so as to make chance differences extremely unlikely.

From what has been said about the web of cause, it follows that causes vary greatly in importance. One must therefore qualify statements indicating a relationship with appropriate quantitation. For example, the most widely used measure of the strength of an association (and thus of the etiologic role played by an exposure) is the risk ratio, or relative risk. It is computed by dividing the risk (rate) in those exposed to the cause or factor in question by the risk (rate) in those not so exposed. It thus represents the factor by which risk is increased under conditions of exposure. A related important measure is the attributable risk, that amount or proportion of the risk to the exposed which is attributable to the exposure in question (as opposed to that proportion caused by other baseline causes operating in the same people). It is calculated by subtracting the risk in the unexposed from the risk in the exposed. As both of these measures neglect the actual prevalence of the exposure itself, a third measure is necessary for estimating the actual impact of an exposure and its resultant diseases upon any given population. The population attributable risk is calculated by subtracting the risk to the unexposed from the risk to the entire population, exposed and unexposed combined. This marginal risk provides an estimate of the maximum impact of a program designed to interdict that cause.

Dependability

Dependability, the fourth important criterion of usefulness, must be judged by the probability with which the observations leading to the statement could have occurred by chance alone. Three important determinants of dependability are: 1) the scales employed to classify the observations, 2) the number of observations, and 3) the form of the expected distribution of results from repeated sets of such observations under the null hypothesis (that is, if the hypothesis being tested is not true). Dependability is thus within the purview of biostatistics and is really beyond the scope of the current discussion.

Even so, it may be worth preparing the reader in one respect. There are two general schools of thought about how such probability statements should be evaluated. The traditional one suggests that if the chance probability is high (the finding is not significant) then the information is not dependable and the world has not been enriched. The more modern (Bayesian) view is that no finding should be classified as dependable or undependable, but that the consumer of information should put the finding and its corresponding chance probability into his personal computer and allow it to affect his personal understanding of truth. With that method, observations which could have occurred by chance in 5 percent of such studies affect one's opinion only slightly more than studies which could have occurred by chance in 6 percent of such studies.

SUMMARY OF QUANTITATIVE ASPECTS OF INFORMATION

Quantitation may appear in informational items in a variety of ways and, because it is the most confusing aspect of the evaluation of information, a brief review may facilitate orderly thinking.

1. The scope may be limited by a quantitation constraint:
   Among those boys under 15 years of age, the tall ones are fat.

2. One or more of the subject variables may be quantitatively scaled:
   Among the boys, tall ones weighed 150 pounds or more.
3. The frequency of units in a given category reported may be quantitated:
   Among the boys, many of the tall ones are fat.
4. The frequency of studies, samples, or sets of data may be quantitated:
   In many samples, tall boys have been found to be fat.
5. The degree of association or correlation may be quantitated:
   Among the boys, height was very highly correlated with weight.
6. The probability, from the sample observations, of the truth of the correlation or association may be quantitated:
   From these observations, there is a high probability that height is associated with weight in boys.
7. The probability that a future individual or sample of units will fall into a given category can be quantitated:
   In the boys to be processed, it is highly likely that height will be associated with weight.

And if that were not complicated enough, there are a number of variations on each theme.

1. Each quantification can be expressed on any scale above a nominal one.
   Ordinal scale: lesser, greater, higher, highest
   Interval scale: few, some, many, a lot
   Ratio scale: most, a fraction, about half, the vast majority
   Probability scale: usual, unusual, extreme, average, likely, unlikely, probable, improbable
2. Most quantifications can be recorded on a discrete or continuous scale.
   10 years, 2.74 months of age
   173.42 pounds
   83.25 person-years
   14 samples
   4.73 relative risk of fatness
   .0007 probability of occurring by chance
   53.7 times out of a hundred
3. For each quantitation which is an estimate, as opposed to those which are directly observed, a second quantitation may provide a measure of the reliability of the estimate.
   Estimated mean height of 73.497 inches, with a probability of .99 that the true mean falls within 73.497 ± .321 inches.

THE PRODUCTION OF INFORMATION

Information may be produced in the laboratory, in the clinic, in the community, or indeed in the library. To summarize the preceding section, any useful piece of information, irrespective of origin, should display the following properties:

1. The scope should be broad enough to permit the anticipated decisions. Ideally, the conditions and population studied would be identical to the conditions and population for which the most far-reaching decision is anticipated.
2. The subject variables should be specifically defined in keeping with the anticipated problem. The classifications chosen should provide all necessary details and no more.
3. The relationship should not be tautological. If there is an interest in causality, a) the sequence between exposure and outcome variables should be clear; b) bias and confounding should be eliminated; and c) the association should be described quantitatively.
4. The dependability of the information should be maximized and described in probabilistic terms.

Epidemiologists' contributions to knowledge are most commonly made in response to a problem associated with some specific disease. The first three steps in formulating a response involve making decisions concerning the problem itself; the other seven are closely related, affect several of the qualities of ideal study, and must be made more or less simultaneously.

Suppose that a problem with high priority is the etiology of the large number of deaths from multiple sclerosis which occur in Massachusetts. An investigator setting out to solve that problem should proceed implicitly or explicitly in the following order:

1. *Assignment of priority of the problem.* The importance of multiple sclerosis mortality and morbidity in Massachusetts should be evaluated and compared to mortality and morbidity from other causes. The likelihood that a study would produce useful information should be estimated. A rank should be assigned and the problem taken up in its turn.
2. *Search for demonstrated associations.* One should review both available morbidity and mortality data from Massachusetts and previous epidemiologic studies of multiple sclerosis in all populations. If no descriptive information is available, descriptive surveys may be warranted, the variables to be chosen on the basis of their availability, broad signifi-

cance, and special theoretical significance. Clinical studies of multiple sclerosis and laboratory studies of multiple sclerosis and related animal diseases should be reviewed.

3. *Hypothesis formulation.* An exhaustive set of hypotheses should be specified. From this list, the only hypothesis which is likely to represent the most useful information should be selected. Suppose, in this instance, that the hypothesis chosen is "Exposure to a virus of domestic cats causes multiple sclerosis."

   The next step is to put the hypothesis into a form suitable for testing. This means that the two variables and the hypothesized relationship must be more precisely defined for operational purposes: Daily physical contact with domestic cats is causally associated with the appearance, at any time in life after one year of exposure, of a fatal disease characterized by neurologic symptoms and displaying microscopic pathology thought by trained pathologists to be consistent with multiple sclerosis. (Note that the hypothesis defines precisely, both qualitatively and quantitatively, outcome, exposure, and the nature of the relationship, including the interval between the purported cause and the purported effect.)

4. *Testing the hypothesis.* This testing can be broken down into its component parts; the first three have to do with choosing the subjects to be studied and the others are concerned with the methodology to be employed:
   a) Choosing the population. Keeping in mind the site of any eventual decision, we choose the population of Massachusetts.
   b) Choosing the unit. Because the problems of multiple sclerosis are individual, and because the most probable method of preventing the results of exposure would be on an individual basis, an individual person is the most logical unit.
   c) Choosing the size of the sample. This choice determines the dependability of the information gained; the credibility of the results is dependent upon the strength of the association and the frequency of exposure and outcome. Because this is to be an ideal study, let us plan to study at least 1,000,000 people, a number chosen to exceed by far the minimum number necessary.

The next seven decisions are related and must be made more or less simultaneously:

   d) Choosing the method to identify individuals.

e) Choosing whether to make a comparison within a group identified by a single method, or between two or more groups identified by separate methods.
f) Choosing whether to first identify persons with the outcome condition or persons having suffered the exposure.
g) Choosing whether to provide an experimental exposure.
h) Choosing how to measure the exposure.
i) Choosing whether to stratify in the design, and what other measurements to record.
j) Choosing whether, in the event that the exposure is to be provided, to assign persons to the exposure by chance or by some systematic method.

The method of identifying the 1,000,000 persons from Massachusetts who will be studied could greatly alter the scope of the resulting statement. Presumably they should be representative of all persons in Massachusetts who would fall within the same categories as defined by the scales of exposure and outcome. The validity of the study would not depend on its scope, however.

If the study and comparison groups are identified separately, it is possible that some unplanned difference in definition would introduce bias and thus cast doubt on the causality of the association.

The possibility of bias is also affected by the sequence of the measurements and by the chronologic position of the investigation in relation to both the exposure and outcome. If the exposure is measured before the outcome has occurred, the only bias that can enter into its measurement comes from a knowledge of predictors of outcome that might already be available. If both phenomena have already occurred at the time of measurement, no matter which is measured first, risk of bias accrues to each measurement. Bias may appear when the second of the two sets of measurements is made, regardless of whether outcome or exposure was measured first.

The choice of a method of measurement of the exposure will affect the information obtained. The scale providing the most information for the money should be selected, with the realization that it can later be degraded (e.g., days of cat exposure per year degraded into cat exposure—yes or no). A number of factors which might not at first appear quantifiable can indeed be quantified. For example, exposure to an infectious cat could be quantified in terms of physical proximity (in meters), in terms of the social intimacy of the exposure, or in terms of the length of time exposed. Genetic inheritance can be quantitated in terms of the probability of genes in common (no relation, in-laws, first degree relatives, second degree relatives, and so on). If the investigator chooses to provide the exposure himself, he may still introduce bias, but he has the advantage of being able to better classify and quantitate the exposure. He has the further advantage of being able to deploy the strongest tool against confounding, randomization.

Whether or not randomization is possible, decisions about whether to stratify the subjects and about whether to record additional items of information will depend upon a consideration of the potential problems with confounding.

In our proposed study, we might choose to select randomly, by a single method, 1,000,000 persons, to randomly assign them to one of two equal groups, to record all items of information, describing known or suspected confounding factors, and to arrange for the members of one group to be exposed to ten cats, for twenty-four hours per day for ten years. Weekly interviews might be scheduled for the purpose of recording the daily amount of contact actually experienced.

k) Choosing the interval between the two measurements. An intervening time interval is necessary if sequence is to be determined. The length of the interval depends upon the specification of the hypothesis, and if the interval is inappropriate, the study may be transformed into a good test of the wrong hypothesis.

The longer the interval between the two measurements, the easier it is to eliminate bias in the second measurement—both that bias which originates with the investigator and that which originates with the subject. On the other side of the coin, the longer the interval of follow-up, the more probable that losses to follow-up will occur. If study and comparison groups lose subjects at the same rates and for the same reasons, the net effect is simply a decrease in the size of the study. If the reasons differ for the two groups, however, the losses may result in noncomparability between the two groups and invalidity in the study because of bias.

l) Choosing the measure of outcome. Double blind studies are those which truly hide the results of the first measurement from both measurer and measured at the time of the second measurement. Thus in our proposed study the measure of outcome, an interpretation of microscopic pathology, cannot be directly influenced by the subject; information about cat exposure will also be withheld from the pathologist who makes the interpretations.

Not all bias is eliminated by such measures, however. If the diagnosis of multiple sclerosis is made only on the basis of microscopic examination of autopsy specimens and if the pathologist knows that only the families of cat fanciers permit autopsies, a bias toward the hypothesis will result. For this reason it is frequently useful to list every step in the chain of events which has led an individual member of the population to be symbolized by a number in a table, and to examine each of these steps for bias.

In our ideal study, let us plan to follow all subjects for life by planning to make the final measurement of outcome status at the autopsy table after the death of each subject.

5. *Analysis of the data.* This process also includes several steps.
   a) Redefinition of the study population may be necessary after all opportunities for losses of data have passed.
   b) A different set of variable scales from that originally planned may have to be used in the analysis. This may depend not only on the original intent, but on the completeness with which detailed observations were obtained, and on the distributions of the actual values for each variable. Scale reductions may be necessary, and continuous scales may need to be converted to a discontinuous form for computer analysis.
   c) Stratification of the data in the analysis may be necessary for purposes of eliminating confounding, but should be avoided if possible since each division reduces the number of values available and thus diminishes statistical power. Further analysis may then occur only within the individual strata; analytic techniques may be applied which attempt to evaluate complex associations of multiple variables; or methods of analysis may be used which attempt to summarize a relationship examined simultaneously in many subgroups.
   d) Methods must be chosen for testing the dependability (significance) of new information. The procedure is usually as follows:
      1) Explicitly state the hypothesis and its alternatives. As it is easy to logically disprove a rule by demonstrating an exception, but impossible to validate a rule by demonstrating an example, the actual hypothesis tested is the null hypothesis—the hypothesis of no association. Thus when other alternatives to the proposed hypothesis and the null hypothesis exist, that is, when other (confounding) factors would reasonably explain the presence of an association, the test of significance becomes relatively meaningless.

2) Choose that quantitative element which best distinguishes between alternative hypotheses, that value which would clearly differ in the present circumstance depending on which hypothesis is true.
3) Choose the best single (observed) estimate of that quantitative element, the point estimate.
4) Decide which probability model (binomial, Poisson, normal, nonparametric, and so on) describes the chance variability of estimate.
5) Calculate the actual value of the test statistic, using the family of test statistics which is most indicative of that chance variability.
6) Qualify the point estimate by describing the degree of uncertainty, the predicted variability in hypothesized replications of the same study—the interval estimate.
7) In view of that uncertainty, quantitate the probability that the data are consistent with a hypothesis other than that proposed.

In the case of our example, let us presume that we do not need to redefine the study population, and that we decide to use simple dichotomous nominal scales, i.e., disease-no disease and exposure-no exposure. We might decide to divide the study into two strata on the basis of whether the exposure began in childhood or in adulthood, and to report the results separately. The best measure of association, the risk ratio, would also be that measure which best distinguishes between the hypothesis of association and the null hypothesis of no association. We would therefore calculate the point estimate of the risk ratio, the interval estimate around that point, and the probability that the point estimate was compatible with chance under the hypothesis of no association. We then might calculate the attributable risk, the population attributable risk for Massachusetts, and possibly further describe or graph the data in order to facilitate a complete understanding of its significance.

SHORTCUTS IN DESIGNING AN EPIDEMIOLOGIC STUDY

If an ideal study like this could be designed and executed for every hypothesis that needed testing, life would be much easier but infinitely more boring. Practical considerations rarely permit such large, randomized trials.

Many exposures simply do not lend themselves to study by an investigator. Some examples would include lifelong exposure to varying levels of background radiation, or to maternal deprivation during childhood. Ethical considerations are important constraints; no exposure to a treatment believed by responsible experts to decrease morbidity can be withheld, randomization or no randomization. No exposure generally believed to be dangerous can usually be provided, randomization or no randomization. The cost in time and money of making the observations may be prohibitive, or the number of subjects needed for useful information may not be available. There may not be enough time available before the information is needed.

For these reasons, investigators must be satisifed with less reliable methods of producing information. While each of the following shortcuts may be generically less reliable, a given design may be just as reliable as a test of a specific hypothesis in a specific circumstance. In practice, many epidemiology man-hours are spent considering the pros and cons of such compromises.

1. *Choice of a more feasible study venue.* In most investigations a population is chosen for convenience, with the explicit or tacit assumption that the information obtained will be broadly useful. Care is taken to avoid any obvious limitations upon future generalizability. In those subject areas most influenced by changes in the cultural or geographical milieu, the decision maker must often confirm a hypothesis himself, under the actual conditions of the proposed decision, rather than proceeding on the basis of bargain information.

2. *Choice of a smaller number of subjects.* Simple economics restricts the number of subjects studied and, in many circumstances, so does the number of available cases or persons exposed. Generally one admits as many subjects as can be studied with the given limitations of time and money. If the number of subjects needed to provide solid information is clearly larger than the number available, a decision must be made about the value of the information that would be provided by small numbers. Especially when economic or ethical issues demand that therapeutic evaluation be no more extensive than necessary, a sequential design may be of use. Termination of the study may then occur at a point determined by the appearance of dependable findings rather than by the inclusion of a fixed number of subjects.

3. *Choice of a different study unit.* Data may sometimes be easily available for families, for communities or for countries, but not for individuals. Because a history of individual consumption may be

difficult to obtain, the consumption of a given product by a community or by a nation instead might be available. However, the larger the unit of study, the fewer the number of units usually available, and thus the more difficult it may be to obtain dependable, valid results.

4. *Choice of information already collected for other reasons.* Obviously, the use of someone else's information saves money and, equally obviously, its chief liability is inflexibility. Still, many hypotheses can be summarily rejected on the basis of easily available information, and if larger political units are of use as study units, specific information may be available in detail. (Sources of such data are appended to this chapter.)

Census information provides demographic detail by geography, sex, age, race, and certain other economically useful characteristics. Birth and specific mortality statistics are also usually available, as are other vital statistics such as those of marriage and divorce. Unfortunately, morbidity information is available only for certain diseases of public interest, such as communicable diseases. Even then such information may be very unreliable. Cancer registries, both public and private, may contain information about cancer morbidity in restricted geographic areas. The United States National Center for Health Statistics regularly conducts morbidity and health care surveys which are painstakingly reliable, but because they can only cover relatively small samples, they are most useful for evaluating common conditions. Lastly, some data gathered for other reasons are available on various exposures. Some examples include federal air and water pollution information, marketing surveys, tax receipts, or manufacturers' sales data providing estimates of regional cigarette sales.

5. *Choice of a different scale or scales.* Precise detail must often be relinquished for reasons of feasibility. When testing the association between a drug and a physiologic reaction, the best study would result in an examination of the severity of the reaction compared with the dose of the drug. If it is felt that those being asked to provide the information would simply refuse to respond if such detail were requested, the demonstration of an association between a history of the drug and a history of the reaction, in qualitative terms only, may be still worthwhile.

6. *Choice between the natural and the experimental exposure.* Most hypothetical exposures do not lend themselves to the experimental method; that is, they cannot be provided by the investigator,

either because of technical infeasibility, or ethics, or both. This simple fact, because it decrees that randomization cannot always be used as a method of maximizing validity, is responsible for much of the complexity of study designs. In addition to being necessary in many instances, observational (nonexperimental) studies are often preferable by virtue of their rapidity, simplicity, and thus, economy. In such studies the study and control groups are more likely to have undesirable differences between them, and more care must be taken to ensure comparability by minimizing confounding and bias.

Observational studies permit a number of other shortcuts, among which are the following:

7. *Choice of a cross-sectional over a longitudinal study.* Time and money can be saved by classifying on both scales at the same time, as in a survey, thus eliminating the expense of processing each subject twice and eliminating losses to follow-up. The disadvantages of cross-sectional studies are several. Only longitudinal studies permit a reliable judgment about sequence, because all subjects previously experiencing factor number 2 can be excluded at the time of first measuring factor number 1. Cross-sectional studies are particularly dangerous in this respect when prevalent (currently existing) conditions, such as status with respect to some inherited trait, chronic disease, or socioeconomic class, are being measured instead of such incident (new) events as first cancer symptoms or familial exposure to a case of communicable disease. The act of recording both factors simultaneously is particularly vulnerable to bias, because there is a simultaneous awareness of both factors on the part of both the subject and the person doing the measuring. More valid results are obtained from serologic or other laboratory surveys, in which objective results are unaffected by such knowledge, than from opinion surveys. Lastly, if there is interest in events rather than in conditions, it is unfortunate that availability of survey information is usually dependent upon the memory of the subject, which may be a source of bias. For these reasons, cross-sectional studies are best done for objectively measured conditions which can be assumed to appear in a given sequence.

8. *Choice of a retrospective rather than a prospective investigation.* Particularly when the interval between exposure and outcome events is long, the documentation of an association may be perfectly feasible except for the time that must pass in follow-up. One

solution to this problem is to identify a cohort of subjects who have been exposed in the past and to examine from records their subsequent outcome experience, together with the experience of a group who were not exposed. One obvious difficulty with such retrospective[2] studies is the rarity with which such a roster of persons is available; another is the ease with which bias can enter into the results, either because of losses to follow-up which are beyond the investigators' control, or because the exposure status cannot be hidden from those who are measuring the outcome. In addition, such studies permit an investigation of only one exposure at a time, a constraint which inhibits the study of diseases of unknown etiology because alternative exposures cannot be studied simultaneously.

9. *Choice of a comparison group of subjects using separate criteria.* Even when intervention is not intended, it is advantageous to identify both study and comparison subjects at the same time, by the same means, later separating them into exposed (study) and nonexposed (comparison) categories for purposes of analysis. This is true because bias is avoided on two counts: 1) the groups comprise a single population, and 2) the exposure status can be kept secret until after the outcome is measured. This population selection process is another common feature of community surveys. Its disadvantage is that when there is an interest in a rare disease, a very large number of subjects must be studied in order to obtain useful numbers. Consequently, most population studies deal with common diseases, and the shortcut of choosing a separate comparison group is usually adopted for studies of rare events.[3]

10. *Choice of identifying study subjects on the basis of the outcome variable rather than on the basis of the exposure variable.* When study and comparison subjects are identified separately, the method analogous to experimentation is to choose first the exposed, along with a control, and then later to measure outcome. The reverse can be done, choosing subjects first on the basis of outcome,

[2]Notice here that the word retrospective is used to refer to the point of view of the investigator, not of the study subject.

[3]There is a compromise method which combines the advantages of both extreme methods, but it is only possible when a roster of study subjects from a defined population can be obtained without the expense of processing all the nonexposed in that population. Then a random sample of the nonexposed members of the defined population can be selected as a comparison group, maintaining, with high probability, the advantages of a single identification process but without incurring the expense of processing large numbers of persons.

selecting a control, and then measuring their respective exposures.

This alternative is probably the most useful and at the same time the most misunderstood option open to the investigator. Such studies are often ambiguously termed retrospective studies because they are retrospective from the point of view of the subject, as well as from that of the investigator. However, they may be done prospectively from the point of view of the investigator, by identifying the cases as they are diagnosed and studying them one by one. For these reasons, they are best termed case-control studies, as opposed to cohort studies, in which subjects are identified with respect to a common exposure. Case-control studies have the time and cost advantages of retrospective cohort studies. They have the additional advantage of permitting the simultaneous evaluation of several alternative hypothesized causes of the same disease (and the mirror-image liability, i.e., several hypothesized diseases from the same exposure cannot be easily studied). It is possible to select by a single criterion a defined population, to divide it into case and control subjects on the basis of a common disease, and then to measure the exposure to one or more possible causes. However, in most such population studies, the analysis proceeds on the alternative assumption that the population was divided into exposed and unexposed components.

Case-control designs are perhaps most distinctive and useful when rare diseases are studied with the use of a separate comparison group. A roster of cases can easily be obtained from one or more clinical facilities and a comparison group chosen, either from the same facility or from another source. If the population from which these cases are derived can be defined, it may be possible to select comparison subjects randomly from a sampling frame of the non-cases in that population.

Two disadvantages of this method are often cited. Bias, as in any study, may affect the initial selection of cases (only cases known to be exposed might be admitted to the hospitals) or the measurement of exposure (subjects known to be cases may be questioned more thoroughly and may be more willing to respond to questioning). The second disadvantage is that a measure of the strength of the association (relative risk) must be estimated rather than calculated directly from the data obtained. The difference between the two methods of calculation can be seen from Example 1. Unless the disease affects a significant proportion of the population, however, this estimation is sufficiently accurate for practical purposes.

Example 1.

Cohort Study

Outcome	*Exposure* *Yes*	*No*
Yes	10	100
No	20	870
Total	30	970

Risk Ratio (Relative Risk) =

$$\frac{\frac{\text{cases exposed}}{\text{total exposed}}}{\frac{\text{cases not exposed}}{\text{total not exposed}}} = \frac{\frac{10}{30}}{\frac{100}{970}} = 3.23$$

Case-Control Study

Outcome	*Exposure* *Yes*	*No*	*Total*
Yes	10	100	110
No	20	870	890

If the disease is uncommon, then the *cases* in each category are negligible compared to the noncases. The *distribution* of exposure among noncases is equivalent to that among the mass of the population from which the cases come. (If it is known to be different, confounding is present and the relative risk itself must be invalid.) This estimate of relative risk is called *relative odds*, and is an overestimate when the actual relative risk is greater than unity.

$$\text{Risk Ratio (Relative Risk)} = \frac{\frac{\text{cases exposed}}{\text{total exposed}}}{\frac{\text{cases not exposed}}{\text{total not exposed}}} = \frac{(\text{cases exposed}) \times (\text{total not exposed})}{(\text{cases not exposed}) \times (\text{total exposed})}$$

$$\text{Odds Ratio (Relative Odds)} = \frac{(\text{cases exposed}) \times (\text{non-cases not exposed})}{(\text{cases not exposed}) \times (\text{non-cases exposed})} = \frac{(10)(870)}{(100)(20)} = 4.35$$

MISCELLANEOUS EPIDEMIOLOGIC TASKS

Not all problems appear in the form of a specific hypothesis to be tested. A number of other epidemiologic services should be mentioned.

1. *Hypothesis formulation.* The detailed distribution of a disease of unknown etiology may provide clues to its etiology; an understanding of epidemiology greatly aids in the interpretation of such data. The information used to generate a hypothesis cannot, of course, be used to test it. A list of useful and available descriptive variables would include:

Time: secular trend (decades); season (months, weeks).

Person: age, sex, birth cohort, birth order, parity, race, religion, occupation, income, education, marital status, residence, citizenship, travel and migration history.

2. *Outbreak investigation.* The epidemiologist is often asked to assess the origin and significance of a sudden epidemic cluster of cases. Three steps are generally required: First, the hypothesized presence of an unexpectedly high frequency of disease must be verified. The pattern of frequency in the community must then be reviewed for purposes of hypothesis formulation. This step requires a detailed knowledge of empiric epidemiology, since various forms of exposure (air or water ingestion, droplet inspiration, venereal contact, and so on) may be manifested in reproducible patterns. Lastly, the most likely hypotheses must be tested using material other than that used to develop them.

3. *Management of disease control or eradication programs.* Whether formally administered by an epidemiologist or not, programs which are directed by repeated tactical (as opposed to long-term policy) decisions are highly dependent for their success upon constant employment of two techniques—surveillance and cluster analysis. Surveillance refers to the process of gathering routine data for the purpose of identifying and responding to outbreaks. Cluster analysis is a commonly used method of detecting the presence of outbreaks or clusters. The presence of such phenomena implies an environmental and time-restricted causal element in the etiologic web. Examples of such programs would include malaria and smallpox eradication, polio and measles vaccination, and lead poisoning prevention campaigns. Available data are gathered and hypotheses formulated in explanation of the pattern of disease or of program coverage. Specific remedial efforts are designed to fit the circum-

stance, surveillance reinstituted, and another cycle of tactical program management begun.

4. *Natural history investigation.* Clinicians must generally rely on the study of self-selected patients whose disease beginnings and terminations may or may not be observed depending upon the whims of the medical care system. Consequently, the prodromata and outcomes of diseases are often poorly understood. The epidemiologist has several tools which can be used to advantage in studying these problems.

Entire populations may be surveyed, or they may be screened; either way, the usual care system exigencies are avoided. Record systems may be used to advantage for follow-up, particularly if record linkages permit individuals to be followed across geographic boundaries and personal transitions. Measures of outcome, such as case fatality ratios (deaths/cases or mortality rate/incidence rate), complication and residual abnormality rates, disease infection ratios, and five-year survival rates, need to be calculated with careful avoidance of confounding.

Disease models permit useful estimates of dimensions which cannot be directly measured. For example, as incidence rate = persons diagnosed/population/unit time, and prevalence rate = diseased persons at a given point/population at the same point; then, if the disease is stable and in equilibrium (with constant incidence and prevalence), prevalence rate = incidence rate times the duration of disease in units of time. Therefore, if a survey measures the prevalence of undiagnosed intraepithelial carcinoma of the cervix (in situ), and the incidence of the same condition is measured either by periodically reexamining known negatives or by extrapolating from the incidence of symptomatic disease, the average duration of the condition prior to diagnosis can be calculated.

5. *Assessment of therapy.* As in natural history studies, careful evaluations of therapeutic efficacy are often difficult in a clinical setting, either because of the number or special nature of the available patients, or because of the clinician's inability to painstakingly follow up patients or to overcome problems in ethics or bias. Epidemiologists are increasingly called upon to provide study designs which reduce these problems with the use of such techniques as randomization, blind assessment, linked record searches, and sequential design. Commonly, sample size is increased by enlisting several geographically separate institutions in a common study design and centrally coordinating the assignment of subjects and the follow-up.

6. *Evaluation of programs.* Even when a therapeutic service is

effective, the program delivering it may have no impact, whether because of deficient scope, appeal, or thrust, or because of the effectiveness of alternative solutions to the same problem. Program evaluation may be very difficult for several reasons. Outcome criteria may be difficult to specify, for the system of intervention may retard health in some respects, just as it advances health in other respects. In addition, the program itself may confound the usual measures of outcome. For example, screening programs detect disease earlier than would normally occur and those cases tend, of course, to be milder at time of diagnosis. Because an increment ("lead time") has thus been added to the observed disease duration, the average 5-year survival will seem to be increased even if the program has no effect. Similarly, the case fatality ratio will temporarily seem to decrease as an increment of mild cases is added to the total number thought to be at risk of dying. In such circumstances it may be necessary to rely upon age-specific mortality or morbidity from the disease in question, or even upon age-specific mortality or morbidity from all causes.

In addition, it is usually difficult to find a comparable population for the purpose of obtaining a source of expectation under the null hypothesis of no program effect. Randomization is rarely possible, and time trends and geographic comparisons are often highly confounded. The use of such stable outcome indices as age-specific mortality further complicates matters. Because decisions must be made, however, such problems demand the most careful epidemiologic examination, rather than the superficial attention that seems warranted by the quality of the data. This complex area will be discussed in a later chapter.

SUMMARY OF OBJECTIVES FOR THE READER

It is hoped that the study of this chapter will result in behavioral changes in the readers. They should henceforth be able to:

Accept the notion that epidemiologists are a heterogeneous collection of diverse investigators, but that the subject of epidemiology itself is fundamental to biology, to the health sciences in particular, and especially to health decision making.

Understand that decision making is an act which requires both qualitative and quantitative information, and that neither decision making nor its quantitative aspects can be avoided.

Expect biologic information, like other human products, to be of variable quality.

Develop the habit of examining the scope, the relevance of the actual subject variables, the nature of the implied relationship, and the dependability of each piece of information.

Understand the subjective aspects of the scope and of the relevance of classifications, of scales, and of adjustments.

Understand and differentiate between the various quantitative elements found in informational items.

Understand the concept of multiple causation.

Understand that while hypotheses may be rejected, they never can be verified. They may be rejected by finding that no association can be demonstrated, or that a demonstrated association is either attributable to chance, or not valid, or not causal.

Understand the probabilistic nature of any scientific conclusion.

Understand the general procedure for evaluating the dependability of a piece of information.

Be prepared to specify, without invitation when necessary, what potentially useful information is not available.

Be prepared to recognize when epidemiologic skills can be useful.

Be aware of the efficiency and validity implications of various study designs so as to discourage waste and increase the overall level of information quality.

It is also hoped that, having studied this chapter, readers will discourage any future tendencies to:

Accept dogmatic information, classifications, causal ideas, study design caveats, or management rules without justification.

Assume a sufficient expertise in epidemiology, biostatistics, study design or decision theory to preclude useful consultation or search in the sources comprising the appended bibliography.

BIBLIOGRAPHY

For a more complete understanding of study design, or of other epidemiologic topics, the reader is directed to the following source materials:

Armitage, P. *Statistical methods in medical research.* Oxford: Blackwell, 1971. Best single volume on biostatistics.

Clark, D. W., and MacMahon, B. *Preventive medicine.* Boston: Little, Brown & Co., 1967. A general text with useful descriptive epidemiology and vital statistics sections.

Fox, J. P., Hall, C. E., and Elveback, L. R. *Epidemiology: Man and disease.* New York: The Macmillan Co., 1970.

Hill, A. B. *Principles of medical statistics.* New York: Oxford University Press, 1971, 9th ed. Most readable introduction to biostatistics.

Hurst, J. W., and Walker, H. K., eds. *The problem-oriented system.* New York: MEDCOM, 1972.

Ipsen, J., and Feigl, P. *Bancroft's introduction to biostatistics.* New York: Harper & Row, 1970, 2nd ed. Good, oversimplified introduction to biostatistics.

Lusted, L. B. *Introduction to medical decision making.* Springfield, Ill.: Charles C Thomas, 1968.

MacMahon, B., and Pugh, T. F. *Epidemiology: Principles and methods.* Boston: Little, Brown & Co., 1970. Best guide to study design.

Miettinen, O. *Evaluation of cause-effect relationships in epidemiology.* WHO Monograph, 1972. Best guide to analytic issues in epidemiology.

Oldham, P. D. *Measurement in medicine.* Philadelphia: J.B. Lippincott Company, 1968.

Raiffa, H. *Decision analysis. Introductory lectures on choices under uncertainty.* Reading, Mass.: Addison-Wesley, 1968.

Snedecor, G. W., and Cochran, W. G. *Statistical methods.* Ames, Iowa: Iowa State University Press, 1967, 6th ed. Most comprehensive textbook of biostatistics.

APPENDIX—SOURCES OF DATA

I. U.S.A. NATIONAL

A. *Vital Records*—Vital Statistics of the U.S. USDHEW (until 1945 Dept. of Commerce), National Center for Health Statistics (until 1963, National Office of Vital Statistics). Annual volumes, several years behind. Source: Birth, Death, Marriage, Divorce Certificates.

1. Birth Tabulations: State of occurrence, residence, month, color, sex, plurality, weight, maternal age, maternal nativity, gestation, birth order, legitimacy, urban-rural.
   a. Birth Rates: State, month, color, maternal age, birth order.
2. Death Tabulations: State, institution, place, residence, county, summary of time trend, month, age, color, race, sex, autopsy, cause of death—ISC 3-digit and 4-digit code. Selected causes (in 1967 lists of 258, 60, and 15) with more detail.
   a. Death Rates: Age, color, sex, cause of death (60—list). Infant, fetal, and accident mortality covered separately.
3. Other Vital Statistics: Marriage, Divorce, Life tables.
4. Miscellaneous inclusions: Population summaries and intercensal estimates, methods, etc.
5. Before 1963: Special reports on mortality, natality, trends, etc.
6. Monthly Vital Statistics Report: Current (2-3 months) information.

B. *Morbidity*—U.S. National Health Survey. USDHEW, N.C.H.S. Several series of topical reports. Source: Households, physicians, and medical records.

1. Before 1963: PHS publication #584—Health Statistics from the U.S.N.H.S.
   - Series A. Program description, survey designs, definitions.
   - Series B. Results by topics.
   - Series C. Results for population groups.
   - Series D. Development and evaluation reports.
2. After 1963: PHS Publication #1000—Report for Vital and Health Statistics.
   - Series 1. Programs and collection procedures.
   - Series 2. Data evaluation and methods research.

Series 3. Analytic studies (including international comparisons).
Series 4. Documents and committee reports.
Series 10. Data from the Health Interview Survey.
Series 11. Data from the Health Examination Survey.
Series 12. Data from the Institutional Population Surveys.
Series 13. Data from the Hospital Discharge Survey.
Series 14. Data on health resources, manpower, and facilities.
Series 20. Data on mortality.
Series 21. Data on natality, marriage, and divorce.
Series 22. Data from the National Natality and Morbidity Surveys.

3. 1928-1931: 9000 randomly selected families. Perrott, G. St. J. et al. Publ. Health Reports 54:1663–1687, 1939.

C. *Population*—U.S. Census. U.S. Dept. of Commerce, Bureau of Census. Decennial. Source: Household interview.
   1. Characteristics of the population for 57 states and territories.
      a. Number by state, city, county, size of community, urban-rural.
      b. Number by sex, age, marital status, color, race, relationship to head of household.
      c. Number by nativity, parentage, state of birth, country of origin, mother tongue, previous residence, education, employment status, occupation group, income.
   2. Subject Reports: Selected detail for such subjects as national origin, fertility, marital status, migration, education, employment, occupation, income.
   3. Selected Area Reports: Selected detail for size of place, economic units, etc.
   4. Housing census.

D. *Notifiable Diseases*—Morbidity and Mortality Weekly Report. USDHEW, CDC. Source: physicians' reports.
   1. Tabulations of current morbidity from 30 specified notifiable (infectious) diseases by week, state, and region.
   2. Tabulations of current mortality (total and infant, 65+, pneumonia and influenza) in 123 U.S. cities.
   3. Brief epidemiologic notes and current epidemics and other epidemiologically interesting events.
   4. Irregular status reports on specified notifiable diseases

and vaccination status reports, etc. (separate).

E. *Cancer*
1. Connecticut: Cancer in Conn., 1935-51. Conn. State Dept. Health, annual reports.
2. Iowa: Cancer Morb. in Urban and Rural Iowa. PHS monograph #37, 1955.
3. New York State (upstate): Bureau of Cancer Control, annual reports.
4. Ten Cities Survey: Incidence data from survey in 1947-48. PHS monographs #29 (1954), #56 (1960), re-survey in progress (1971).
5. End Results Group: Summaries from 3 state registries, 10 large city hospital registries and the VA. NCI monograph #6 (1961) and E.R.G. Report #3, 1968.

F. *Miscellaneous*
1. Vital statistics rates in the U.S. 2 volumes.
   1900-1940: Nat. Off. Vit. Stat. 1947.
   1940-1960: Nat. Cent. Health Stat. 1948. PHS #1677.
2. United States Metropolitan Mortality 1959-61, 1 volume.
3. Historical Statistics of the U.S.; Colonial times to 1957, 1 volume.
   U.S. Dept. Commerce, Bureau of Census, 1960.
4. Health Resources Statistics Annual Summary. USDHEW, NCHS, PHS #1509.
5. Annotated Bibliography on Vital and Health Statistics 1965-1967. USDHEW, NCHS, PHS #2094, 1970.
6. Current Bibliography of Epidemiology (CUBE). APHA, monthly.
7. Statistical Abstract of the U.S. U.S. Dept. Commerce B. of Census, Annual.
8. Vital and Health Statistics monographs. APHA: Accidents and homicide, maternal and child mortality, infectious diseases, fertility, tuberculosis.
9. Current Medical Terminology. AMA, 1970, 3rd ed.
10. National Atlas of U.S. U.S.D.I., Geological Survey, Washington, D.C., 1970. Includes much geographic, meterologic, and economic detail.

II. INTERNATIONAL

A. *Vital Records*
1. Epidemiological and Vital Statistics Reports. Monthly, Notifiable disease, morbidity, mortality. General and

infant mortality. Births. Causes of death (each of 60—list covered at least once annually). Vaccinations, neoplasm incidence, other special subjects covered.

2. World Health Statistics Annual (before 1962: Annual Epidemiological and Vital Statistics). WHO, Geneva.
3. UN Demographic Yearbook—see under *"Population."*

B. *Morbidity*—Not available except for notifiable diseases (see A and D) and individual developed countries.

1. Great Britain: Social Survey 1944-1952. Reported irregularly in Reports of the Ministry of Health, Quarterly Returns of the Registrar General. Also, the Registrar General's Statistical Review of England and Wales for the two years 1950-1951, Supplement on General Morbidity, Cancer and Mental Health, 1955.
2. Canada and Denmark. See National Committee on Vital & Health Statistics—National Morbidity Survey Recommendations. PHS Publ. #333 reprinted in #1000, Series 1, #1, 1963.

C. *Population*

1. UN Demographic Yearbook. Statistical Office of the UN, annual since 1948. Gives world summary, area, population density, population, rate of increase, births and deaths, fetal deaths, marriages, divorces, migrations, rates, and life tables. Special topics in different years.

D. *Notifiable Diseases*

1. Pan American Weekly Epidemiologic Report. PAHO, Washington, D.C. Current incidence of 21 notifiable infectious diseases.
2. Weekly Epidemiologic Record. WHO, Geneva. Current information by locality on 8 internationally notifiable diseases.

E. *Cancer*—Morbidity reports are available for a variety of areas, among them Belgium, Canada, Czechoslovakia, Denmark, Finland, Germany (DDR and BRD), Italy, Netherlands, New Zealand, Norway, Sweden, Poland, U.K., Japan, Uganda, USSR.

1. Cancer on Five Continents. Vol. I (1966) and Vol. II (1970). International Union against Cancer (UICC).
2. Clemmeson, J. Statistical Studies on Malignant Neoplasms. Vols. I, II, III. 1964, 1970 (Monksgaard, Copenhagen).

F. *Miscellaneous*

1. International Classification of Diseases, Adapted. Vols. I & II. Eighth revision, 1968. USDHEW, NCHS, PHS #1693.
2. Medical Research Council Special Report Series #1-320+. A complete listing of the Series may be found in the dictionary catalogue of the London School of Hygiene and Trop. Medicine. Library Vol. 2.
3. Registrar General's Statistical Review of England and Wales. Her Majesty's Station. Office, London, Annual since 1839. Vital Statistics, census estimates, morbidity surveys, cancer registration, special investigations, deaths and death rates, births and birth rates, commentary. Supplements on general morbidity, cancer, and mental health (1949-1955), hospital inpatient statistics (1949-1955), cancer (1952-1964), mental health (1952-1960), and decennial supplements.
4. Studies on medical and population subjects. Occasional publications since 1948. Her Majesty's Station. Office, London.
5. WHO Technical Report Series 1-500+: Summary publications by expert committees.
6. Bull Hyg and Trop Dis Bull: Systematic annotated bibliographies monthly.
7. UN Statistical Yearbook. UN Statistical Office, New York. Annual.

4

Health Services Research: Asking the Painful Questions

Charles E. Lewis

Health services research can be viewed as the epidemiology of the health care system, when this system is conceived in its broadest terms. Whereas conventional epidemiology deals with the distribution and determinants of disease, health services research (HSR) focuses on the factors which impinge on results of disease, especially those mechanisms mounted by society in an effort to alter the course of disease. Put another way, HSR is evaluative research which may examine all or any part of the health care system.

The business of health services research is to study: 1) the workings of a system—including all subsystems (traditional and nontraditional) by which people perceive needs and try to meet these needs through some form of care (whether it be from herbalist, youth clinic, or cardiologist); 2) the subsequent adventures between doctor and patient, or nurse and patient; 3) the utilization of goods, commodities, and facilities; and 4) the piling up of costs. HSR studies the process by which we do something to people, and may even include studies to determine whether or not those things we do achieve any change in health status.

In this sense, HSR is part of a continuum that begins with epidemiology's focus on the causes of illness in a population. Viewed from the HSR perspective, these illnesses may be labeled needs, but needs as defined by whom? The provider? The consumer? Needs are in the eye of the beholder.

Needs give rise to the decision to demand care. This demand is based upon: 1) being aware of some problem; and 2) translating this awareness into a demand (via something called health or illness behavior, depending upon whether the demand is to maintain health or to treat sickness or illness). The demand for care results in utilization of services; and utilization of services results in processes of care which, in turn, lead to outcomes.

Perhaps this chain of events is best considered as a series of questions. The problem-oriented approach to health services research helps one to understand the organization of health services. Why do people become ill? Who's sick? Where are they sick? Who makes the demands? What kinds of services are provided? Who does what to whom? How much does it cost? Who pays for it? What are the results of these services? By asking such a series of questions, one can develop some designs for studies to examine the bits and pieces.

The Scope of Health Services Research

Health services research is a fascinating field because it is a smorgasbord of many academic disciplines. A good project may involve a biostatistician to facilitate the derivation of a sample. In all probability, it will require a computing center or computer backup. It will utilize the talents of the epidemiologist to help adjust for those things in the population that can't be controlled. If it is like many investigations, it will range into the social sciences—anthropology, sociology, psychology, and economics. It will also draw on the talents of the clinician. It can involve people in schools of theology or law. (It may even involve psychiatrists to take care of the people who do this kind of research!)

It is a fascinating field for generalists. The research applications one reviews reflect the fact that in conducting HSR one needs access to almost everyone in the university (although not necessarily to do any one piece of research). Basically, it is multidisciplinary research involving some disciplines whose practitioners not only don't talk to each other, but sometimes don't even like each other. Health services researchers look at preventive, environmental, and other types of health services which are not necessarily intended to cure disease or illness.

Some examples may illustrate the breadth of health services research. Figure 1 outlines several of the components in the health care system. The decision to seek care is an interesting one. In spite of many studies, very little is known about the factors that influence some individuals to see a doctor for low backache, while others assume that this discomfort is rather normal (1). Often a visit to the

Figure 1

COMPONENTS OF HEALTH CARE SYSTEM

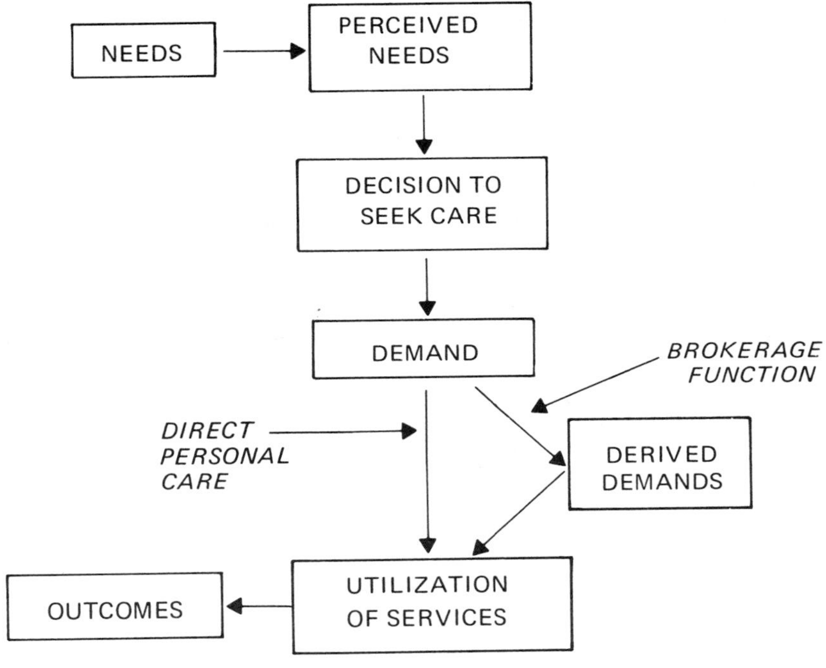

physician constitutes one's initial entry point into health care. The physician performs a brokerage function. He decides to take the patient's money or his proxy for money (insurance). With it he buys so many shares of x-ray or laboratory service, public health nursing, or occupational therapy. The physician is the source of derived demands by almost everyone in the health business, including himself. Up to 70 percent of the physician's patients are in that office because of the doctor's request that they return; physicians are thus the primary initiators of patients' return visits (2).

Although the physician can and does provide direct personal care, one of the important areas for both research and education is the physician's brokerage function in securing the professional services of other groups to whom he may never have been exposed in medical school. In care teams or any other form of comprehensive care service, the extent to which certain physicians are aware of and can define the role of the occupational therapist, the speech therapist, and other supportive professionals is often a determinant of the extent to which he utilizes those services for the care of his patients.

Figure 2

PATIENT CARE SYSTEM

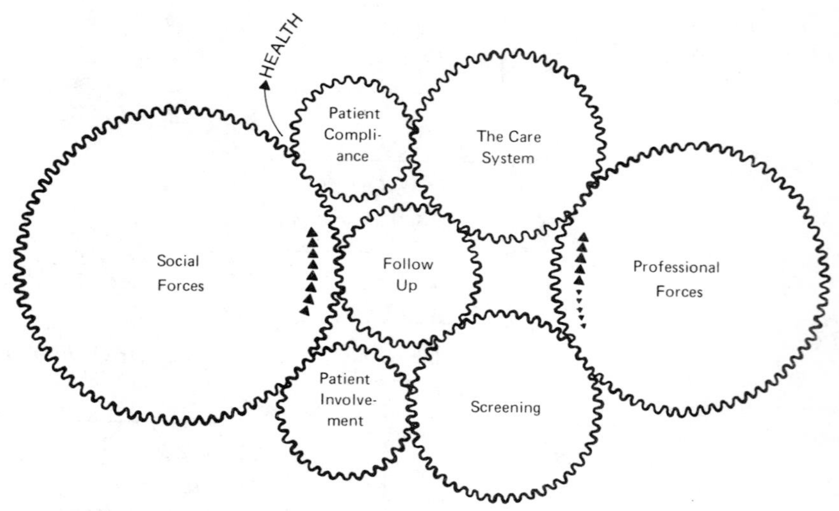

But the trend for the physician to furnish the initial pathway by which the patient enters the care system is beginning to break down. Nurses are involved in giving primary care; social workers are seeing patients directly; occupational therapists are seeing patients without referrals from physicians—so are psychologists. The system seems about to rupture completely, and permit patients direct access to a large variety of health professionals and disciplines.

There is a tendency for those who discuss health services research to oversimplify the subject and to confuse research itself with the consequences of research. Figure 2 offers a schematic representation of our present patient care system. Patient involvement is the initial step. For example, the first problem in setting up a multiphasic screening program is obviously to get the patients in. Not all patients show up; the epidemiologist can identify bias in the order of their coming into care. The screening process is probably the simplest thing we do. It requires simply having the patient lie down, doing certain things to him, and letting the machines run. The real problem begins with the follow-up of abnormal conditions revealed by these screening procedures. Even then, getting the patient into the care system for definitive diagnosis and therapy implies the return of the system to the patient's control as far as his compliance with follow-up is concerned.

One can break this system into those forces which are related to professional issues—that is, screening, making a diagnosis, and prescribing treatment—and those which are totally related to the social forces in our society (the extent to which the medical care is delivered is dependent upon the patient—his social class, his education, his ability to comply, his own version of whether or not tomorrow is worth living for). These latter forces are perhaps not within the direct control of the medical profession as it is now structured, yet it is fascinating to find physicians talking about equity of care, equality in health services, and so on, without some degree of separation of social and professional responsibilities.

If one looks at infant death rates (deaths of infants over 28 days of age and less than 1 year of age), one finds that a social class gradient is evident. As a matter of fact, there seems to be a social class gradient in everything. If one were inclined to overgeneralize, one could say that in education and health services nothing makes as much difference as the social class of one's family and one's peers. A study which is rarely cited in the literature, but which involved 1.5 million people in England and Wales after the institution of the National Health Service, looked at factors influencing infant death rates (3). One of the issues was the extent to which housing, age of mother, and other social factors, including the quality of mothering, were important to the survival of babies. These are the kinds of questions HSR has to deal with, that is, it studies how processes work to influence care.

EXAMPLES OF HSR

Nurse Clinicians

Health services research may be concerned with questions of manpower. Can alternatives be found to replace or supplement professionals in short supply such as physicians? An example of this type of experiment is the nurse-clinic program established at the University of Kansas. It seemed logical to the investigators that certain nurses, particularly those with a high degree of competence, who had worked on inpatient services or were experienced as public health nurses, and who were capable of working independently, would have the skills needed to care for chronically ill ambulatory patients. In 1964 a protocol was drafted for transferring to nurses the care of a group of chronically ill patients who were in a fairly static phase of their illness, and plans were made to evaluate this program in terms of what it accomplished. At this time everyone in the institution was very favorably disposed toward the project—the chief of medicine, the head of nursing services, and the hospital administrators.

The program was established with a grant in 1965. Patients were selected according to certain criteria (those with hypertensive cardiovascular diseases, arteriosclerotic heart disease, and so on). All patients were interviewed to discover their past experiences with medical care, other places they had received care, and their images of physicians and nurses; they were asked which things they preferred to have done by doctors and which by nurses. After the patients had been pretested, and after the nurses and the physicians had written objectives for their care, we randomly allocated half of them into the nurses' clinic and half to the medical clinic, the control situation. The group sent to the nurses had the proposal explained to them: from that time on, they would be treated primarily by a nurse; two physicians would review their records and would see them any time the patients wanted to be seen (they would be seen periodically anyway), but generally they would be seen by a nurse in her office at her scheduled time; she would initiate their care. There were no refusals. After this program had run for one year, we retested and added the following findings to observations made en route (4,5).

One of the first things we were concerned about was the extent to which certain people will not let certain other people do certain things to or for them. So the patients were asked about this. In the beginning, they preferred to have the doctor perform all functions except for giving instructions about diet and for changing dressings. At the end of a year, those patients who had been seen by nurses were asked this question again, and every function that they had previously reserved for the doctors had been transferred to the nurses: the patients had reversed themselves. Many of the perceptions of what professionals feel patients will not accept seem to be projections of the professionals' images of professionals.

Every patient completed a structured interview questionnaire which included: the past history of their disease, whether or not the patients were pro-doctor or pro-nurse in general, the frequency of their complaints, the extent to which they would have sought medical attention for complaints, and their preference for doctors over nurses. A comparison of the study and the control groups before and after revealed virtually no change in the experimental group except in two areas: 1) in the area of declared illness behavior, the nurses' patients reported a decrease in frequency of complaints and stated that they would less often seek attention for the complaints; and 2) in the area of preference, they preferred having a nurse perform clinical functions formerly left to the physician.

A time and motion study of how the patients spent their time in the control clinic and in the nurses' clinic showed that the control group spent 57 percent of its time in waiting, versus 9-10 percent for the nurses' clinic group; 5 percent versus 6 percent in clerical activities; and 38 percent versus 84 percent receiving professional care. This study illustrates how one can borrow industrial engineering techniques to examine what's going on in health care agencies.

Major interest in this study centered around the nature of the care processes provided by the nurses and whether or not they made any difference in terms of outcome. These outcomes are commonly classified under a series of D's—death, disability levels, disease severity levels, discomfort, dissatisfaction, and so on. Clinicians tend to be more interested in process and focus on factors within it, such as the number of tests performed, the number of things done, the number of items used. As a general rule, if a process can be measured without any trouble, it probably yields process information. If the measurement takes more time, it probably yields outcome information.

Using a critical incident technique which Paul Sanazaro and John Williamson (6) had employed with internists, we measured what the nurses were doing in their clinic. The nurses described what they did that they felt made a significant difference in the care of a particular patient; this information was classified in a taxonomy which ranged from ordering a procedure, to providing a certain kind of support, to involving a community agency. These process data were then juxtaposed against D's in the two study groups. To sum it up, there were no differences in death rates, or in disease levels; but the patients cared for by the nurses had a significantly lower disability level after a year of care than those cared for in the medical clinic. The soft outcomes—discomfort, dissatisfaction in terms of broken appointments—were also different, but most significant was the difference in disability.

In many ways, this study represented a lot of work to prove something everyone knows. When someone focuses on chronically ill patients, without trying to cure them (which is impossible) but trying to improve their quality of life—getting them back to work, getting them a job, getting them moving in activities of daily living—they improve. Aiming at the target more specifically *ought* to result in better outcomes. However, the failure to implement this concept early testifies to the need for careful documentation of any innovation, no matter how obvious it may appear.

Continuing Education of Physicians

To illustrate the varied scope of HSR it may be helpful to review another but very different study of health manpower. Continuing education for physicians has become increasingly popular. Currently there is debate about requiring it for relicensure. The University of Kansas has an interesting continuing education program which began as courses for health officers in the 1920s. Over the years, a number of circuit courses were developed, i.e., courses on various topics were conducted off campus. Other courses and symposia were offered at the medical center. Some programs were designed for practitioners who came to the center for in-residence training.

We decided to look at what had gone on in continuing education during the decade 1956-65 (7). This presented the problem of determining just who was at risk—who had been exposed to the "treatment" of continuing education. Data from all medical directories, the obituary columns of the medical society, and county medical society directories were collated. In about four different ways, all physicians who had been in practice in Kansas during that ten-year period were listed, along with the dates on which they entered and/or left practice any time during that period. The average length of exposure was less than ten years, revealing a substantial amount of movement among physicians entering, leaving practice, and dying. After securing this information for all 2,090 physicians who were in practice, we analyzed their characteristics.

A big problem in HSR is related to the way records are kept, not only on patients, but on everything. The records for the continuing education program consisted of two closets full of shoeboxes filled with slips of paper on which the names of physicians had been written as they had enrolled for every course that had been given. It took an enormous amount of effort to collate all of these slips of paper for all 2090 physicians. As can be seen in Table 1, the average number of hours the physicians spent in circuit courses and non-circuit symposia during this ten-year period was impressive. The average time per physician at risk per year was 7.5 hours in internal medicine, but 6.5 percent of the physicians took half of all the hours of continuing education offered.

The cost of this educational program was quite high, coming to several million dollars. This included the estimated cost of physicians' time and travel and the operational costs of empty physicians' offices. The cost to the university over the ten-year period

Table 1
Experience of 2090 Physicians in Private Practice (1956–1965)

Type of Program	Average Hours/ Physician	Hours/Physician/ Year at Risk	Percentage of Physicians Accounting for 50% of All Hours
Circuit*	49.1	7.3	6.5
Non-circuit symposia:	35.7	5.3	9.1
Medicine	11.6	1.7	3.6
Surgery	6.1	0.9	2.4
Pediatrics	3.2	0.5	1.8
Obstetrics	2.6	0.3	1.9

* Excludes physicians in regions without access to program.
Source: reference 7.

approximated $13.5 million plus or minus one or two million dollars—or an annual tuition rate of about $650 per physician per year.

Because Kansas includes regions with different characteristics, data were grouped according to where these physicians were in practice and by their specialty—general practice, surgery, or medicine. Certain regions provided the most problems in health care: the fewest physicians, the oldest physicians, the fewest new physicians, the oldest population, and the highest infant mortality rates. These same regions had the lowest involvement in continuing education.

There was a relationship between continuing education and type of practice. Physicians specializing in medicine took the highest number of symposia hours—50 percent of the internists were involved in some activity of this type as compared with 38 percent of the general practitioners. On the other hand, 32 percent of the internists took some circuit course, versus 44 percent of the generalists.

We compared some data on medical care with these educational process figures. The tonsillectomy and adenoidectomy (T & A) rates (per 10,000 at risk) for Blue Cross subscribers' children under 14 years of age were compared with postgraduate education data. In the two regions that had the highest T & A rates, no physician took any otolaryngology postgraduate education course during the ten-year period.

Table 2 demonstrates the relationship between elective surgical

Table 2
Relationship between Rates for Four Elective Surgical Procedures and Continuing Education in Surgery

Region	Average Hours Continuing Education in Surgery/M.D.	Rank[1]	Rate for Elective Surgery[2]	Rank[3]
1	2.45	11	—	—
2	7.41	8	101.3	8
3	10.31	4	75.3	10
4	4.96	10	125.1	6
5	15.96	1	152.2	5
6	13.81	2	187.4	3
7	10.96	3	204.6	1
8	8.57	7	192.4	2
9	10.06	5	177.2	4
10	6.51	9	111.1	7
11	9.93	6	84.7	9

[1]Ranked so that 1 = highest number of hours/M.D.
[2]Rate—Total number of hernia repairs, + hemorrhoidectomies, + varicose vein strippings, + tonsillectomies per 10,000 Blue Cross subscribers during 12 months (1965-1966).
[3]Ranked so that 1 = highest rate of surgical procedures.

procedures—in this case T & A, hernia repair, hemorrhoidectomy, and varicose vein stripping—and physicians' average hours of continuing education in surgery. No significant associations were found. This lack of association also held in comparing perinatal death rates by region with participation by physicians in obstetrics and pediatrics courses.

Examination of the maternal death rate by regions and by physicians' educational experiences revealed some interesting findings. The area with the next to lowest physician participation in postgraduate education had the lowest maternal death rate. This is not the way it is supposed to be!

Discriminant function analysis was used to characterize those doctors who took the highest and lowest number of hours. The "discriminators" for noncircuit courses were younger physicians and specialists who practiced outside the metropolitan areas. Incidentally, these rates had no relationship to rank in medical school class on graduation. One of the interesting byproducts of this study was the opportunity to look at all the class ranks for Kansas University graduates. During the period studied the school was ranking every student so that it was possible to place every graduate in the state and know whether he ranked first or one hundredth in his class. There was no relationship between participation in continuing education and class rank.

EVALUATIVE HSR

Evaluation research is a growing type of HSR. The term itself implies values; someone has to declare what is and what is not important. Several efforts are being made to evaluate health service programs. Some evaluative studies describe end results. A national halothane study showed a 27-fold difference in the postoperative death rates among a variety of institutions in the United States (8). After adjustments for age of patients and so forth, this difference dropped to 10-fold, and when the severity of operation factor was controlled it was down to 3-fold. Nonetheless, this is an example of an end result that shows differences of some magnitude between hospitals in regard to the survival of patients (standardized by operation, by age, and so on). In this case, the results were merely descriptive without judgment or prescription for change.

Another study examines whether or not something happens to someone. For example, Leon Gordis looked at teenage pregnancy prevention programs; the end result of this study was whether the girls got pregnant (9). Such a study looks at the outcome as a function of patient characteristics. Many studies reported in the literature have used various outcomes, results, events, or deaths as their end results. In general, these outcomes can be divided into those with favorable results and those which did not come out well.

Other process studies merely describe how things are done. The process of providing surgical care differs from one hospital to another. If one utilizes normative standards to conduct quality of care audit measurements, one can show a difference in performance level among groups. Another group of studies merely points out that the processes were different. In the University of Kansas study, the utilization of continuing education in Kansas over a ten-year period was different; it was a function of certain physician characteristics. Finally, there are other studies in which one simultaneously looks at a process and describes an end result. Again, the continuing education study represents one attempt to link these two types of data.

RESEARCH TECHNIQUES AND METHODOLOGY

The Kansas study illustrates the importance of identifying the right question. One can't get away from the fact that the most important procedure in HSR is to ask a good question; that is, a question which is both important and precise. The literature in this field is replete with reports of studies on trivial questions. Health services research of any analytical nature requires an epidemiologic stance. Without a sample drawn from a known population at risk, and without adequate control groups, one encounters a great deal of trouble achieving anything except rhetoric.

Health services research requires valid and precise measurements of "it," whatever "it" is, at time zero and at end-result time, as well as accurate measurements of what is really being offered as treatment. There are more phantom treatments in this world than anyone could dream of—treatments that never reach patients. In one classic paper of this type the investigators concluded that mental patients referred to public health nursing service showed no difference in terms of relapse rates as compared with those not referred (10). The investigators were disappointed; but they didn't fall back on the best criterion they had—they neglected to measure what the nurses actually did to or for the patients. Until we standardize treatment measurements, we will continue to work in a black-box business.

Laboratory research is very different from HSR. One works on animals or excretions, publishes papers, and occasionally insults some person's intelligence, but nobody ever gets mad. Health services research is a hazardous business—researchers raise such questions as: Do you really do anything for patients? Is the medical clinic functioning? Why are the lines so long? What happens to your patients after they go home? Why is your operative rate for appendectomies three times as high as anyone else's? The answers to these questions may insult people's sense of their own integrity.

One can do little about changing systems unless one measures both process and end results. Most studies that ask significant questions raise issues of change, and thus threaten prestige and organizational integrity. There is a large mass of social experimentation from the 1960s which has never been evaluated, because no one considered how to measure the process. It is very difficult to sell negative outcome results that suggest the need for major change unless one can specify how he got those results and what might be changed to provide different results. One must be prepared to offer several alternatives by which to institutionalize the program under study, together with a sequenced schedule for proposed changes.

The foregoing remarks may sound anti-intellectual and unscientific, but there is a primary issue involved. Is evaluation simply a statistical dry run, or is it designed to do what it's supposed to do; i.e., provide mechanisms for change? Evaluation includes guidance, experience, and surveillance procedures for organizational maintenance and change. At times it may even include organizational destruction. Unfortunately, much of what is done in evaluation appears to be very destructive. Sometimes we fail to examine the consequences of our evaluations and to look for ways of softening the blow.

Consider the problems facing people working in renal dialysis today. They began with a procedure that achieved dramatic results; they saved lives. Now they are the victims of their own success; they cannot get money for process-oriented research into the problems of membrane transport, choice of media, and the like. They have been unable to attract basic science support because they already have end results. This is exactly what the "end-result people" will claim—end results are usually so overwhelming that if you really want to get something done, show end results. But if you anticipate negative end results and hope to change things, you will need a process-oriented approach as well to find out where or how things go wrong.

Good HSR that sets out to achieve end results usually fulfills these criteria. It specifies the treatment; it measures the treatment; and it measures the processes en route. As with any experiment one hopes to reproduce in other settings, what happened needs to be described in detail.

Many instruments are needed for HSR but one vital tool is a good record system. Record systems should be designed to provide information the physician wants but they should also meet the needs of the people who are evaluating processes and trying to effect change, neither of which can be accomplished in the absence of an adequate and appropriate record system. It is hard to imagine how one might evaluate ambulatory care without problem-oriented records.

Part of the difficulty in basic HSR planning and evaluation arises from the tendency to separate the groups involved. Too often, the evaluators, planners, and policy makers are isolated from those delivering health care on a daily basis. One group is thinking great thoughts, planning great evaluations, and making plans for health services. Then they deliver these to a department of medicine or pediatrics and expect to see them carried out. There is little chance of accomplishing operational programs or change through such procedure. The only way to make planning meaningful and evaluations of any consequence is to require early involvement of those who deliver the care; two-culture approach is untenable. A truly adequate record system is achieved only when the records meet the needs of those who use them as well as the researcher's needs. A sense of trust must be developed between the evaluator or researcher and the purveyor of care.

The work of some investigators who do a lot of research in which they isolate themselves from those who deliver health services is not accepted by medical schools, hospital associations, or other organizations. These evaluators appear intent upon proving something wrong, i.e., medicine is in a bad state, doctors cheat, and so on. Many protocols are drafted with a priori assumptions, for example, that multiphasic screening is the superior way of delivering care or that it has no place in the health care system. Although intellectual juggling of data may be necessary for planning and other purposes, the setting up of an hypothesis that can be disproved is fundamental to HSR. This procedure presents problems for many who see such statements as overtly critical of the project under study. Health services research demands a posture of concerned neutrality; maintaining one's credibility is essential to remaining effective.

IMPLICATIONS OF HSR FOR MEDICAL EDUCATION

What do all these ideas mean to medical education? How can they be taught? Is HSR relevant? Does it have any worth for medical students? It would seem that medical students certainly should know something about the way the system works, but how is that best taught? Studies of the type described here present some problems for the institution in which they are conducted and for those who carry them out.

Medical students fit basically into three categories. There are 1) the pragmatists who basically want to know how to do something and don't really want to know why; they usually go into certain specialties; 2) the abstractionists who are very comfortable with such concepts as compliance, cognitive dissonance, and other things—ego structure, ego trips, for example; they often go into psychiatry or community medicine; and 3) the activists who seem just plain anti-intellectual; they want to DO, they don't care to know HOW TO DO; they don't want to study the community, they want to save it.

Several years ago we looked at the specialty interests of all medical students, the results of their personality tests, and their ability to function cognitively in either abstract or concrete dimensions (11). We found that the pragmatists (who frequently become surgeons) see things in black and white. They should be taught medical care and community medicine on the wards where these are tangible and visible. The abstractionists are the ones we like to teach in seminars. They want to talk, want to think; we like to give them papers to read. We want to talk about methodology with them. These are probably the people who are going to join us in HSR. The activists learn in only one way—by being personally *involved* in the health care system. One method that proved successful in reaching this group was tried out in an elective course in applied community medicine at Harvard Medical School. Most of the students in the course had been active in community organization work. They organized themselves into several task-force groups—one on private practice, one on institutions, another on consumer groups, another on mental health, and so on. Then, they received a reading list which consisted of the names, addresses, and telephone numbers of the people who "owned" Roxbury, the ghetto around the medical school. The task for each group was to get out and discover what was going on in their sector. Seminars on any topic would be held whenever the students requested them. At the eighth week they began meeting to present reports on what they had found.

The students reported with enthusiasm. Many remained active in community groups and continued working with them. The instructor served two roles: 1) that of facilitator in a nondirective, almost objectiveless course; and 2) that of provider of psychiatric interpretations of what some of them had really been describing, at times when the students were ready to hear them.

There was general enthusiasm about the experience and probably some significant learning. It took the students ten afternoons (and many of them worked evenings) to learn what could have been presented in a two-hour lecture. But, because they had learned it themselves, through participation and observation, they believed it.

How can we organize experience of this type? Perhaps medical care may best be taught by allowing the students to self-select themselves into groups in which the same content is taught in three different ways—through patient care material, through seminars and readings, and through relatively unstructured community experiences. The medium is indeed the message in the teaching of medical care.

Although psychological tests and the cognitive function tests are fairly valid, it might be unwise to classify students on the basis of any paper-and-pencil tests. The students should have the opportunity to group themselves after the objectives have been described in some detail. When this approach is taken, one must be careful to match the right faculty with each student group. It takes a certain kind of person to run an activist session. Not all of us feel very comfortable in a loosely structured setting, and not all of us can play encounter games without getting hurt. Not all of us know the literature well. Some of us are comfortable only in a more contemplative role. Thus, a diversified faculty is required to match these different types of students.

The concept of three categories of students introduces the subject of criteria for admission to medical school. Do we want one-third of each? How will we identify them? In 1966 we developed a registry of activist students in order to follow them prospectively. We collected a fascinating set of data on the 140 medical students in the registry. They were what Kenneth Kenniston would describe as the young radicals—young men on the cutting edge of the new frontier in medicine. Many were firstborn sons of well-to-do families. More often than not they had majored in the humanities; they were mostly single. They had many other common characteristics. For example, almost all had been involved in the civil rights movement. The question of admissions screening might thus be answerable, at least in part. One could approach a medical school and offer information which would allow for identification of the activists among the candidates a little more accurately than can be done under current admissions procedures.

Finally, we must contend with the political implications of health services research. When one operates with uncertainty and makes mistakes, one is forgiven. If one gives the admissions committee information that says, "If you avoid these students, you will not get certain young men you may want; on the other hand, if you load your class with these men and they burn down the clinic, the legislature may be angry," one has in essence put the responsibility not on "chance," but on the backs of the admissions committee. Some people don't want data that will help them make decisions. They prefer to select those who are capable in the predictive, certain sciences and, sure enough, they do well in medical school—a nice self-fulfilling process.

This brings us full circle to the point where we began. Health services research is value laden. It asks questions and may provide information that not everyone is prepared to accept. Probing into the core of the complex system we use to deliver health care requires a combination of firm adherence to basic research principles and discretion in the dissemination of information. It offers insight for those medical students attracted to it, but may prove equally intimidating to those who lean toward pragmatism.

REFERENCES

1. Mechanic, D. Social psychologic factors affecting the presentation of bodily complaints. *New England Journal of Medicine,* 1972, *286,* 1132-1139.
2. Lewis, C. E., and Keairnes, H. W. Controlling costs of medical care by expanding insurance coverage: Study of a paradox. *New England Journal of Medicine,* 1970, *282,* 1405-1412.
3. Lewis, C., Neumann, C., and Breslow, L. The health care system —maligned or malignant? *Annals of Internal Medicine,* 1971, *74,* 746-757.
4. Lewis, C. Nurse clinics and progressive ambulatory patient care. *New England Journal of Medicine,* 1967, *277,* 1236-1241.
5. Lewis, C., Resnik, B., Schmidt, G., and Waxman, D. Activities, events and outcomes in ambulatory patient care. *New England Journal of Medicine,* 1969, *280,* 645-649.
6. Sanazaro, P. J., and Williamson, J. W. End results of patient care: A provisional classification based on reports by internists. *Medical Care,* 1968, *6,* 123-130.
7. Lewis, C. Continuing medical education—An epidemiologic evaluation. *New England Journal of Medicine,* 1970, *282,* 254-269.
8. Moses, L. E., and Mosteller, F. Institutional differences in postoperative death rates. Commentary on some of the findings of the National Halothane Study. *Journal of American Medical Association,* 1968, *203,* 492-494.
9. Gordis, L., Finkelstein, R., Fassett, J. D., et al. Evaluation of a program for preventing adolescent pregnancy. *New England Journal of Medicine,* 1970, *282,* 1078-1081.
10. Taybeck, M., and Scally, L. An evaluation of community nursing services in the care of the mentally ill. *American Journal of Public Health,* 1963, *53,* 1260-1268.
11. Lewis, C., and Easton, R. E. Personality characteristics, career interests, observed health behavior and the teaching of community medicine. *Archives of Environmental health,* 1970, *21,* 99-104.

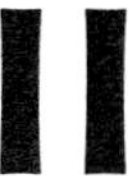

Medical Care Organization

Among the general population there is a common tendency to equate medical care with health. The chapters in this section will examine some of the ways the medical care system can be viewed and how it can be utilized to improve the health of a community. The first chapter by Powles will dissect the limitations of modern medicine in arriving at solutions for the health problems of today. Assumptions of causal relationships and intuitive acceptance of medical benefit are challenged as the reader is provoked to question his own tenets regarding the health care system.

In a similar vein, the role of medical care in preventing illness and disability is examined in Chapter 6. Several major preventive programs are reviewed in the light of current technology and its implications for medical care delivery. Community medicine has its roots firmly planted in the soil of preventive medicine and public health. The pattern of disease has changed, and our methods for controlling diseases must adapt. It seems appropriate to examine some of the major approaches to disease control currently being advocated.

Both the professional and the lay public hold their own conceptions of what the medical care system should be doing. From an economist's perspective, these concepts represent the difference between needs and demands. As the cost of medical care persists as a major national concern, the response of the public to various proposals will depend upon finding ways to bring these separate concepts of needs and demands closer together. Jeffers offers a framework which explains the implications of these differences.

Demands represent the viewpoint of the consumer. In many instances, community medicine represents the interface between the medical care system and the community. Community implies people and people mean political and social power. Consumers have become an increasingly potent force in health planning. Depending upon the setting, they have been used or abused. The chapter by Kane and Kane deals with the role of consumers in decision making in medical care issues.

5
On the Limitations of Modern Medicine

John Powles

One of the more striking paradoxes within modern medical culture lies in the contrast between the enthusiasm associated with current developments and the reality of the decreasing returns to health for rapidly increasing efforts. As this paradox involves both the technical and nontechnical aspects of medicine, any attempt to unravel it must involve an exploration of both. It must also investigate the whole medical culture, encompassing as it does a complex web of explanations and activities accepted by both doctors and their patients.

In this chapter we shall attempt to explore the origins and dynamics of this paradox. In demonstrating that the paradox is real, the argument will move to an assessment of the current status of modern man's efforts to gain technical mastery of disease. It will then go on to explore the complex interaction of the technical and nontechnical aspects of modern medicine.

DIMINISHING RETURNS

It seems unnecessary to demonstrate the optimism that underlies contemporary confrontation with disease. News stories of fresh battles won are frequently relayed through the mass media to a public that has grown to expect such victories. More frequent still are stories of new and more powerful weapons that will ensure future

Abridged from the original article which appeared in *Science, Medicine and Man*, 1973, *1:* 1–30.

Figure 1
Mortality Trends over the Last Century, England and Wales (with Recent Expenditure Trends)

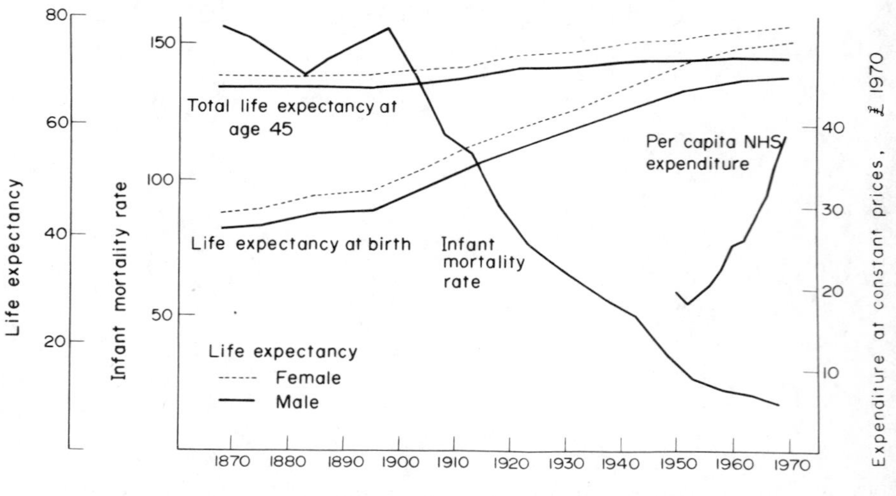

Source: See reference 6.

conquests. While most are aware that cancer and heart disease remain to be subdued, few doubt the ultimate outcome.

Nor is it necessary to document in detail the rapid pace of medical inflation—especially in the last two decades. In England and Wales the number of hospital workers increased by 70 percent over the two decades up to 1969 (1). By comparison, the increase in total workforce was only 10 percent (2). In the Soviet Union in the period 1940 to 1968, the number of physicians in relation to population increased more than threefold and the number of days spent in hospital in relation to population increased more than two and a half times (3). In the United States, per capita health expenditures rose from $79 to $324 in the two decades up to 1969/70 (4). This was an increase of 310 percent over a period in which the consumer price index rose only by around 60 percent (5).

What has been the result of these redoubled efforts? Do they provide grounds for optimism to a purely rational man? Figure 1 shows the trends in the major mortality indices in England and Wales for the 100 years up to 1970. Note that it is precisely during the last two decades—when scientific medicine is alleged to have blossomed and when the quantity of resources allocated to medical care has been rapidly increased—that the decline in mortality associated with industrialisation has tapered off to a virtual zero.

Whilst it is true that female life expectancy is continuing to increase marginally, the picture for men is very sobering. Although more are surviving the infectious diseases of childhood in England and Wales than was the case three decades ago, their prospects once they have reached adulthood are hardly better. The gap between male and female life expectancies has widened with marked social consequences. This can be shown by trends in a national "mean period of widowhood" (figures for England and Wales) (7,8). Thus the slight gains in female life expectancy are serving to increase the number of lonely old women. Such gains are a mixed blessing.

	1930–1932	1948–1950	1966–1968
Mean difference in age at marriage	2.58	3.39	2.63
+	+	+	+
Mean difference in life expectancy at age of marriage (say 25)	3.01	4.10	5.62
=	=	=	=
"Mean period of widowhood"	5.59 years	7.49 years	8.25 years

The major technical failure of modern medicine has been its inability to reduce premature death in men. In several countries, male death rates in middle age have actually been rising; in others, they are failing to decline (9,10). In England and Wales it is the poor who seem to have gained least. The age-specific death rates for unskilled workers over the age of 50 were probably higher in 1959-63 than they had been in the depression years 1930-32 (11). Nearly twice as many men as women currently die in middle age in England and Wales, and 90 percent of this excess mortality in men can be attributed to heart disease, lung cancer, and bronchitis (12).

Some will object that there is more to life than the avoidance of death and that trends for lethal conditions may not be reflected in trends for nonlethal illness. Death statistics are, however, the most reliable figures that are comparable over time. In England and Wales the best information on trends in illness are returns for the employed male population on sick-leave from work. Morris has reviewed these from the 1920s to the early 1960s and concluded that "sick absence rates in men show no improvement" (13). He made a more detailed examination of trends in the 1950s which showed "an appreciable rise of chronic sickness among men in their late fifties, and a very substantial one, amounting to 30 percent in men in their early sixties" (14). More recent figures for the period 1962/3 to 1968/9 show an overall increase of 20 percent in days lost, with the most marked increases in absence attributed to cardiovascular disease, respiratory diseases (other than bronchitis and tuberculosis), diseases of the musculoskeletal system, and accidents, poisoning, and violence (15). Whilst these figures may be reflecting an increasing tendency not to work when feeling unwell, trends by disease category are broadly parallel to known mortality trends. At the very least, these data fail to support an optimistic interpretation of the recent health experience of middle-aged men.

Two final qualifications to this critical review of the recent gains from medical technology need to be made. First, technology exists not only to prevent and cure illness but also to help sick people cope with their illness. There have been many gains in symptom relief—the anti-allergy, asthma-relieving, and pain-killing drugs are obvious examples. Second, given the close relationship in the long term between the regulation of population and health, oral contraceptives, intrauterine devices, and improved abortion techniques are significant gains.

However, the overall outcome of the recent contest with disease is hardly the success story it is so widely believed to be. It is now necessary to enquire why this has been so.

THE HUMAN EXPERIENCE OF DISEASE

What is the nature of the contemporary disease burden? What has been the relative impact on it of changes in life style and medical activities? Is the current medical strategy appropriate to the task it faces? For at least 99 percent of the duration the genus *Homo* has inhabited the earth, he has lived by hunting and gathering. This way of life was presumably also shared by the preceding prehominids. Of the 50,000-odd generations in the last million years of human history, only about 400 have lived since agriculture was first adopted. With agriculture came dramatic changes in diet, population density, and patterns of daily life. These exposed the human organism to stresses that were, in evolutionary terms, novel. It is unlikely that there has been any major biological change in man since the Neolithic revolution (16). Such genetic change is even more highly improbable with respect to the more recent adoption of urban and advanced industrial patterns of life. The selection pressures associated with hunting and gathering were predominant in determining man's genetic constitution. It is therefore reasonable to take the functioning of the human organism under such circumstances as the baseline in discussing the impact of civilisation and medical technology on the health of man. While it may be argued that behavioural flexibility provides the very basis of man's success as a species, it is man's biological adaptability that is being questioned here. It must be recognised, however, that the two interact.

Infection

At first glance, it is the infectious and parasitic diseases whose decline has been so evident in recent times. Together they constitute a group of diseases where modern man seems clearly to have "improved on nature." What, however, was the baseline situation? Can we know anything with confidence about the impact of infection on hunter-gatherer man?*

There are several reasons for believing that the burden of infection was considerably lighter on hunter-gatherer man than in advanced agricultural civilisations such as preindustrial Europe. First, birth spacing seems to be wider (three to four years as compared to two to three) and completed family size smaller (three to five compared to four to six) (17). Smaller family size means a smaller proportion of infants and children dying before reproductive age. The second consideration is that population sizes and densities would usually not have been sufficient to sustain those infections specific to man that conferred lasting immunity. This assumption, based on theoretical epidemiological considerations, is confirmed by the frequently reported vulnerability of contemporary hunter-gatherer populations to introduced infections of this kind. Fenner has suggested that cholera, measles, smallpox, poliomyelitis, and many viruses invading the upper respiratory tract are post-Neolithic developments (18). Low population densities and shifting camps would also have reduced the contagiousness of bowel infections such as those caused by the salmonellae. A third factor pointing to a lesser burden of infection is the higher host resistance likely to have been conferred by the generally better nutritional status of hunter-gatherers when compared to advanced agricultural populations. The good nutritional status generally enjoyed by hunter-gatherers has frequently been noted (19,20). Whilst population numbers are likely to have been ultimately regulated by food supplies, there generally appears to have been a good measure of "reserve capacity." Under hunting and gathering conditions, a diverse and usually well-balanced diet re-

*For a more complete discussion of the data on primitive man see the full version of this paper in *Science, Medicine and Man, 1:* 1-30, 1973.

sults. Brothwell has noted that a single pair of tibiae are alone suspicious of deficiency disease in the very large number of prehistoric skeletons that have been examined. By contrast, 7 percent of the 233 skeletons in the St. Brides Church series (London c. 1750 to 1850) show some degree of rickets (21).

In summary, the transition from hunting and gathering to agriculture almost certainly led to a significant increase in the burden of infectious disease. With industrialisation this burden has largely been abolished. Virtually all of the decline in the death rate in England and Wales in the second half of the last century was in deaths registered as being due to infection—half of them to tuberculosis (22). Thus it is to the changes that led to a decline in infections that we largely owe our current standard of health. McKeown has endeavoured to assess the probable causes of this decline since it first began in the second half of the eighteenth century (22). Medical treatments available then were unlikely to have altered for the better the course of many illnesses. Two other major factors would appear to have been general environmental conditions and nutrition. While the sanitary reforms of the mid-nineteenth century led to a decline in bowel infections, it is difficult to see how other environmental changes could have worked to reduce infection. The concentration in the new industrial cities would appear to have favoured the transmission of tuberculosis. McKeown therefore settles for improved nutrition as the factor most likely to have been operating to reduce deaths in the period since that reduction first began in the second half of the eighteenth century. This is consistent with known increases in agricultural productivity at that time. Perhaps the starchy cereals on which the population had long been dependent were now supplemented by more vegetables and meat. The dietary balance that had been forfeited with the Neolithic revolution was restored. However, improvement in living standards could only have been sustained by birth control:

> If the birth rate in England and Wales had remained at the level of 1870, the population today would be 140 million instead of 46 million, with effects on the standard of living and health that can be imagined. . . . Although the improvement in health was initiated by increased food supplies, without limitation of numbers the advance would soon have been eliminated. Viewed historically, the balance between food and population size on which health depends owes less to increase of food than to control of numbers (23).

It is ironical that the single measure that was to prove most critical for the sustained improvement of the health of the British people—birth control—was not merely overlooked by the medical profession, but was vigorously opposed by them (24).

The contribution of medical intervention in individuals—both preventive and curative—is much more difficult to assess. Razzell has argued for the importance of vaccination against smallpox (25) but the proportion of the total decline in mortality that could be attributed to this one disease is unlikely to be great. In McKeown's assessment, the contribution of clinical medicine was not significant until the second quarter of this century (23). By this time the larger proportion of the total decline in mortality had already been achieved.

It is widely believed that the introduction of antibiotics and effective immunisation campaigns marked a dramatic breakthrough in the fight against infectious diseases. Whilst this may have been true in particular cases—for example, immunisation against diphtheria—their contribution to the total decline in mortality over the last two centuries has been a minor one. Most of the reduction had already occurred before they were introduced and there was only a slight downward inflection in an otherwise declining curve following their introduction. (See Figure 2.)

Figure 2
Deaths of Children under 15 Years Attributed to Scarlet Fever, Diphtheria, Whooping Cough, Measles (England and Wales)

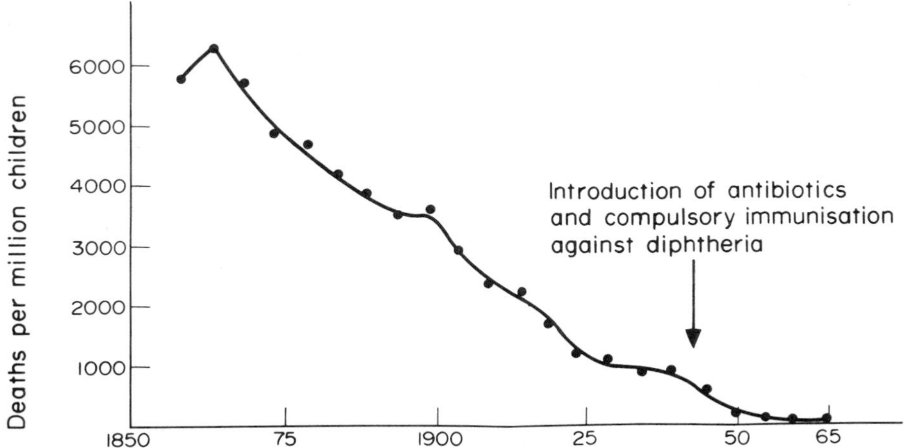

Source: Porter, R. R. The contribution of the biological and medical sciences to human welfare. *Presidential Addresses of the British Association for the Advancement of Science,* Swansea Meeting, 1971. Published by the British Association, 1972, p. 95.

This account of the changing impact of infectious disease throughout the three main phases of human history—hunting and gathering, agricultural, and industrial—has demonstrated the major importance for health of man's interactions with his environment. The provision of food, sanitary control, and the regulation of births have been the three central factors.

This is not to underrate the recently acquired capacity to intervene in individuals by means of immunisation and antibiotics. But it does put that capacity into perspective.

The Diseases of Civilisation

> In industrialised countries cardiovascular diseases and neoplasms account for two-thirds of total mortality in both sexes, and in Japan for 50 percent (10).

Those diseases which appear to have increased relative to the posited natural state of man will now be considered. A central issue is whether this increase is a real one or simply the result of people living long enough to succumb to degenerative processes. In other words, are they the universal consequences of the aging of the human organism or are they, in large measure, the consequences of changes in behaviour associated with economic development? There is also the related issue of whether the way of life affects the overall rate of aging as distinct from the development of particular diseases. However, the evidence on this latter issue would be very difficult to obtain, so this analysis will be concerned with particular categories of disease.

Cardiovascular disease of a degenerative kind is manifested by two principal changes that progress with age—degeneration of the arterial walls and rising blood pressure. These two changes tend to occur together but need not do so. The underlying causal mechanisms may well be different in each case and so may the final lethal event. Kuller and Reisler have attempted to explain these interactions (26). High levels of arteriosclerosis combined with hypertension tend to produce a high incidence of both heart attacks and strokes (as in U.S. Negroes). Arteriosclerosis without high blood pressure tends to be associated with a high incidence of heart attacks and an intermediate level of strokes (as in U.S. whites). Hypertension unaccompanied by high levels of coronary arteriosclerosis tends to be associated with a high incidence in strokes but not heart attacks (as in Japan).

Table 1
Some Data on Signs of Degenerative Cardiovascular Disease in Hunter-Gatherers

		Systolic Blood Pressure		Serum Cholesterol		
Groups	Authors	Level at age 40	Increase with age?	Level	Increase with age?	Comments
Australian aborigines	Casley-Smith (27) (review) Abbie & Schroder (28) Schwartz & Casley-Smith (29) Schwartz & others (30)	<120	slight	low to moderate	no	Exception is high blood pressure recordings from groups on Gulf of Carpentaria by Croll (27).
Malayan aborigines	Polunin (31)	(low)	no	—	—	
Bushmen (Kalahari)	Kaminer & Lutz (32) Bronte-Stewart & others (33) Truswell & Hansen (34) Tobias (35)	c.115	no	low	no	Circumstantial evidence of arteriosclerosis and sudden death with chest pain in (33). See text.
Hadzas (Tanzania)	Barnicot & others (36)	c.120	slight	low	no	Most had adopted a settled way of life within the previous 3 years.
Pygmies (Congo)	Mann & others (37)	c.130	slight	low	no	Contact with agricultural Bantus. Plantain, sweet potato and rice prominent in diet.
Amerindians of the Brazilian Mato Grosso	Neel & others (38) Hugh-Jones & others (39) Lowenstein (40)	<115	no	low	slight	

Reliable information on the prevalence of arteriosclerosis is only available by direct examination of the arteries at autopsy, but indirect evidence is provided by the level of serum cholesterol. Information on blood pressure is more readily available. Some of these data for contemporary hunter-gatherers is listed in Table 1 (27-40). Evidence for former hunting and gathering groups who have changed their way of life is not included. While it would be unwarranted to conclude from this evidence that hunter-gatherers are free from degenerative cardiovascular disease, the evidence certainly points towards its incidence being low. It is also interesting to note that in most of these groups blood pressure and serum cholesterol do not tend to increase with age.

There is now a very large body of data on the epidemiology of ischaemic heart disease which shows a general tendency for it to increase with increasing economic development (41,42,43). There has been a very substantial rise in the age-specific death rates in many industrial countries in recent decades (10). While many of the way-of-life factors responsible have been identified, the full sequence and interrelation of causal events remain to be clarified. The pattern with hypertension seems a little less clear-cut and there are exceptions to a simple association with economic development (44,45,46,47).

In summary, there are grounds for believing that the marked degeneration of arterial walls and the rise in blood pressure with age that are typical of industrial populations are much less prominent features of aging under natural (hunting and gathering) conditions. Therefore, these degenerative processes may be characterised as diseases of maladaptation in the sense that they arise "because our earlier evolution has left us genetically unsuited for life in an industrialised society" (42). They constitute a large and growing component of the contemporary burden of disease.

In Table 2 an attempt has been made to identify the relative impact of the major categories of disease in contemporary Britain, as indicated by different measures (48-52). The relative impact of the killing disorders may be assessed by calculating the years of a national "total life" (say to age 85) that are lost from each cause. In England and Wales in 1968 more than 20 percent of such "total loss" was due to cancer. In males, 40 percent of this loss was in turn due to one cancer—cancer of the lung (48). This is almost entirely caused by tobacco smoking (53). Cancer of the colon and rectum is the second commonest cancer in men and a major one in women in many industrialised countries (54). Burkitt has noted that its incidence appears to increase with economic development (55). The incidence in U.S. Negroes is comparable to that for U.S. whites and is around 10 times greater than that estimated for rural Africans. The removal of dietary fibre and a high intake of refined carbohydrates that is typical of diets in industrialised countries is associated with a much slower transit of food through the gut. Burkitt argues that this may be significant not only in the aetiology of large bowel cancer but also for other large bowel diseases associated with economic development—for example, appendicitis and diverticulitis (56,57). If this were so they would all fit neatly into the category of diseases of maladaptation.

For many cancers, however, the picture is less clear-cut. Cancer of the cervix and stomach have both been declining in many industrialised countries. Doll has reviewed the geographical distribution of cancer (54) and has recently commented:

> The marked differences in cancer incidence in different countries and the changes that have been noted in the experience of migrant groups when they move from one country to another are among the many pieces of evidence suggesting that most cancers are due to environmental factors. It follows that most cancers are, in principle, preventable (58).

Higginson of the International Agency for Cancer Research has estimated that 80 percent of all cancer has its aetiology in man's relation to his environment (59). There is little information on cancer incidence in hunter-gatherers.

So far an attempt has been made to show that diseases of maladaptation are probably responsible for a major proportion of premature deaths in industrial populations. Disease of this kind may also be responsible for a good deal of morbidity and discomfort. Upper respiratory infections spread much more easily where large numbers are gathered together (18). Smoking and air pollution are responsible for much chronic bronchitis (53,60). The chemicalisation of the human environment may well be leading to further untoward effects which are not yet apparent (61). Diabetes (62) and dental caries (21) both appear to be associated with a diet rich in refined carbohydrates. Even varicose veins appear to be associated with industrialisation (63). It will be seen from Table 2 that mental and nervous disorders are major causes of general practitioner and hospital utilisation, health service expenditure, and absence from work. Much inappropriate and distressing anxiety and depression result from the stresses of modern life (64). Recent research has also linked greater experience of significant life events (e.g., promotion, marriage, divorce, change of residence and occupation) with greater vulnerability to illnesses, such as ischaemic

Table 2
Major Components of the Contemporary Disease Burden in Britain

	K=Killing D=Disabling	Years of "Total Life" Lost (i.e., to Age 85) (E&W, 1968)		Years of "Working Life" Lost (i.e., Ages 15-64) (E&W, 1968)		Days Certified Sickness Absence (GB, 1969)		N.H.S. Expenditure (E&W, 1961/2)	General Practitioner Consultations (from Fry, 1966)	Hospital Bed Use (E&W, 1968)	
		M	F	M	F	M	F	M & F	M & F	M	F
		%	%	%	%	%	%	%	%	%	%
1. Cardiovascular (including cerebrovascular)	K&D	35	33	21	16	14	9	10	10	10	12
2. Respiratory (including TB)	K&D	15	12	13	13	28	19	10	33	8	5
3. Neoplastic	K	20	23	16	23	1	1	4	—	5	5
4. Congenital and perinatal (including mental handicap)	K&D	10	11	20	23	—	—	5	—	22	14
5. Accidents and violence	K&D	7	4	13	7	7	4	4	—	5	4
6. Mental and nervous	D	—	—	—	—	13	18	15	12	34	35
7. Musculoskeletal	D	—	—	—	—	12	11	4	8	3	4
8. Digestive	D	1	1	1	1	7	5	6	10	5	3

9. Symptoms and ill-defined conditions	D	—	—	—	—	9	12	4	—	3	3
10. Others		12	16	16	17	9	21	38 (including: dental—9 maternity—7)	27 (including: skin—10 preventive—10)	5	15 (including: maternity—9)
Total Rates (100%)		223	141	66	34	16,659	17,586	£665.4m	4–6	6.97	8.46
		per 1,000 population per year			(48)	per 1,000 at risk per year	(49)	attributed to specific diseases out of a total of £900m (50)	per person per year (51)	per 1,000 population	(52)

E&W = England and Wales, GB = Great Britain
Sources: Given under References. Numbers indicated at base of each column.

heart disease (65,66). Although cancer is not usually thought of as a stress disease, the incidence of breast cancer has recently been associated with personality type and past experience of stressful events (67). Findings such as these suggest that a biological and not just emotional price is being paid for the individual mobility which is often regarded as one of the greatest benefits of industrialisation.

Other Diseases

The category of disease in which way-of-life factors do not seem to have major significance is, by definition, a residual one. Its size will depend on the proportion of disease that is deemed neither to be caused by those infections that have decreased nor by those diseases which have increased since Paleolithic times. It is likely to include a significant minority of all cancer, many metabolic disorders, a certain proportion of infection—especially that caused by microbes such as streptococci, staphylococci, and coliforms, which are ubiquitous in the human environment—and most congenital disorders. If organic causes are demonstrated to be predominant in schizophrenia, it also may fit within this category. The question of trauma is a little different. The damage that industrial populations are sustaining from the mechanical violence they have unleashed upon themselves—especially in the forms of the motor car, industry, and mechanised warfare—may lead one to think of this as a disease of civilisation. On the other hand, hunting and other injuries are likely to have been frequent causes of death in Paleolithic times.

To summarise: Industrial populations owe their current health standards to a pattern of ecological relationships which serves to reduce their vulnerability to death from infection and to a lesser extent to the capabilities of clinical medicine. Unfortunately, this new way of life, because it is so far removed from that to which man is adapted by evolution, has produced its own disease burden. These diseases of maladaptation are, in many cases, increasing.

We may now move forward to the following two questions: What has been the strategy for tackling these new diseases? Why has it not been more successful?

THE CURRENT MEDICAL EFFORT

Ischaemic heart disease is the paradigmatic disease of maladaptation; the response to it typifies wider trends within medicine. The major thrust of the medical response to this problem has been towards the hospital treatment of heart attack. This has been elaborated in complex and expensive intensive cardiac care units. For the U.S.A. it has been estimated that 3,000 such units were established by the end of 1971 and that they were using 10 percent of all trained nurses (68). And yet this major effort has been mounted in the absence of convincing evidence of benefit. The only randomised controlled trial which has compared treatment at home with hospital treatment, with which this author is familiar, failed to show any benefit from hospital treatment (69).

A consideration of the natural history both of the acute episode and of the underlying process points to the implausibility of significant gain from the hospital treatment of heart attack. Results from Belfast and Edinburgh indicated that because of the suddenness of death "about 50 percent of fatal heart attacks are outside the possible reach of medical treatment. In such cases hope must lie with prevention" (42). Moreover, the individual who has survived one acute episode is still a coronary-prone individual much more likely than average to succumb to another.

Why then this apparent technological overreach in the response to heart disease? Was it just a simple mistake encouraged by genuine gains in other fields? Or has the perception of the problem been seriously hampered by the character of contemporary medical thinking? If so, in what way is this thinking limited?

Thomas McKeown has noted the extent to which the contemporary medical effort is based on an engineering approach to the improvement of health:

> The approach to biology and medicine established during the seventeenth century was an engineering one based on a physical model. Nature was conceived in mechanistic terms, which lead in biology to the idea that a living organism could be regarded as a machine which might be taken apart and reassembled if its structure and function were fully understood. In medicine, the same concept lead further to the belief that an understanding of disease processes and of the body's response to them would make it possible to intervene therapeutically, mainly by physical (surgical) chemical, or electrical methods (23).

In view of the limited effectiveness of this approach, it is worth examining its origins. At least four things have been important. They are: 1) the nature of the doctor-patient relationship, 2) the limitation of medical theory to the "biology of the individual," 3) the germ theory of disease, and 4) institutional and political factors.

Given the traditional form of doctor-patient interaction, it was inevitable that doctors would strive to get better and better at intervening in their patients' illnesses. This is the historical foundation of the engineering approach. When doctors drew from the emerging biological science of the nineteenth century, they chose that strand which had the most obvious relevance to their ability to treat their patients: They chose what Crombie refers to as the "science of the organised individual" and were singularly uninfluenced by the other strand—"the science of populations." This theoretical bias is the second important factor (70). In medicine this theoretical foundation lent support to the view that it was the doctor's role to intervene chemically (by drugs) or physically (by surgery) in order to restore the patient's disordered system or systems to normal.

The extent to which human population biology—for example, evolutionary theory, historical demography, and medical ecology—has failed to influence medical theory is quite remarkable. The resulting inability to deal theoretically (as distinct from statistically) with biological phenomena at levels of organisation above a single organism has left medical theory seriously deficient. Medicine has deprived itself of the only possible theoretical basis on which criteria for man's biological normality could rest. It hesitates to call progressive health-compromising processes—such as arterial degeneration, rising blood pressure, and the tendency towards diabetes—"diseases," because they are associated with a way of life it feels bound to accept as normal. The limits of normality in blood pressure are endlessly debated. The serious issue of whether a bodily change that is induced by our way of life and predisposes to overt disease should be regarded as pathological has been reduced to the trivial one of whether the distribution of blood pressures in the population is unimodal or bimodal. It hardly needs to be added that the debate gains its significance not from a felt need to prevent the development of the abnormal but from the assumed imperative to knock it into line with drugs.

With little understanding of the way of life to which man is biologically adapted, modern medicine is unable to predict the possible harmful consequences of departures from it. It was surprised to find that the repeated inhalation of tobacco smoke actually harmed the lungs and caused cancer. Until quite recently it was not widely suspected that large bowel cancer, a major cause of cancer death, might be associated with dietary habits that have diverged a long way from those of our forbears. The fourteenth edition of Bailey and Love's famous *A Short Practice of Surgery*, published in 1968, contains 15 pages of discussion on cancers of the colon and rectum (71). Much of it is naturally concerned with operative techniques for the removal of the tumours. In the case of rectal cancer it includes a paragraph and a diagram on the complete removal of all pelvic organs (under the appropriate heading "More Extensive Operations"). In contrast to this readiness to consider drastic attempts at cure there is no discussion of aetiology and there is no acknowledgment of the possibility that these cancers might be caused by our way of life and therefore be preventable.

The limitation of medical theory to the "biology of the individual" also handicaps consideration of the role of genetic factors in disease. Frequently, naive interpretations are placed on the relative contributions of nature and nurture to disease processes. Epidemiological studies, say on ischaemic heart disease, are carried out on populations with an industrial way of life which is implicitly assumed to be normal, and on the basis of the findings a certain weight is accorded to the influence of heredity on the disease. The fact that these inherited characteristics may only become relevant to the aetiology of the condition under stresses that are, in evolutionary terms, novel—and that it is therefore the interaction between the stresses and the inherited variation in body build that is important—is often not acknowledged (72).

The third factor contributing to the dominance of the engineering approach within modern medicine was the rise of the germ theory of disease. It identified discrete, specific, and external causal agents for disease processes which were usually thought of as acute and short-lived. The theory gave support to the idea of specific therapies and failed to emphasise the importance of general resistance to infection. By contrast one could now describe the preindustrial situation with respect to infection (on the basis of McKeown's analysis) as one of chronic predisposition to infection caused by poor nutrition and environmental conditions. Thus the appropriate model for infectious disease need not, as is often suggested, be fundamentally different from that for the degenerative diseases. A fatal infection, like the occlusion of a coronary artery, is often a terminal event to which the individual involved is strongly predisposed by his social experience.

The germ theory also coincided with a high point in the view that progress was to be secured by the mechanical domination of nature. The response to the problem of infection was not thought of principally in terms of the strengthening of the natural forces of defence—for example, improved nutrition and population control. Even the preventive implications were taken up in what were literally engineering terms. Primitive man, it was imagined, lived amongst his own filth. Modern man, by means of sewers, piped water, and antiseptics would cleanse himself of germs.

The fourth group of historical influences on the rise of the engineering approach are professional and institutional ones. Rosenberg has recorded how the American medical profession in the middle of the last century hitched its fortune to the rising star of science (73). The germ theory of disease came just in time to save the faltering public prestige of doctors. Class interest was also important in suppressing an alternative approach. While the well-to-do physicians proffered their clinical skills to the rich, it was social and preventive medicine that was needed most urgently for the poor. Unfortunately, the prestigious physicians dominated the teaching hospitals and medical education and, therefore, the theoretical and practical development of public health and preventive medicine received little encouragement.

This account of the technical side of modern medicine may now be summarised. The engineering approach to the improvement of health has been dominant over an alternative approach which would emphasise the importance of way-of-life factors in disease. Curative medicine has not been very successful in reducing the impact of diseases of maladaptation. While it may be argued that the current strategy still offers the most hope—especially as significant changes in the pattern of life may seem unlikely—the nature of the underlying disease processes involved makes it improbable that curative interventions will be very successful. Nor can there be any guarantee that industrial populations have already exhausted the possibilities in respect to diseases of maladaptation. If technological advances continue to be pursued and implemented with little regard for their impact on man's biology there may well be an additional twenty-first century equivalent of the current epidemic of ischaemic heart disease.

It is therefore concluded that the problem of diminishing returns is a real one. It results from the nature of the contemporary disease burden and the limited front on which medical effort has been concentrated. These technical considerations cannot, however, explain modern medicine's considerable cultural momentum. To do so it will be necessary to explore the relationship between medicine's technical and nontechnical sides.

THE NONTECHNICAL SIDE OF MEDICINE

Medical institutions can be identified by their purpose—they mediate between man and his vulnerability to disease. It is clear that medical cultures differ from one another as radically as do the total cultures of which they are a part. Further, differing medical cultures have a certain internal consistency—that is, the way in which any individual copes with disease is largely socially determined.

Magical medicine is widely regarded as the most primitive element of medical culture. But how is magic to be interpreted? Western rationalism has placed great emphasis on the importance of gaining as accurate a picture as possible of the objective world. Within this approach it is the logical and empirical content of a belief, rather than its function within the mental lives of individuals, which is considered important. Thus magic involves a set of very stupid beliefs from which there is nothing to learn. An alternative and more fruitful approach is to focus on the function of magical beliefs and practices. Levi-Strauss has shown that this is, in fact, what the practitioners of magic do (74). If the members of such a community are presented with empirical evidence which is inconsistent with their magical beliefs, they do not deny the evidence, but the evidence does not weaken their faith in magic. Belief in magic, then, is not critically dependent upon the empirical status of magical propositions. For primitive man, magic helps to impose order on the universe, to reduce ambiguities, and to neutralise and reduce perceived threats and actual misfortunes (75). Communities that are constantly exposed to natural forces that may appear to be random and beyond man's control need means of coping with their incomprehension and vulnerability. Magic is an active response to that need.

Religion and medicine were closely associated in Europe until relatively recent times. In the medieval period, it was the religious orders that maintained the hospitals and infirmaries; this association has continued in some institutions to the present day. Religious interpretations were placed upon illness and relief from suffering was sought in the healing rites of the church. The central theme in the theistic response to man's vulnerability to disease and suffering is resignation to the will of God. Belief in an afterlife helps the sufferer to minimize the cruelties of this earthly realm.

It is worth noting that there was also a fatalistic character to nonreligious interpretations of illness during the medieval period. The movement of the heavenly bodies was widely believed to be responsible for epidemics and for individual episodes of illness. If the social reinforcement of resignation to misfortune is the functional core of religious medicine, then this fatalistic core can be seen to be common also to nontheistic mysticism, such as Buddhism, and even to some atheist philosophies, such as Stoicism.

The emotive mainspring for much of the social response to disease lies in man's capacity for compassion. There are few who are not distressed by the suffering of a fellow creature. Unfortunately, there is another side to the emotive response to the sick: They may be perceived as an unwanted reminder of the vulnerability of the healthy to diseases that they dread, and so evoke apprehension and disquiet. This applies particularly to those whose behaviour is bizarre and unpredictable (the insane) and to those who are physically deformed or mentally handicapped. In these instances, social mediation may well work against the interests of the sick individual—as for example, when they are incarcerated in long-stay hospitals to relieve others of the disquiet that their presence creates. As such incarceration often has an adverse effect on the patient's health (76,77,78), the usual justification—that it was necessary for the effective treatment of the patient's condition—deserves to be treated skeptically.

So far, four modes of mediation between man and his vulnerability to disease have been identified—magic, religion, compassion, and rejection. Together they may be regarded as constituting the nontechnical or helping-to-cope side of medicine. By none of these means is the natural history of disease processes within individuals predictably and specifically changed for the better. That has been the achievement of the fifth mode—the technical mastery of disease. All medical cultures can be regarded as being made up of these five elements (79). For some centuries in the West, the technical mode of response has become increasingly manifest. There has been a progressive increase in the understanding of the structure and function of the human body and, to some extent, of the nature of disease processes within it. Disease has been described in increasingly scientific terms. But it needs emphasising that until very recently indeed, doctors could do little to alter the natural course of events (23). Thus the response to disease came to be described in technical terms well before the technical capacity to master disease became significant. The vocabulary and activities changed, but the functional content of doctor-patient interaction remained that of the helping-to-cope side of medicine.

In recent decades, and especially since World War II, scientific medical technology of an engineering kind has gained overwhelming dominance in the mediation between industrial man and disease. The situation of the sick is increasingly defined in scientific terms and, by this means, ambiguities and uncertainties are reduced. Major crises are responded to in a confident and surehanded manner. The victim of a heart attack is taken to an intensive cardiac care unit; the victim of a car accident, to an accident and emergency unit; the cancer patient "has to go to hospital for an operation." And the minor illnesses too: For upper respiratory infections, there are antibiotics; for depression and anxiety, psychoactive drugs.

The technical response to disease pervades the whole of contemporary medical culture—the organisation of medical care, the education of doctors, and the character of doctor-patient interaction. The costs of this style of medicine are not limited to its considerable and rapidly rising resource demands. It concentrates the medical effort in the large acute hospitals while the ordinary citizen finds access to primary care ever more difficult. It concentrates resources on patients with technically interesting conditions while the insane, the handicapped, and the elderly are frequently left to live out their lives in overcrowded and unpleasant conditions. Medical education detours doctors from the areas of greatest need by emphasising technical challenges rather than moral ones. Concentration on the technical (biological) problem deflects attention from the emotional and existential significance of disease.

And yet, in spite of deficiencies of this kind, discontent with health services does not usually lead to criticism of the basic characteristics of contemporary medicine. The system is strongly legitimised. This position is strengthened by medicine's consonance with the wider culture of which it is a part. Its technical aspects are themselves consonant with the general pattern of interaction between industrial man and his environment. So too is the idea of progress. Progress is seen to be the simple sum of what are taken to be its component parts. Thus, if the hospital treatment of heart attack really did show a significant, if marginal, improvement over treatment at home, this would be regarded as progress. An increase from, say, 50 to 70 percent in patients surviving 5 years after treatment for cancer would be regarded as further evidence of medical progress. So also in economic life: a + b cars per thousand population is better than a cars; x + y television sets better than x, and so on. But in terms of real human welfare, neither whole is the simple sum of parts as these. There is as little reason for believing that the health of the population is being significantly improved as there is for believing that the material conditions for human life are becoming more favourable.

The original paradox remains: Enthusiasm for the system has outpaced its concrete achievements and its indirect costs tend to be underplayed. Despite the evidence to the contrary, it is widely believed by both patients and their doctors that industrial populations owe their higher health standards to scientific medicine, that such medical technology as currently exists is largely effective in coping with the tasks it faces, and that it offers great promise for the future. To unravel this paradox it is helpful to explore further the complex and subtle relationship between the truly technical, the apparently technical, and the nontechnical elements of modern medicine. This will be done by focusing on the nature of the interaction between the sick and the purveyors of high technology medicine in two typical cases—first, the hospital treatment of heart attack and, second, the treatment of upper respiratory infections with antibiotics.

A heart attack is one of the gravest threats that faces middle-aged men of the industrial world. The sure-handedness of the technical response to this problem and its elaboration in coronary care units has already been noted. This technical response seems both impressive and credible. And yet, as noted earlier, there is no convincing evidence that this energetic intervention secures any more favourable an outcome than simple treatment at home.

What is notable in all this is the preoccupation with an engineering style of response and the reluctance to compare outcome with that from a low technology (home treatment) response. The scientific testing of this high technology response was widely regarded as unethical until the publication in August 1971 of the study by Mathers and others (69) which failed to show any benefit from it. Despite this, specialists have been willing to encourage massive expenditure on intensive cardiac care. Some of this expenditure would almost certainly have secured much greater reductions in mortality if it had been used to persuade people to change those elements in their way of life (such as smoking and overeating) which increase their risk of heart disease. (Skeptics see 80.)

The development of coronary care units has far outpaced what would have been justified in terms of a rational programme to reduce the toll from ischaemic heart disease. It has a momentum which is almost separate from considerations as rational as this. How different, *functionally,* are the activities involved from the rituals of the magicians of old? Both are active responses to forces threatening well-being. In neither case is there much enthusiasm amongst the operators for the empirical testing of the effectiveness of their treatment.

One of the recurrent annoyances of urban life is upper respiratory infections which frequently cause one to feel miserable. Patients, therefore, expect their doctor to "do something." Now most of these infections are viral and nearly all doctors, if questioned at a scientific meeting, would admit both that antibiotics are ineffective in altering the course of viral infections and that they should not be used indiscriminately. Yet the prescription of antibiotics is now widely expected by patients when they go to their doctor with an upper respiratory infection—and most doctors oblige.

The argument therefore is that the almost exclusive concentration, within modern medical culture, on the technical mastery of disease is more apparent than real. For in addition to countering the challenges to human well-being on the biological level, this technology is also being used to cope with the emotional and existential challenges that disease involves. The problem of disease cannot be reduced to the purely technical one of prevention and correction of biological malfunctioning. Nor is it sufficient just to add on the dimensions of emotion or of symptomatology. For in addition to the distress that disease causes directly and to such emotional distress as is itself regarded as a disease, there is the threat that disease poses to the individual's sense of his own integrity and well-being. This existential challenge, in the ultimate, is the threat of oblivion.

At this point it is desirable to clarify, in the terms of this analysis, the nature of symptomatic treatment. Such treatment may serve to counter disease on all three levels: First, there are medical interventions which relieve symptoms by means of specific and predictable physiological effects. The use of aspirin in a muscular sprain is a good example. Second, there are nonspecific but nonetheless physiological responses that cannot be predicted from the known properties of the drug. This is frequently referred to as a placebo effect and may be observed, for example, in the effect of dummy tablets in lowering blood pressure or relieving tension and anxiety. Third, there are those doctor-patient interactions which do not alter the observable course of events but which both parties nevertheless feel to be worthwhile. By means of explanation, ritual, and symbol, such interventions are serving principally to counter the existential threat. The patient's situation is defined, ambiguity is reduced and reassurance—as doctors frequently call it—results. Psychotherapy and much prescribing behaviour would appear to serve this objective.

In this attempt to explore the interrelation of the technical and nontechnical aspects of modern medicine, two sets of distinctions have been drawn: First, five different modes of mediation between man and disease have been identified—magic, religion, compassion for the suffering, rejection of the abnormal, and the technical mastery of disease. The first four of these may be taken as constituting the nontechnical or helping-to-cope side of medicine. Second, it has been argued that disease challenges well-being on three main levels—biological, emotional, and existential. Clearly, these two sets of factors are interrelated. Thus, the technical mastery of disease is serving to reduce biological malfunctioning. Further, the helping-to-cope side of medicine principally serves to reduce the emotional and existential challenge. But the essence of this argument is to point out that these interrelationships are not simple or self-evident. And most important of all, that which appears to be about the technical mastery of disease is not necessarily serving merely to counter biological challenges to well-being. To an increasing extent medical technology is serving as a mask for nontechnical functions. It carries a large symbolic load. The more attention within medicine is focused on the technical mastery of disease, the larger become the symbolic and nontechnical functions of that technology. This process has been intensified by the decline of theistic religion.

THE FUTURE OF MEDICINE

It has been suggested that the character of a medical culture is largely determined by the character of the total culture and that the medical beliefs and behaviour of individuals are largely socially determined. It would be wrong, however, to ignore the possibility for change. For one thing, current developments do not always fulfill past expectations. Thus strains are created, both in the sphere of practice and the sphere of theory. The old ways of seeing the world are fractured and through the cracks the real world becomes more visible. The scope of human freedom expands. Within the wider sphere of productive life, as indeed within medicine, the most serious emerging strains derive from industrial man's relation to the natural world.

It is clear that the increase in human numbers and the increase in material consumption per capita must reach limits in a finite world. This is not a problem that will go away if it is ignored, and an increasing awareness of it is likely to lead to a fundamental reassessment of the wider constraints on human action. As ecology is central to health, it would be surprising if such a reassessment did not also involve reexamination of the assumptions underlying modern medicine. In any case, medicine is facing its own crisis of diminishing returns.

How then might medicine respond to these emerging strains? In which direction will thinking need to develop if it is to reorient itself within these newly recognised constraints? Because the technical side of medicine involves fewer conceptual problems, it will be considered first. The problem is to identify those means of increasing biological well-being that are not dependent on measures (such as continued economic growth) which are likely to aggravate the wider ecological problem. This will almost certainly involve a switch away from the increase in highly technical clinical interventions towards an emphasis on the importance of way-of-life factors in disease. For medical theory to meet this challenge it will need to broaden its scientific base. Lessons relevant to the improvement of health will need to be learned from human evolution; from the study of the health consequences of the transition from hunting and gathering to agriculture and from agriculture to industry; from historical demography and the debate about the regulation of numbers in animal populations. The health aspects of the relationship between human communities and their environments need much more detailed study. There is a need for good comprehensive epidemiological studies on groups with widely differing ways of life. The critical importance of an understanding of health and disease in hunter-gatherers deserves urgent recognition—especially because many groups are being subject to rapid acculturation (20).

It would be unrealistic however to expect all doctors to be expert in comprehending biological phenomena at both an individual level and a population level. The principal concern of the clinician will continue to be the treatment of the sick. It is understandable that clinicians, in their day-to-day practice, should take for granted the usual way of life of the community and judge the significance of behavioural factors in individual illness against that background. But if the burden of the maladaptation diseases is to be reduced by changing those elements of our way of life that are most to blame (and this is the most effective strategy currently available for these diseases) then clinicians need to have a much more sophisticated understanding of the relationships between behaviour and disease. Human population biology is essential to that understanding.

The greatest theoretical challenge within contemporary medicine lies with those responsible for the health of communities—specialists in public health or community medicine. Such specialists cannot afford to take any way of life for granted. They will need a comprehensive understanding of the experience of disease in different human communities with differing ways of life—that is, they should be experts in the biology of human populations. Unfortunately, there is, as yet, little recognition of the need to develop the theoretical basis of community medicine in this way.

When health problems are perceived differently, they may be responded to differently. For example, despite health propaganda efforts that have been very modest in comparison to the promotional activities of the tobacco interests, tobacco consumption per adult British male had fallen by 1971/2 to its lowest level since 1916 (80). Anti-smoking propaganda does seem to be having an effect —given its low intensity it would have been unreasonable to expect more. The current rates of decline in tobacco consumption are likely to prevent several thousand premature deaths each year (80). Their impact on health is therefore of an order of magnitude that bears comparison to major hospital-based activities.

Much of the impact of diseases of maladaptation may be reducible by changes in our way of life that are not too onerous. Habits can be changed. It is relatively easy to increase the amount of high residue food in the diet and, although we've become accustomed to helping ourselves to more and more sugar and salt, it is possible to wean oneself back down to more modest intakes without loss in the palatability of food. If a reduction in the intake of saturated fats is shown to reduce the risk of heart disease, then the substitution of polyunsaturated margarine for butter and the avoidance of fatty meat need be no great hardship. Avoiding obesity and keeping fit both have their own immediate rewards as well as the long-term one of improved health. The fundamental task is to change thinking about disease and what can be done about it. Given that, significant further gains in health may well be possible. In Victorian times there was a happy synergism between the germ theory of disease and the wider puritan culture which led to the successful war against the germs. That battle has been largely won. Is it too much to expect a similar future interaction between specific advice on changing health-damaging habits and a wider culture which is increasingly sensitive to the need for man to treat the natural world with respect?

None of this is meant to imply that the improvement of biological well-being should take automatic precedence over other human goals. Individuals and the wider community may well choose to pay a biological price for the achievement of competing objectives. But such choices should be both deliberate and well informed. At the moment, they are usually neither.

A switch in strategies away from complex, technological hospital medicine may have a major impact on the nontechnical side of medicine. The placing of deliberate constraints on the further development and deployment of such technology would seem to deny its potential for the alleviation of human suffering. One line of defence—especially against the existential challenge of illness—would be weakened. Such a change would, however, make possible other major gains on the nontechnical side. With a more realistic assessment of the capabilities of medical technology, there might be less of a tendency to interpret the problem of illness in purely technical terms. The emotional and existential aspects of its challenge to well-being could be given more open recognition. It has often been argued that a more balanced response to illness is more effective. By being more sensitive to the patient's situation, doctors are likely to obtain better information about the problem, provide more relevant advice and treatment, and secure more cooperation.

Little has been said so far in this chapter about the very large categories of people whose illnesses and disabilities have not (and often could not have been) prevented and who cannot be easily restored to health—those with congenital and acquired handicaps, the mentally ill, the chronic sick, and the disabled elderly. This is because the argument has been principally concerned with the major forces at work in the evolution of contemporary medical culture. Meeting the needs of these handicapped groups for humane care and rehabilitation has not been a major objective in practice (81,82). Resources and energy have been directed elsewhere—to the high technology, short-stay hospitals; to the patients with interesting conditions for whom something (i.e., a technical something) could be done. The needs of the handicapped comprise a large and growing proportion of the work load of the health services. Within a more balanced medical culture, there would be less need to translate their frequently nontechnical needs into technical ones. The challenge that they pose to the compassion of the healthy could be confronted and responded to more directly. And the resources to improve their lot can only be made available by carefully constraining the further development of expensive high-technology medicine. There is, in fact, a growing recognition that the care function of health services is in direct competition for resources with the cure function and that, hitherto, cure has had more than its fair share (83).

One of the most important preconditions for improving the care of the mentally ill is an increased tolerance on the part of the normal for bizarre and unpredictable behaviour. Given such tolerance the need for institutionalisation and its attendant harm to the patient is reduced. Currently, it is often felt necessary to represent this essentially ethical problem as a technical one—to try and make mental illness respectable by insisting that it is just like other illness and needs treatment just the same. The problem would benefit from a more direct and honest confrontation.

CONCLUSION

In much discussion of the current state of medicine the broader concept of medical culture is often accepted as a given. This acceptance confers an unnecessary aura of inevitability to current ideas about how to improve health and about the relationship between the technical and nontechnical aspects of medicine. Medicine is a product of man and can be as he chooses to make it. It is, in any case, possible to argue that there have always been two conflicting approaches within medicine itself—one emphasising the potency of clinical intervention, the other the importance of way-of-life factors.

Medicine may be expected to come under increasing pressure from the wider culture, which is in turn likely to change as a result of increasing confrontation with material and biological constraints on human action. With a rising proportion of illness evidently man-made and with increasing restrictions on the further increase of resource consumption for medical care, medicine seems bound to move in another, holistic direction.

If it does, biological well-being may be expected to benefit. Emotional problems in relation to illness may be increasingly respected. But the sense of exposure of the existential threat that disease represents may, by contrast, be heightened. It will be more difficult to say such things as "Don't worry, doctor. By the time I get lung cancer they'll have a cure for it." Faith in the effectiveness of society's defences against death might be weakened. With less confidence in his ability to master nature, man will have to learn to live more openly with his vulnerability to forces he cannot control and with the frailty of individual human existence. Man's domination of nature has been the central impetus of modern industrial culture. Further pursuit of this within the already industrialised countries is likely to be self-defeating and could well be disastrous. Could it be that man will return instead to the development of his inner life?

Mary Douglas has characterised the primitive world view as one which interprets the universe in terms of human needs (75). The belief that expansionary economics and technical advance will solve the most pressing human problems often contains the unsupported assumption that the material and biological worlds will help sustain the drama of human expansion—by supplying virtually unlimited raw materials and energy sources, by absorbing pollutants, and by allowing the constraints implicit in man's biological constitution to be easily transcended. Such thinking might be considered to be interpreting the universe on the basis of human needs—as being primitive. Rather, the thinking of modern man should be directed towards identifying his best available options in a universe indifferent to his welfare, but sensitive to his insults.

REFERENCES

1. Department of health and social security. *Digest of health statistics, 1970.* H. M. S. O., 1971. Table 3.2.
2. Central Statistical Office. *Annual Abstract of Statistics* for 1952 and 1970.
3. Popov, G. A. *Principles of health planning in the U.S.S.R.* Public Health Paper No. 43, World Health Organisation, Geneva, 1971. Figure 5.
4. Rice, D. P., and Cooper, B. S. National health expenditures, 1929-70. *Social Security Bulletin,* U.S. Department of Health, Education and Welfare, January 1971. Table 1.
5. Klarman, H. E., Rice, D. P., Cooper, B. S., and Stettler, H. L. *Sources of increase in selected medical care expenditures, 1929-1969.* U.S. Department of Health, Education and Welfare, Social Security Administration, Office of Research and Statistics, Staff Paper No. 4, 1970, Table 2.
6. Life expectancies from Office of Population, Censuses and Surveys, *Registrar-General's statistical review for England and Wales for the year 1970,* Part II, Tables Population, H. M. S. O., London, 1972, Table B2. Infant mortality rates from the same source, Part I Tables Medical, Table 3. N. H. S. expenditure for the United Kingdom by calendar years from Office of Health Economics, Information Sheet No. 15, December 1971. Expenditure standardised using consumer price index from Central Statistical Office, *National Income and Expenditure,* 1971, H. M. S. O., London, 1971, Table 16. As costs within the health service increase more rapidly than consumer prices generally, the graph will over-state the true rise in real expenditure—perhaps by 20 to 30 percent.
7. Central Statistical Office (United Kingdom), *Annual Abstract of Statistics,* 1938-1950, 1950, 1969 (for life expectancy).
8. Office of Population, Censuses and Surveys. *Registrar-General's statistical review of England and Wales for the year 1969,* Part II. (For mean age at marriage.)
9. U.S. Department of Health, Education and Welfare. Leading components of upturn in mortality for men, United States 1952-67. *Vital and Health Statistics,* Series 20, No. 11, September 1971, Tables 1 and 2.
10. de Hass, J. H. Geographical pathology of the major killing disorders. Cancer and cardiovascular disease. In *Health of mankind,* G. Wolstenholme and M. O'Connor, eds., Churchill, London: Ciba Foundation 100th Symposium, 1968.
11. *The Registrar-General's Decennial Supplement, England and Wales, 1961,* Occupational Mortality Tables, H. M. S. O., 1971. Tables D4 to D8 and Diagram 2.

12. Central Statistical Office (United Kingdom), *Social Trends,* No. 2, 1971. Table 58.
13. Morris, J. N. *Uses of epidemiology,* 2nd ed. Edinburgh: Livingstone, 1964, p. 8.
14. Morris, J. N. Ibid., p. 11.
15. Department of Health and Social Security. *On the state of the public health, the annual report of the Chief Medical Officer . . . for the year 1970,* H. M. S. O., London, 1971. Table II.7.
16. Rendel, J. M. The time scale of genetic change. In *The impact of civilisation on the biology of man,* S. V. Boyden, ed., Canberra: Australian National University Press, 1970, 27-47.
17. Birdsell, J. B. Some predictions for the Pleistocene based on equilibrium systems among recent hunter-gatherers. In *Man the hunter,* I. De Vore and R. B. Lee, eds., Chicago: Aldine, 1968, 229-240, and the following discussion, 241–249.
18. Fenner, F. The effects of changing social organisation on the infectious diseases of man. In *The impact of civilisation on the biology of man,* S. V. Boyden, ed., Canberra: Australian National University Press, 1970, 48-76.
19. Barnes, F. The biology of pre-Neolithic man. In *The impact of civilisation on the biology of man,* S. V. Boyden, ed., Canberra: Australian National University Press, 1970, 1-26.
20. Dunn, F. L. Epidemiological factors: Health and disease in hunter-gatherers. In *Man the hunter,* I. De Vore and R. B. Lee, eds., Chicago: Aldine, 1968, 221-228.
21. Brothwell, D. R. Dietary variation and the biology of earlier human populations. In *The domestication and exploitation of plants and animals,* P. Ucko and G. Dimbleby, eds., London: Weidenfeld and Nicholson, 1969.
22. McKeown, T. *Medicine in modern society,* London: Allen and Unwin, 1965, 21-58.
23. McKeown, T. A historical appraisal of the medical task. In *Medical history and medical care,* G. McLachlan and T. McKeown, eds., London: Oxford University Press for the Nuffield Provincial Hospitals Trust, 1971, p. 36.
24. Banks, J. A. Family planning and birth control in Victorian times. Paper read at second annual conference of the Society for the Social History of Medicine, Leicester University, July 1972. Abstract in Bulletin No. 8 (September 1972) of the Society for the Social History of Medicine (183 Euston Road, London).
25. Razzell, P. E. Population change in eighteenth century England: A re-appraisal. *Economic History Review, XVIII,* 1965.
26. Kuller, L., and Reisler, D. M. An explanation for variations in distribution of stroke and arteriosclerotic heart disease among populations and racial groups. *American Journal of Epidemiology,* 1971, *93,* 1-9.

27. Casley-Smith, J. R. Blood pressures in Australian aborigines. *Medical Journal of Australia,* 1959, *1,* 627-633.
28. Abbie, A. A. and Schroder, J. Blood pressures in Arnhem Land aborigines. *Medical Journal of Australia,* 1960, *2,* 493-496.
29. Schwartz, C. J., and Casley-Smith, J. R. Serum cholesterol levels in atherosclerotic subjects and the Australian aborigines. *Medical Journal of Australia,* 1958, *2,* 84-86.
30. Schwartz, C. J., et al. Serum cholesterol and phospholipid levels of Australian aborigines. *Austral. J. Exp. Biol. Med. Sci.,* 1957, *35,* 449-456.
31. Polunin, I. The medical natural history of Malayan aborigines. *Medical Journal of Malaya,* 1953, *8,* 62-167.
32. Kaminer, B., and Lutz, W. P. W. Blood pressure in bushmen of the Kalahari Desert. *Circulation,* 1960, *XXII,* Part 2, 289-295.
33. Bronte-Stewart, B., et al. The health and nutritional status of the Kung bushmen of South West Africa. *South African Journal of Laboratory and Clinical Medicine,* 1960, *6,* 187-216.
34. Truswell, A. S., and Hansen, J. D. L. Serum lipids in bushmen. *Lancet,* 1968, *2,* 684.
35. Tobias, P. V. The peoples of Africa south of the Sahara. In *Biology of human adaptability,* P. T. Baker and J. S. Weiner, eds., Oxford: Clarendon Press, 1966.
36. Barnicot, N. A., et al. Blood pressure and serum cholesterol in the Hadza of Tanzania. *Human Biology,* 1972, *44,* 87-116.
37. Mann, G. V., et al. Cardiovascular disease in African pygmies; a survey of the health status, lipids and diet of pygmies in Congo. *Journal of Chronic Disease,* 1962, *15,* 341–371.
38. Neel, J. V., et al. Studies on the Xavante Indians of the Brazilian Mato Grosso. *Human Genetics,* 1964, *16,* 52-140.
39. Hugh-Jones, P., et al. Medical studies among the Indians of the Upper Xingu. *British Journal of Hospital Medicine,* March 1972, 317-334.
40. Lowenstein, F. W. Blood pressure in relation to age and sex in the tropics and subtropics. *Lancet,* 1961, *1,* 389-392.
41. Jones, R. J., ed. *Atherosclerosis: Proceedings of the Second International Symposium,* New York: Springer-Verlag, 1970.
42. Rose, G. Epidemiology of ischaemic heart disease. *British Journal of Hospital Medicine,* March 1972, 285-288.
43. Tejada, C., et al. Distribution of coronary and aortic atherosclerosis by geographic location, race and sex. *Laboratory Investigation,* 1968, *18,* 5.
44. Stamler, J., Stamler, R., and Pollman, T. N., eds. *The epidemiology of hypertension,* New York: Grune and Stratton, 1967.
45. Kean, B. H., and Hammill, J. F. Anthropopathology of arterial tension. *Archives of Internal Medicine,* 1949, *83,* 355.
46. Becker, B. J. P. Cardiovascular disease in the Bantu and Coloured

races of South Africa. *South African Journal of Medical Science*, 1946, *11*, 1-34 and 107-120.

47. Shaper, A. G., Wright, D. H., and Kyobe, J. Blood pressure and body build in three nomadic tribes of Northern Kenya. *East African Medical Journal*, 1969, *46*, 273-281.
48. General Register Office. *The Registrar General's quarterly return for England and Wales*, Quarter ended 30th June, 1969, H. M. S. O., London, 1969, Appendix B.
49. Department of Health and Social Security. *Digest of Health Statistics for England and Wales*, 1971, H. M. S. O., London, 1971, Table 11.3.
50. Office of Health Economics. *The costs of medical care*, London (162 Regent Street), 1964, Table A. Twenty-five percent of the hospital costs of "mental, psychoneurotic and personality disorders" have been allocated to the mentally handicapped and transferred to category 4 in Table 2.
51. Royal College of General Practitioners. *The present state and future needs of general practice*, 2nd ed., London (14 Prince's Gate S.W.7), May 1970, Table XIX.
52. Department of Health and Social Security. *Digest of Health Statistics for England and Wales*, 1971, H. M. S. O., London, 1971, Tables 11.6, 9.2, 9.7, 9.9. The maternity beds rate has been recalculated per one million females. Mental handicap inpatients have been divided into male and female in the same proportions as admissions (Table 9.9).
53. Royal College of Physicians of London. *Smoking and health now*. London: Pitman Medical, 1971.
54. Doll, R. The geographical distribution of cancer. *British Journal of Cancer*, 1969, *XXIII*, 1-8.
55. Burkitt, D. P. Epidemiology of cancer of the colon and rectum. *Cancer*, 1971, *28*, 3-13.
56. Burkitt, D. P. The aetiology of appendicitis. *British Journal of Surgery*, 1971, *58*, 695.
57. Painter, N. S., and Burkitt, D. P. Diverticular disease of the colon: A deficiency disease of western civilisation. *British Medical Journal*, 1971, *2*, 450-454.
58. Doll, R., and Kinlen, L. Epidemiology as an aid to determining the causes of cancer. Cancer Research Campaign (2 Carlton House Terrace, London SW1Y 5AR), *49th Annual Report*, 1971, 42-46.
59. Quoted in Department of Health and Social Security, *On the state of the public health, the annual report of the Chief Medical Officer . . . for the year 1970*, London, H. M. S. O., 1971, p. 5.
60. Royal College of Physicians of London. *Air pollution and health*. London: Pitman Medical, 1970.
61. Boyden, S. V. The human organism in a changing environment. In *Man in his environment*, R. T. Appleyard, ed., Perth: University of Western Australia Press, 1970, 1-20.
62. West K. M., and Kalbfleisch, J. M. Influence of nutritional factors on prevalence of diabetes. *Diabetes*, 1971, *20*, 99-108.

63. Mekky, S., Schilling, R. S. F., and Walford, J. Varicose veins in women cotton workers. An epidemiological study in England and Egypt. *British Medical Journal*, 1969, *2*, 591-595. (Reviews other epidemiological studies.)
64. Levi, L., ed. *Society, stress and disease: The psychosocial environment and psychosomatic diseases.* London: Oxford University Press, 1971.
65. Mims, C. Stress in relation to the process of civilisation. In *The impact of civilisation on the biology of man*, S. V. Boyden, ed. Canberra: Australian National University Press, 1970, 167-189.
66. Syme, S. L., Hyman, M. M., and Enterline, P. E. Some social and cultural factors associated with the occurrence of coronary heart disease. *Journal of Chronic Diseases*, 1964, *17*, 277-289; Syme, S. L., Borhani, N. O., and Beuchley, R. W. Cultural mobility and coronary heart disease in an urban area. *American Journal of Epidemiology*, 1966, *82*, 334-346.
67. Personal communication, C. Bagley, member of Research Team, Courtauld Research Unit, Kings College Hospital, London.
68. Holland, W. W. Clinicians and the use of medical resources. *The Hospital* (London), July 1971, 236-239.
69. Mather, H. G., et al. Acute myocardial infarction: Home and hospital treatment. *British Medical Journal*, 1971, *3*, 334-338.
70. Crombie, A. C. The future of biology: The history of a program. *Federation Proceedings*, 1966, *25*, 1448-1453.
71. Bailey, H., and Love, M. *A short practice of surgery.* London: H. K. Lewis and Co., 14th ed. 1968, 918-924 and 1014-1021.
72. See for example: Sonksen, P. H. Aetiology and epidemiology of diabetes. *British Journal of Hospital Medicine*, February 1972, 151-156; Kannel, W. B., Castelli, W. P., McNamara, P. M., and Sorlie, P. Some factors affecting morbidity and mortality in hypertension, the Framingham study. *Milbank Memorial Fund Quarterly, XLVII, 3*, Part 2, 1969, 116–142.
73. Rosenberg, C. E. The medical profession, medical practice, and the history of medicine. In *Modern methods in the history of medicine*, E. Clarke, ed., London: The Athlone Press of the University of London, 1971, 22-35.
74. Levi-Strauss, C. The sorcerer and his magic. In *Magic, witchcraft, and curing*, J. Middleton, ed., New York: Natural History Press, 1967.
75. Douglas, M. *Purity and danger.* Harmondsworth: Penguin, 1970.
76. Barton, R. *Institutional neurosis.* Bristol: John Wright, 1966.
77. Lieberman, M. A. Relationship of mortality rates to entrance to a home for the aged. *Geriatrics*, October 1961, 515-519.
78. Aldrich, C. K., and Mendkoff, E. Relocation of the aged and disabled: A mortality study. *Journal of the American Geriatric Society*, March 1963, 185-194.
79. I have derived this analytic model from that used by Mark Field. To his four types of "societal response" I have added "rejection." See:

Field, M. The health care system of industrial society: The disappearance of the general practitioner and some implications. In *Human aspects of biomedical engineering.* E. Mendelson, J. Swazey, and I. Taviss, eds., Cambridge: Harvard University Press, 1971, 156-180.

80. It is often suggested that health education has little effect. However tobacco consumption has recently been falling at around 5 percent per year *(The Times,* 1/12/1972). The Chief Medical Officer of the Department of Health and Social Security has estimated that there are approximately 100,000 premature deaths due to smoking in the United Kingdom each year (Department of Health and Social Security. *On the state of the public health; The annual report of the Chief Medical Officer . . . for the year 1969,* H. M. S. O., London, 1970, p. 9). As the health damage from smoking is roughly proportional to the quantity of tobacco consumed (Royal College of Physicians of London. In *Smoking and health now.* London: Pitman Medical, 1971), the current decline may be saving around 5000 premature deaths each year. And this is the result of a small-scale campaign. The Health Education Council spent £120,000 on its smoking and health campaign in 1970-71 (The Health Education Council, United Kingdom, *Accounts, 31st March, 1971,* Appendix IV. Middlesex House, Ealing Road, Wembley). By contrast the tobacco industry spent £52 million on sales promotion in 1968 (Royal College of Physicians of London. *Smoking and health now.* London: Pitman Medical, 1971).
81. Mead, T. W. Medicine and population. *Public Health* (London), 1968, *LXXXII,* 100-110.
82. Department of Health and Social Security, Information Division, Intelligence Section. *National Health Service Notes, 13* (figures for 1949-50) and Department of Health and Social Security. *Digest of health statistics for England and Wales, 1971,* H. M. S. O., 1971, Table 2.3 (figures for 1969-70).
83. See for example, McKeown, T. *Medicine in modern society.* London: Allen and Unwin, 1965, 104-142; Cochrane, A. L. *Effectiveness and efficiency, random reflections on health services.* London: Oxford University Press for the Nuffield Provincial Hospitals Trust, 1972, 70-77.

6

Disease Control: What Is Really Preventable?

Robert L. Kane

Traditionally, preventive medicine and public health have been concerned with the control as well as the eradication of disease. Developments in such areas as sanitation both consciously and inadvertently produced marked changes in the patterns of diseases available to afflict us. Vaccines were hailed as miracles by one generation and accepted as commonplace by the next. Gradually, many preventive functions became incorporated into clinical medicine, particularly in the field of pediatrics. Organized public health turned its efforts to large-scale attacks on specific and, usually, infectious disease entities such as tuberculosis or venereal disease. By default, it also assumed responsibility for disease control among certain otherwise ignored populations, usually the indigent. Community medicine, on the other hand, derived from a synthesis of several disciplines, including clinical medicine; the history and traditions of the discipline of public health have had relatively little influence on its development. Accordingly, it offers a more contemporary perspective on disease control.

Everyone is familiar with the avoirdupois equivalent of an ounce of prevention. The sixteen-to-one ratio may not miss the mark by far when it comes to health, depending upon the specific problem in question and what is meant by prevention. When we are able to use prevention to intervene effectively in the disease process, the savings can be enormous, not only in direct costs of care but also in the indirect costs of productive man-years that would otherwise be lost (1).

With encyclopedic omnipotence, the classifiers of prevention describe a spectrum from avoidance through rehabilitation. Traditionally, they recognize four types of prevention. *Primary prevention* consists of taking steps that actually prevent a disease from occurring; it includes a variety of environmental actions or interventions, the most familiar of which is vaccination against smallpox. *Secondary prevention* includes early action that minimizes the possible seriousness of a disease process; for example, active screening programs may result in early detection of a disease such as tuberculosis, and the institution of effective therapy. *Tertiary prevention* actually consists of preventive actions that are often labeled clinical medicine; the purpose here is to minimize the complications of an established disease process. *Quartan prevention* is prevention only to the extent that rehabilitation may discourage the development of sequelae which lead to further deterioration following the arrest of a disease process.

PRIMARY PREVENTION

Clearly the most effective type of prevention is primary prevention—that which alters some factor in individuals or in the environment so that the disease never develops. Indeed, many of the celebrated and most of the heralded breakthroughs in modern medicine have occurred as the result of primary prevention tactics. Malaria's infamous position as world-champion killer could only be challenged by an assault on the environment; curative treatment would never have stemmed the tide of death and disability from this disease. John Snow (1813-1858), the father of modern epidemiology, successfully halted the ravages of cholera in London by removing the handle from the Broad Street pump, thus rendering the contaminated water unavailable. Although the bacteriology of cholera was then unknown and chemotherapy had not been heard of, Snow was able to intervene in the progress of a frightful epidemic in a remarkably effective manner.

Primary prevention has great flexibility of approach and can attack at a variety of points. For example, control of the environment may offer a potent means of preventing the spread of a given disease. The use of DDT to control the mosquito population is more effective than the administration of quinine in controlling malaria. Most of the parasitic diseases, such as hookworm, have been brought under control in similar ways. Another viable route may be a direct assault on the causative agent of a disease. Perhaps the best example of this is the prevention of malnutrition by making food available. In an opposite kind of attack, a noxious substance can be removed from the environment to prevent its undesirable effects on health.

Increasingly, primary prevention has begun to focus on the host. Since the time of Edward Jenner, we have appreciated the potential for artificially stimulating the human body to resist disease through immunization. In general, we tend to concentrate our immunization efforts on diseases for which no therapy is available. Since the discovery of antibiotics, these have been primarily viral diseases. However, we are beginning to reconsider the need for additional immunological approaches to the control of bacterial diseases. For example, investigators are now studying the feasibility of reemploying the pneumococcal vaccines as a major preventive modality against otitis media and pneumonia among the Navajo Indians, in whom, despite the availability of modern chemotherapy and antibiotics, the incidence of these conditions remains alarmingly high. In this instance, the barriers to implementing meaningful therapy indicate a need to reconsider a primary preventive focus.

Today, we seem on the verge of accepting genetic intervention as a preventive modality; we anticipate the deletion of specific traits of susceptibility either by genetic counseling or by chromosomal surgery. As modern medical technology makes possible the alteration of the genetic substance of an unborn individual to remove deleterious traits, we shall open yet another Pandora's box. The technology of genetic surgery has developed more rapidly than its morality. Genetic counseling raises many concerns about the potential implications of genocide, particularly since several of the traits we expect to alter or delete are restricted to specific racial or ethnic groups. Certainly, we are as yet philosophically ill prepared to grapple with the questions of who will decide what should be done to whom. Equally certainly, we must begin to solve these dilemmas before the actuality outstrips the morality of the situation.

Unfortunately, the diseases of today may not be as amenable to the interventions of primary prevention as were infections such as malaria and tuberculosis. Enmeshed in multifactorial matrices of causes and interactions, the control of present-day chronic diseases appears to demand major behavioral changes at both individual and societal levels. No simple injection exists for the control of chronic degenerative diseases. We are aware of a variety of risk factors which, if brought under control, might reduce or eliminate the ravages of a variety of health problems, but we have not yet found the means of acting effectively against them.

The complexity of causal interactions may be partially responsible for this state of impotence. We know that poverty, with all its social, economic, and psychological concomitants, is associated with a high incidence and prevalence of a wide variety of disease-producing conditions (2), but we are not as well informed about how to sort out the individual role of each causative factor. While many have noted the relationships between illness and living conditions, a study by Wilner et al. suggests that merely altering the housing of a family will not substantially change the rates of physical illness among its members, although the incidence of mental illness can be markedly reduced (3).

Alcoholism is a major health problem about which we seem able to do little. The national social experiment of prohibition produced confusing results. Although some available data suggest that the incidence of cirrhosis dropped following this period of enforced sobriety, the rate of drunkenness apparently continued or even increased (4). There is an abundance of well-documented scientific data to link cigarette smoking to a variety of lethal outcomes (5), but cigarette consumption continues to rise.

Then too, Americans are literally eating themselves to death. Increased morbidity and mortality from excessive consumption of diverse foodstuffs run the gamut from dental caries to myocardial infarction. Statistics compiled by life insurance companies reveal that men who are 20 percent overweight have a 25 percent increased mortality rate; for those as much as 30 percent or more overweight, the increase in mortality rises to 40 percent (6). It would seem that most of the world is dying from a maldistribution of food; half the world suffers from too much and the other half from not enough.

The apparent inability of the average person to take responsible action to preserve his own health has encouraged some pragmatists to focus their efforts on those portions of the risk factors which can be attacked in other ways. Automobile accidents are a major cause of loss of life and economic productivity. Substantial reductions in this loss could be achieved if people drove more slowly and more carefully, but the automotive population continues to drive unbridled and unbuckled and, too often, unsober. Efforts have therefore been directed toward making safer cars which are easier to handle and which increase the chances of survival once an accident has occurred (7). If we are to achieve any significant measure of primary prevention, we would do well to focus less on the foibles of people and more on those links in the chain of causation that are most susceptible to attack.

Increasingly, we note an attitude of dependence on external forces to control our behavior. We cry for stricter controls on environmental pollution but continue to smoke cigarettes. We expect the Food and Drug Administration to check any food substance for possible toxicity but make no effort to control our gluttony. Federal controls could be quite productive if we were prepared to permit our private lives to be still further manipulated. For example, the rather well-established deleterious effects of cigarette smoking might be countered to some extent by heavier taxation on cigarettes. Similarly, it would be possible to enact laws that would prohibit the interstate transportation of saturated fats in certain types of foodstuffs. This federal mechanism has proven relatively effective in controlling the milk industry even at a local level. Such a law would markedly alter American dietary patterns and reduce a major risk factor in coronary artery disease (8).

Needless to say, these proposals have not been implemented —for a variety of reasons. Powerful industrial lobbies, coupled with a general reluctance to interfere in what we think of as a free society, mitigate against such actions. We need only recall the brief tenure of prohibition to appreciate the complexity of social engineering problems. Nor is the public of one mind. Despite the fact that the addition of small quantities of fluoride to water supplies has been established as an effective means of reducing the incidence of dental caries, a significant proportion of our towns and cities still oppose this service.

Advertising media exploit our human foibles for commercial ends which may be either deleterious or beneficial to our health. The implied relationship between virility and fast, powerful automobiles can only increase the potential for self-destruction on the highways. On the other hand, one would be safe in attributing a general desire for leanness to the current well-publicized association between slimness and sexual attraction. The children of the Pepsi generation may well be less obese than their parents.

Primary prevention may be realized as a means of controlling a major killer, coronary heart disease, at least at a theoretical level. The Inter-Society Commission for Heart Disease Resources has recently stated, "the research findings on risk factors strongly indicate the possibility of effective primary prevention of atherosclerotic diseases, particularly premature coronary heart disease" (9). They recommend a strategy with three major goals: 1) changes in diet to reduce hyperlipidemia, obesity, hypertension, and diabetes; 2) elimination of cigarette smoking; and 3) pharmacologic control of elevated blood pressure.

The question that remains unresolved is, What commitments of money and manpower are we prepared to make in our pursuit of these desirable and perhaps attainable ends?, and What are we willing to forsake in lieu of these efforts? Thus far our answer has been, Not much.

SECONDARY PREVENTION

A frame of reference must first be established in order to assess the effectiveness of early detection on the course of a disease process. Hutchison (10) has developed a model for evaluating secondary prevention (see Figure 1). In order to be useful, a screening procedure must be able to detect disease while the patient is still asymptomatic and when intervention can alter the course of the disease process.

After reviewing the many screening tests currently available, Wilson (11) developed the following criteria for a good test:

1. The condition sought should be an important public health problem.
2. There should be an acceptable treatment for patients with recognized disease.
3. Facilities for diagnosis and treatment should be available.
4. There should be a recognizable latent or early symptomatic stage.
5. There should be a suitable test or examination.
6. The test should be acceptable to the population.
7. The natural history of the condition, including its development from latent to declared disease, should be adequately understood.
8. There should be an agreed-upon policy on whom to treat as patients.
9. The cost of case-finding (including diagnosis and subsequent treatment of patients) should be economically balanced in relation to the possible expenditure on medical care as a whole.
10. Case-finding should be a continuing process and not a "once and for all" project.

In brief, a test should be simple, cheap, accurate, and capable of uncovering a disease for which an effective remedy is available. The utility of a test is determined by its sensitivity and specificity. By sensitivity we mean the probability that someone with the disease in question will have a positive test result. Specificity refers to the likelihood that someone who is found to be positive really has

Figure 1
Points of Intervention in the Disease Process

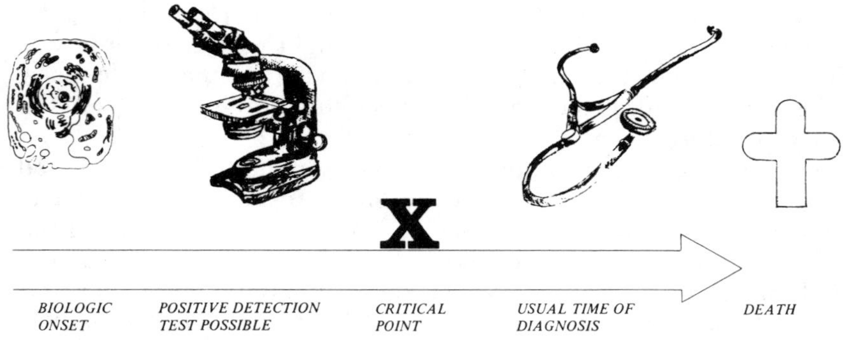

Source: Adapted from G. B. Hutchison. Evaluation of preventive services. *Journal of Chronic Diseases,* 1969, *11,* 497-508.

the disease; in more operational terms, we talk of the probability that someone without the disease will be found negative. In general, one can affect the sensitivity and specificity of a test by manipulating the threshold level for a positive result. When this is done there is a trade-off of increased sensitivity for less specificity, or the opposite. Unfortunately, we rarely have been able to find the ideal point to maximize both. Data on persons (or animals) with the disease, particularly in early stages, and with screening tests are scarce (12). The usefulness of a screening test can be illustrated by applying Bayes's theorem to a set of hypothetical data. If we consider the case of a test with a sensitivity of 95 percent and a specificity of 95 percent for a disease which occurs in five out of every 1000 in a population, the probability that a person who is found positive by the screening test actually has the disease is only 8.7 percent, i.e., in only 8.7 percent of the cases in which the test gives a positive result and asserts the disease to be present is it actually true that the disease is present! (Note that this proportion will vary with prevalence of this disease.)

In a careful review of current efforts in screening, a group of British scholars concluded, by criteria similar to those developed by Wilson, that mass screening could be economically justified for only a very small number of diseases (13). Of ten commonly screened conditions,* screening procedures for six were seriously deficient in one or more of the following: knowledge of the natural history of the disease, methods of diagnosis and treatment, opera-

*Bacteriuria in pregnancy, breast cancer, cervical cancer, deafness in children, diabetes mellitus, glaucoma, iron deficiency anemia, phenylketonuria, pulmonary tuberculosis, and rhesus hemolytic disease of the newborn.

tional procedures, and cost-benefit assessment. Even among the four tests for which the investigators thought mass screening was justified (cervical cancer, iron deficiency anemia, pulmonary tuberculosis, and rhesus hemolytic disease), there were gaps in the relevant information.

Perhaps the greatest controversy over screening has developed in connection with the Papanicolaou smear test for the early detection of cervical cancer. This procedure would appear to be a logical, efficient, and relatively economical means of detecting a potentially fatal disease at a treatable stage. Numerous reports have extolled its value in detecting new cases (14). However, reports of population studies have not always reflected the same optimism. The initial optimistic reports of a mass cervical cancer screening program in British Columbia aroused a furious controversy which has still not been resolved (15). Such debate serves to emphasize the confusion which results from lack of adequate data on the effectiveness of screening efforts.

However confusing the picture may be in regard to the feasibility of a single screening procedure, technology has helped to increase the chaos through the development of automated multiphasic screening. It is now as easy and as inexpensive to perform a dozen laboratory analyses as one. The ease of performance cannot, however, be equated with utility.

The tremendous volume of information generated by such procedures may be so overwhelming as to remain unused by the physician. Bates and Mulinare found that physicians vary in their use of and attitudes toward screening tests in the symptomatic patient. Many felt that they were too expensive and inconvenient. These authors suggest that physicians' dependence on clinical indication and their fear of losing medical control of the patient may reduce the utilization of such screening tests (16).

With such batteries of tests being performed, the odds of finding at least one abnormal result are proportionately greater, particularly if the sensitivity of each test is set to maximize the detection of any disease. Where the normal values are set so that 95 percent of the determinations fall within the normal range, obviously 5 percent of the determinations will then have abnormal values. In a situation in which 12 constituents are measured simultaneously, one can expect over half the patients to have at least one abnormal value on a battery of screening tests (17).

Evidence for the utility of multiphasic screening can be presented on both sides of the case (18). There are those who see it as a potential point of entry into the health care system, a portal to the efficient handling of the "worried well" (19). Data are available on the cost per positive test (20), but the vital question of what impact these findings will have on the health of the populations screened remains unsettled. Collen and his colleagues have calculated the cost per positive test for a variety of procedures. They indicate, however, that these costs are much lower than the cost per "true" positive case, which would require follow-up confirmatory procedures. In the example of mammography the difference was fivefold. It is this second cost per true positive case that is the economically decisive one. Moreover, neither calculation allows for the economic equivalent of a sense of well-being from a clean bill of health, or for the impact of unnecessary health concerns related to false positives.

It is not uncommon to come across glowing reports of large numbers of abnormal findings (21); it is more difficult to find instances where these screenings have been shown to identify patients with potentially correctable or reversible illnesses at an asymptomatic stage (22). One area which appears to hold promise is the treatment of asymptomatic hypertension. The reports of the Veterans Administration Cooperative Study suggest that adequate control of elevated blood pressure is feasible and that such control will reduce morbidity and mortality from hypertension and its sequelae, including heart failure and strokes (23). However, certain caveats can be raised. This study was limited to a particular restricted patient group in terms of age and sex. (A more broadly representative community sample is currently under study by the National Institute of Health.) More importantly, the costs of a program to maintain asymptomatic patients in a compliant state may prove prohibitive. We have yet to discover efficient means for motivating people to follow long-term regimens, particularly when they are feeling no symptoms from the malady.

One potential method for maximizing the benefits of such automated testing is the "health-hazard appraisal" developed by Robbins and his coworkers (24). Risk factors calculated for a given patient on the basis of social, historical, and laboratory data are used as a basis for counseling and patient management. This approach promises to result in greater motivation to take the steps necessary to improve one's health.

The question of the effects of screening on health remains unclear. Early studies could show few positive effects (25); however, more recent evaluations using life table analyses have been more positive (26). Preliminary reports from the Kaiser-Permanente group indicate a favorable impact of screening on at least one group, namely males over 45 years of age, in terms of reduced disability rates, increased work time, and lower utilization of medical services (27).

Despite the lack of convincing evidence for the efficacy of mass screening, there are situations in which such procedures can be readily justified. These occur when there is a decision available about the appropriateness of assigning an individual to a given task. The armed forces have long recognized the need to reject for military service individuals with certain physical or psychological problems. Industries regularly screen employees to match a man's job to his physical competence, particularly where there is a need for strength or an exposure to high risk. Employers of such workers as airline pilots and bus drivers have set up stringent regulations designed to eliminate anyone who has a health problem that might cause him to act so as to endanger the lives of others. Screening before employment is different from clinical screening in that a definitive action can be taken independently of the patient's concurrence. The vital role of patient behavior modification in the utility of multiphasic screening remains one of the major areas to be adequately explored.

TERTIARY PREVENTION

While we generally think of tertiary prevention as the treatment of disease already manifest, there are examples of its more clearly preventive aspects. For instance, rheumatic fever patients may be placed on a regimen of prophylactic penicillin to prevent streptococcal infections and subsequent recurrences of rheumatic fever with resultant sequelae. Effective treatment of symptomatic illness can be an important preventive modality. To the extent that therapy itself is efficacious, its effectiveness is directly proportional to the accessibility and availability of care. A variety of models have been proposed to explain the use of medical services by various populations (28). The study of the factors which impede appropriate care and the design of programs to overcome them are, then, legitimate concerns of community medicine.

The analysis of people's use of health care services generally hinges on what are called "needs." These needs may be recognized by the individual (felt needs) or they may go unheralded (unfelt needs). When they are expressed in action, these needs become demands. A person's actions will depend upon the extent to which he recognizes a problem as a threat to him, his knowledge of the resources available to him, and the number of obstacles which stand in the way of his having the problem treated. Impediments may vary from a matter of inconvenience to the threat of financial catastrophe (29).

The inaccessibility of medical facilities, especially when transportation services are inadequate, is a common barrier to care. The logistics of transportation often produce conflict between consumers and providers of health care. The patient who is dependent on a driver may arrive at the doctor's office or a care facility at inappropriate hours or only after his disease has progressed to an advanced stage. Such patients have likely experienced a physician's rebuke for delaying treatment to the point of complications. Ironically, they may also have been chastised, when they have obtained a ride, for bothering the doctor with minor complaints.

Although the obstacles of cost, distance, and limited hours for obtaining service affect all patient populations, they converge with greatest force on indigent families. Many of the health programs designed for the indigent have attempted to minimize these obstacles. Neighborhood health centers provide care close to home at moderate to no cost. Outreach workers decentralize care still further by educating residents in health matters and performing case-finding (30).

The difficulties of gaining access to the health care system may often generate inappropriate utilization of certain resources. Persons of all social classes have come to utilize emergency rooms as sources of primary care. While generally accessible, emergency rooms are expensive to operate, and are not designed for providing comprehensive care. Some institutions have responded to this situation by establishing evening clinics, thus freeing the emergency facilities for true emergencies.

Another impediment to obtaining care is the fear that the symptoms may indeed represent the onset of a dreaded disease. In an all too human way, we may avoid treatment for fear that it will confirm our expectations (31). These fears may be alleviated to some extent when patients have confidence in the treatment resources. Certainly one's feelings about the potential value of treatment are culturally determined. Not only does our culture dictate, in some measure, our feelings about an institution, it may also influence our ability to utilize it effectively. For someone with a language problem the technological morass of the modern hospital may present insurmountable barriers (32).

For the general public, poverty has become synonymous with inadequate care (33). The life style of the poor seems to embrace all of the obstacles to care in an environment which is itself detrimental to health. Despite major efforts to mount a war on poverty, there is little evidence that we are winning many battles (34).

One area of concern to those interested in improving the delivery of health care is the inappropriate training afforded health professionals, especially physicians. Those who are trained in medical centers that deal with esoteric disease tend to emerge woefully unprepared to cope with the more common health problems (35). Moreover, medical students' orientation is more toward the advanced stages of complicated diseases than the early presenting signs of the more common illnesses (36). A variety of potential solutions have been put forward to counteract this trend, ranging from the reorientation of medical curricula to the development of new cadres of such personnel as physicians' assistants and nurse practitioners.

REHABILITATION

The increasing emphasis on medical science has threatened to divorce medicine from its original point of reference—the patient. Increasingly, as the quality of care is called to scrutiny, attention focuses on the result of care. Such concern must inevitably lead to recognition of the vital role of rehabilitation. Along the spectrum of prevention, rehabilitation represents the final effort oriented toward preventing further deterioration of function and toward increasing the potential for restoration of lost capacity.

With the shift in modern patterns of illness toward the chronic degenerative diseases, the approach to medical care has, of necessity, changed. Medical spokesmen now speak less of cure and more of containment. Whole new therapeutic vistas have been opened by the use of transplantation and artificial organs. Critics of modern medicine, its cost in particular, are quick to point out that these developments have done little to increase longevity (37). Indeed they have not; what advances have been achieved are reflected in decreased disability and improved coping with chronic conditions.

The prevalence of chronic disease has forced a reexamination of a number of health care activities. The rapidly increasing cost of care has provoked a search for more efficient means of delivering care. Ambulatory programs are being substituted for hospital care whenever possible. Perhaps the most successful efforts in this direction have been in the field of mental health. The development of community mental health centers, together with the availability of new medications, has virtually emptied many mental hospitals. Patients previously condemned to indefinite hospitalization are now functioning in their communities (38). To a lesser, but nonetheless welcome extent, comprehensive ambulatory medical care shows promise of reducing hospital utilization (39).

The growing concern with the cost of health care has inevitably led to the application of cost-benefit analysis to health (40). For example, the various modalities of treatment for chronic renal disease yield differing survival rates. The yield from each can be compared to the cost of providing that form of care to net a measure of efficiency of return on the investment (41).

Attention to the relative benefit of different modalities of care causes us to reexamine the entire chain of events in the medical care process. If we use the analogy of a chemical reaction, the rate-limiting step is the effective application of therapeutic measures. Despite the emphasis placed on diagnosis as a primary medical skill, its role is important to patient care only to the extent that it influences the choice of treatment. A vital link in the care process is the cooperation of the patient. Patient compliance may indeed be the most overlooked element of medical practice.

In the ambulatory situation, one readily appreciates the importance of patient cooperation in effecting positive outcomes. The outcome of treatment is dependent upon the patient's willingness and ability to cooperate. Often, treatment failures may not represent inadequate diagnostic or therapeutic skills, but rather the failure to establish a relationship with the patient that will ensure his knowledge of his problem and his confidence in his therapist (42).

The need for patient compliance extends as well to the more controlled situation of the hospital. Perhaps the most critical area for this cooperation is the field of rehabilitative medicine. Without a firm working relationship between the patient and the therapeutic team, there would seem to be little likelihood of success in achieving any significant restoration of function and/or adjustment.

In some ways, our concern with rehabilitation brings us full circle to the problems faced in contemplating primary preventive measures. We must consider not only the physical and economic resources available to patients but also the nonmedical social, political, and psychological issues involved. To illustrate the multidimensional aspects of rehabilitative medicine, consider a major target of rehabilitative efforts, the general area of geriatric care. Here the goal is clearly to prevent, or at least retard, further deterioration. While physical medicine has made great progress in retaining and restoring function, advances in geriatrics are threatened by our lack of a social system which provides a meaningful role for older persons. Rapid obsolescence of skills and experience have made these people more of a liability than a resource in contemporary life. The political furor over Medicare legislation and the failure to provide an adequate social security system to permit aging with dignity betray a lack of commitment to support the elderly in our society. This ambivalence is understandable. Even today the elderly represent a relatively small proportion of the population that is expensive to maintain. The escalating costs of care have been acutely felt in nursing homes and other types of maintenance programs.

Ironically, rehabilitation is also acute in terms of the very young, particularly the large group of mentally retarded children whose complex problems require that the patients be institutionalized. The growth of sophisticated knowledge and skill in rehabilitating these children raises similar social and political questions as to how much society is willing to invest in efforts to help them. We have within our grasp the potential to prevent their further deterioration and to maximize their abilities through specific individualized rehabilitation programs, including vocational and recreational modalities, but these will require broad social measures and substantial commitments of both fiscal and social resources.

COMBINED APPROACHES

The arbitrary division of prevention into four stages is no doubt intended as a taxonomic convenience to describe the broad range of available approaches to maximizing health. Clearly, in practice these divisions are not strictly followed. One draws simultaneously upon all potential means to attack the problem at hand.

For example, lead poisoning in children is a health problem in urban ghettos. Screening projects for body lead identify those who have ingested significant quantities. Additional psychomotor screening may find those who betray evidence of significant lead poisoning. Those found can be put on appropriate medical regimens to remove the lead accumulated, but for some the condition has advanced to the point where rehabilitative efforts are necessary. These efforts would include physical therapy, special education, psychotherapy and, for some, institutionalization. Health education programs designed for both parents and children caution about the dangers and early signs of lead poisoning. For the most part, lead-based paints have been removed from the market, but the

Figure 2
A Systems Approach to the Problem of Lead Poisoning

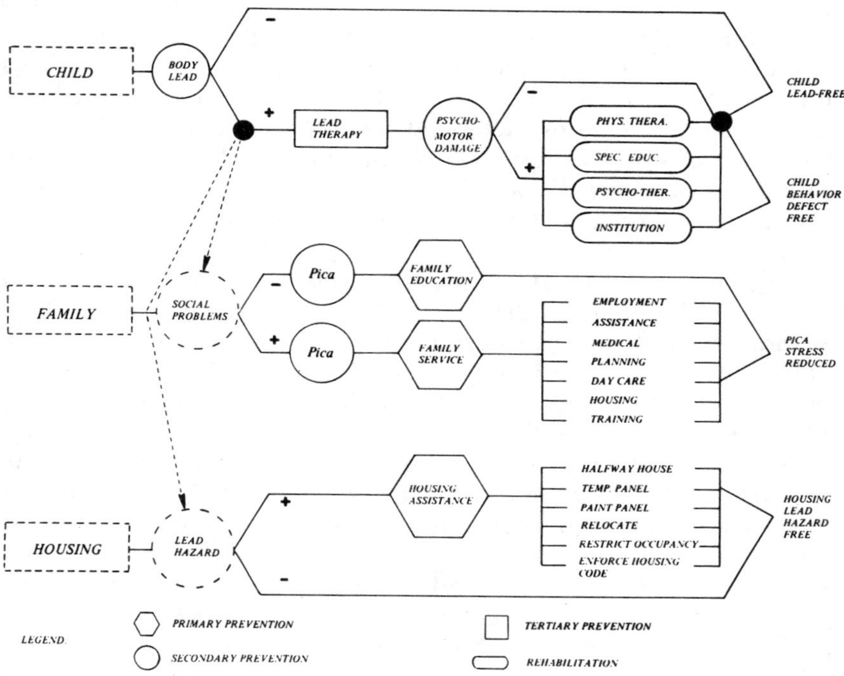

demolition of old slum dwellings remains a major challenge to urban planners.

Primary preventive efforts against lead poisoning would include an attack on housing problems, ranging from revision and enforcement of building codes to restricted occupancy of blighted dwellings, repaneling of walls still coated with lead-based paints and, when necessary, relocation of families. Pica has become regularly associated with lead ingestion. In turn, pica has been found most prevalent in families beset by social stress (43). Thus a program to prevent lead poisoning may have to involve itself in employment, day care, and family counseling. Figure 2 represents a systems approach to the menace of lead poisoning. Several points of intervention are indicated in terms of the appropriate level of prevention which might be applied.

The control of venereal disease was at one time considered accomplished. The availability of potent antibiotics offered a tool for definitive treatment. However, VD is once again a major national health problem. Faced with resistant strains and often resistant population groups, preventive programs must rely on multiple points of attack. Case-finding programs, carried out by public health departments or private physicians, can provide early detection and treatment, but successful primary prevention depends upon thorough follow-up to reach the reservoir of infection. This type of follow-up requires maximal cooperation from those contacted, and this is rarely achieved. Venereologists have advocated treatment of any person who *might have* contracted gonorrhea (so-called "epi treatment") as one means of overcoming this lack of cooperation. Perhaps the only workable solution to control venereal disease lies in the development of vaccines against it.

It is not unusual today to find ourselves in the position of having a useful test to detect a disease but few tools available with which to intervene effectively. A current example of this dilemma is sickle cell anemia which affects approximately one in every 600 American Negroes (44). Although we have reliable and inexpensive means for identifying those with the full-blown disease or the heterozygous trait, there is little we can do to treat them beyond providing symptomatic relief. One form of primary prevention that is available is genetic counseling to inform those with the disease that they risk passing it on to future generations. This approach requires a synthesis of talents, pooling the efforts of geneticists and behaviorists who are attuned to the potential social implications of such advice.

The modern plague threatening our nation today is the misuse of addictive drugs. It is an affliction all the more terrible because it is self-induced. There are major parallels between this contemporary epidemic and the infectious diseases of the past. In this case the vector is human and is responsible for the person-to-person transmission of misery and suffering. With no vaccine in sight we must turn our attention to other forms of prevention. Secondary and tertiary prevention have not been impressively successful to date. Rehabilitative efforts have yielded equivocal results in many ways similar to those achieved with alcoholism. Primary preventive efforts may require major manipulations of both the physical and the social environment.

CONCLUSIONS

The concept of controlling disease varies enormously with the context. From the perspective of community medicine, it is appropriate to consider the multiplicity of means extending far beyond those traditionally employed by public health. We have tried to concentrate on examples which might be most appropriate to the health professional. Consideration of these problems should extend over all four stages of prevention. Increasingly, we note a growing unification of the activities of public health and curative medicine to the point where health departments now operate medical clinics and practitioners offer a variety of preventive services. This unification is a positive trend, for the problems are certainly large enough to permit a variety of solutions. As indicated at the beginning of this chapter, the concept of prevention is so ubiquitous that it must be an integral part of the practice of medicine in general as well as of community medicine.

REFERENCES

1. See Rice, D. Economic costs of cardiovascular diseases and cancer, 1962. PHS Publication No. 947-5. Washington, D. C.: United States Government Printing Office, 1965.
2. Bergner, L., and Yerby, A. Low income and the use of health services. *New England J. of Medicine*, 1968, *278*, 541–46.
3. Wilner, D. M., et al. *The housing environment and family life.* Baltimore: The Johns Hopkins Press, 1962.
4. Terris, M. Epidemiology of cirrhosis of the liver: National mortality data. *Amer. J. Pub. Health*, 1967, *57*, 2076–2088.
5. U.S. Public Health Service Issue 2, monographs on the scientific evidence to support the relationships between smoking and disease: *Smoking and health—report of the Advisory Committee to the Surgeon General of the Public Health Service* (U.S. Government Printing Office, 1964, Washington, D. C.) and *The health consequences of smoking: A public health service review, 1967* (U.S. Government Printing Office, 1968, Washington, D. C.)
6. For women, the corresponding percentages of excess mortality are 21 and 30 percent. These data are derived from the *Build and Blood Pressure Study*, 1959, published by the Society of Actuaries. These findings are summarized in the 1960 *Statistical Bulletin* published by Metropolitan Life Insurance Company.
7. The advocacy approach of Ralph Nader's *Unsafe at any speed* (New York: Grossman Publishers, 1965) may not emphasize both sides of the situation equally but his attempt to improve automobile and highway conditions are positive steps toward preventing death and disability.
8. Milton Terris has advocated a threefold attack on the problems of cigarettes, alcohol, and saturated fats; for each he recommends cessation of advertising, massive public education, and federal subsidies to promote diversification of the industries involved. See M. Terris. A social policy for health. *Amer. J. Pub. Health*, 1968, *58*, 5-12.
9. See the reports of the Atherosclerosis Study Group and the Epidemiology Study Group of the Inter-Society Commission for Heart Disease Resources, "Primary Prevention of Atherosclerotic Diseases" in *Circulation*, 1970, *42*, A55-A95.
10. Hutchison, G. B. Evaluation of preventive services. *Journal of Chronic Diseases*, 1969, *11*, 497-508.
11. Wilson, J. M. G. Principles in practice of screening for disease. *WHO Chronicle*, 1968, 22, 473–483. A more complete presentation is available in Wilson, J. M. G., and Jungner, G. *Principles in practice of screening for disease.* Geneva: World Health Organization, 1968 (Public Health Paper No. 34).
12. For an example of how specificity and sensitivity interact see the data

on tuberculosis in Kane, R. L., and Vandiviere, H. M. The significance of multiple simultaneous tuberculin skin-testing in the prediction of various mycobacterial infections in the host. *American Review of Respiratory Disease*, 1972, *105*, 296–298.

13. McKeown, T., ed. *Screening in medical care: Reviewing the evidence.* London: Oxford University Press, 1968. This collection of essays was designed to assess the efficacy of screening on a mass basis for a variety of commonly sought diseases.
14. Lundin, F. E., Mendez, W. M., and Parker, J. F. Morbidity from cervical cancer: Effects of cervical cytology and socioeconomic status. *Journal of the National Cancer Institute*, 1965, *35*, 1015-1025; McInroy, R. A. Cervical cytology and population screening. *Journal of Clinical Pathology*, 1967, *20*, 218–219; Ranwick, D. H. Statistical methods in the screening program for cancer. *Canadian Journal of Public Health*, 1969, *60*, 267-278; Sall, S., Olivio, E., and Sedlis, A. Mass cytologic screening and the diagnosis of cervical carcinoma in situ. *Cancer*, 1968, *21*, 1180–1183; MacGregor, J. E., et al. Improved prognosis of cervical cancer due to comprehensive screening. *Lancet*, January 9, 1971, *1*, 74-76; Christopherson, W. M., et al. Cervix cancer control in Louisville, Kentucky. *Cancer*, 1970, *26*, 29-38. Most recently see Breslow, L. Early case-finding, treatment and mortality from cervix and breast cancer. *Preventive Medicine*, 1972, *1*, 141-152.
15. The original optimistic report of the British Columbia data by D. A. Boyes, H. K. Fidler, and D. R. Lock (The significance of in situ carcinoma of the cervix. *British Medical Journal*, 1962, *1*, 203-205) was quickly challenged by such people as J. R. S. Douglas (Diagnostic cytology. *Medical Journal of Australia*, 1963, *2*, 598-599) and later by T. W. Lees (Failure of cervical cytology. *Lancet*, 1969, *1*, 1020) and in an analysis by H. S. Ahluwalia and R. Doll (Mortality from cancer of the cervix uteri in British Columbia and other parts of Canada. *British Journal of Prev. Soc. Med.*, 1968, *22*, 161-164). A subsequent report by H. K. Fidler, D. A. Boyes, and A. J. Worth (Cervical cancer detection in British Columbia. *Journal of Obstetrics and Gynecology of the British Commonwealth*, 1968, *75*, 392-404) suggested that the mortality rates appeared to be falling but the trend was yet to be established. A study in Kentucky by W. M. Christopherson, J. E. Parker, W. M. Mendez, and F. E. Lundin, Jr. (Cervix cancer, birth rates and mass cytologic screening. *Cancer*, 1970, *26*, 808–811), reported a major reduction in mortality after a screening program. The issue remains unresolved; for each glowing report of progress there appears to be a rebuttal, for example, see M. Wilson, J. Chamberlain, and A. L. Cochrane, Screening for cervical cancer. *Lancet*, 1971, *1*, 297–298.
16. Bates, B., and Mulinare, J. Physicians' use and opinions of screening tests in ambulatory practice. *J. of American Med. Assoc.*, 1970, *214*, 2173–2180.
17. Daughaday, W. H., Erickson, M. M., and White, W. L. Evaluation of

routine twelve channel chemical profiles on patients admitted to a university general hospital, in *Automation in Analytical Chemistry,* Vol. 1, *Technicon Symposia,* edited by Nichols Biddle Scora. Ardsley, New York: Technicon Instrument Corporation, 1967, pp. 91–98.

18. A good review of the status of automated multiphasic health screening can be found in Volume 45 of the *Bulletin of the New York Academy of Medicine,* December 1969. This volume reports on the 1969 Conference on Automated Multiphasic Health Screening held by the New York Heart Association.
19. See two articles by Sidney Garfield, The delivery of medical care. *Scientific American,* 1970, *222,* 15-23; and Multiphasic health testing in medical care as a right. *New England J. of Medicine,* 1970, *283,* 1087–1089.
20. Morris Collen and his associates have reported the cost of a multiphasic screening program established for Kaiser Permanente group members (Cost analysis of multiphasic screening program. *New England J. of Medicine,* 1969, *280,* 1043–1045). Such cost estimates will vary with the volume of services performed. Collen, et al. Dollar cost per positive test for automated multiphasic screening. *New England J. of Medicine,* 1970, *283,* 459–463.
21. For example, see Breckenridge, R. L. Experience with automated multiphasic health testing. *Industrial Medicine,* 1971, *40,* 18-23.
22. For a discussion of the potentials and pitfalls of multiphasic screening see Ahlvin, R. C. Biochemical screening—a critique. *New England J. of Medicine,* 1970, *283,* 1084–1086, and Thorner, R. M. Whither multiphasic screening? *New England J. of Medicine,* 1969, *280,* 1037–1042.
23. Veterans Administration Cooperative Study Group in Antihypertensive Agents. Effects of treatment on morbidity in hypertension. *J. of American Med. Associ.,* 1967, *202*, 1027–1034, and 1970, *213*, 1143–1152.
24. For more information, see Sadusk, J. F., Jr., and Robbins, L. C. Proposal for health hazard appraisal and comprehensive health care. *J. of American Med. Assoc.,* 1968, *203,* 1108–1112, and Robbins, L. C., and Hall, J. H. *How to practice prospective medicine.* Indianapolis: Methodist Hospital at Indiana, 1970.
25. See, for example, Schor, S. S., et al. An evaluation of the periodic health examination: The findings of 350 examinees who died. *Annals of Internal Medicine,* 1964, *61,* 999-1005.
26. Roberts, N. J., et al. Mortality among males in periodic health examination programs. *New England J. of Medicine,* 1969, *281,* 20-24.
27. Ramcharan, S., et al. Multiphasic checkup evaluation study. 2. Disability in chronic disease after seven years of multiphasic check-ups. *Preventive Medicine,* 1973, *2,* 207-220.
28. For reviews of this issue, see Rosenstock, I. M. Why people use health services. *Milbank Memorial Fund Quarterly* (Part 2), 1966, *44,* 94-127, and Andersen, R. A behavioral model of families' use of health services, Center for Health Administration Studies Research Series No. 25, University of Chicago, 1968.
29. It is interesting to note that the use of services does not vary remark-

ably even between different countries. See, for example, Kalimo, E., et al. Interrelationships in the use of selected health services: A cross-national study. *Medical Care,* 1972, *10,* 95-108. This is one of a series of reports coming out of the World Health Organization's International Collaborative Study of Medical Care Utilization.

30. See for example the description of the Montefiore Neighborhood Medical Care Demonstration Project, *Milbank Memorial Fund Quarterly* (Part 1), 1968, *46.*
31. For examples, see Goldsen, R. K., et al. Some factors related to patient delay in seeking diagnosis for cancer symptoms. *Cancer,* 1957, *10,* 1-7; Aitkin-Swan, J., and Patterson, R. The cancer patient delay in seeking advice. *British Medical Journal,* 1955, *1,* 623–627; Levine, G. N. Anxiety about illness: Psychological and social bases. *Journal of Health and Human Behavior,* 1966, *3,* 30-34.
32. See Samora, J., Saunders, L., and Larson, R. F. Medical vocabulary knowledge among hospital patients. *Journal of Health and Human Behavior,* 1961, *2,* 83, and Seligmann, A., McGrath, N. E., and Pratt, L. Level of medical information among clinic patients. *Journal of Chronic Diseases,* 1957, *6,* 497-509.
33. For example, Chilman, C. *Growing up poor.* Welfare Administration, U.S. Department of Health, Education and Welfare. Washington, D.C.: U.S. Government Printing Office, 1966; The Chamber of Commerce of the United States. *Poverty: The sick, disabled and aged.* Second Report of the Task Force on Economic Growth and Opportunity. Washington, D. C., 1965; Veney, J. E., ed. Medical care for low income families. Proceedings of the Tenth Annual Symposium on Hospital Affairs, Center for Health Administration Studies, University of Chicago. *Inquiry,* 1968, *5,* 1-80.
34. See the editorial by Bryant, T. Goals and potential of the neighborhood health centers. *Medical Care,* 1970, *8,* 93-94, and Moynihan, D. *Maximum feasible misunderstanding,* New York: The Free Press, 1969.
35. To understand the contrast between the illness seen in a primary care practice and that available to the medical center see White, K. L., Williams, T. F., and Greenberg, B. G. The ecology of medical care. *New England J. of Medicine,* 1961, *265,* 885-892.
36. Keith Hodgkin has described this disparity well in *Towards earlier diagnosis.* London: E. N. S. Livingston Ltd., 1966.
37. For a provoking discussion of this issue, see Forbes, W. H. Longevity and medical cost. *New England J. of Medicine,* 1967, *277,* 71-78.
38. Susser, M. *Community psychiatry: Epidemiologic and social themes.* New York: Random House, 1968.
39. One very optimistic projection was reported by Bellin, S. S., Geiger, H. J., and Gibson, C. D. Impact of ambulatory health care services on the demand for hospital beds: A study of the Tufts Neighborhood Health Center at Columbia Point in Boston. *New England J. of Medicine,* 1969, *280,* 808–812.
40. Klarman, H. E. Present status of cost benefit analysis in the health

field. *Amer. J. Pub. Health*, 1967, *57*, 1948–1953; Levin, A. L. Cost effectiveness in maternal and child health: Implications for program planning and evaluation. *New England J. of Medicine*, 1968, *278*, 1041–1047; May, P. R. A. Cost efficiency of mental health care, III. Treatment method as a parameter of cost in the treatment of schizophrenia. *Amer. J. Pub. Health*, 1961, *61*, 127–129.
41. See Klarman, H. E., O'Frances, J., and Rosenthal, G. D. Cost effectiveness analysis applied to the treatment of chronic renal disease. *Medical Care*, 1968, *6*, 48-54.
42. See Francis, V., Corsch, B. M., and Morris, M. J. Gaps in patient-doctor communication. *New England J. of Medicine*, 1969, *280*, 535–540; Bogdonoff, M. D., et al. The doctor-patient relationship: A suggested practical and purposeful approach. *J. of American Med. Assoc.*, 1965, *192*, 131–134; Kane, R. L., and Kane, R. A. Physicians' attitudes of omnipotence in a university hospital. *Journal of Medical Education*, 1969, *44*, 684–690.
43. Meigs, J. W., and Whitmire, E. Epidemiology of lead poisoning in New Haven children—operational factors. *Connecticut Medicine*, 1971, *35*, 363-369.
44. Wintrobe, M. M. The hemoglobinophaties and thalassemia. In *Principles of internal medicine*, Harrison, et al., eds., New York: McGraw Hill, 1966.

7

Health Economics: Wants, Needs, and Demands

James R. Jeffers

"Health is a right, not a privilege." This familiar assertion is often made by both lay persons and health professionals when discussing matters of health care delivery and policy. The statement implies that an all-out effort ought to be made to satisfy the health needs of a community, region, or nation. Yet a fundamental fact of economics is that while people have needs for many things, society possesses only limited means (resources) for satisfying them. Therefore, it is difficult, if not impossible, for an economist to accept such an assertion uncritically. Given that resources are limited, an all-out allocation of the volume of resources necessary to meet the health needs of a given population implies that progress toward satisfying the needs of its members for other things will be inhibited or otherwise unsatisfactory. What is the justification for satisfying health needs while needs for such other things as food, housing, and education go unmet?

An inherent danger which often underlies assertions and discussions about the consumption of certain commodities as a "right" not to be restricted to a "privileged" few is the implication that such commodities can, in some way, be provided virtually "free." Economists, and others, recognize that this is impossible. Free goods of man-made origin, the only kind considered here, do not exist. Commodities that are made available to individual consumers at an explicit price of zero involve costs that, while they are implicit, are nonetheless very real. The real costs of so-called free goods are the values of the goods and services that members of the population could have consumed had the resources (human and material) been used to produce goods other than those commodities provided to consumers at no explicit cost. Thus, the real costs of free health services may be valued in terms of the satisfaction foregone by not being able to enjoy the benefits of more food, housing, and so forth, that could have been obtained with the resources expended in producing free health services. The burden of these costs is often explicitly born, although indirectly, by those collectively underwriting the costs of medical education, the construction and maintenance of health facilities, and the consumption of health care via tax and insurance mechanisms. The truth is that health services, like all commodities, are purchasable and from a social view cannot be regarded as free, no matter how ethically desirable their consumption may be.

Admittedly, economics is a "dismal science," but only because as a discipline it forces us to face up to undesirable realities characteristic of the world in which we live. The fact that resources are scarce relative to the needs and demands competing for them is perhaps the most fundamental of economic realities; indeed, many view it as the cornerstone of economic science.

However, many other basic and fundamental economic concepts are useful to the analysis of health care delivery problems. The appropriate application of these concepts enhances our understanding of many health policy issues. The purpose of this chapter is to carefully define certain economic principles and to show how they can be applied to selected problems of health care delivery. Unfortunately, time and space permit us to deal with only a few problems and economic principles. It is hoped, however, that this brief demonstration will stimulate interest on the part of readers to acquire a greater understanding.

CONCEPT OF A HEALTH SERVICES INDUSTRY

Many are critical of the pattern and organization of our existing health services system. Indeed, the late Walter Reuther called it a nonsystem. Critics believe that a true system involves elements that are lacking in the case of health services as they currently are being produced and distributed in this country. The term system brings to mind a systematic flow of integrated activities. Thus the notion of a health care delivery system suggests an orderly flow of patients through an integrated set of nodes of patient care activity, with patients periodically entering and leaving the system when appropriate.

An Ideal System

Elsewhere I have outlined the essential elements of an ideal health care delivery system along the following lines:[1]

1. Numerous entry points that are readily accessible to patients.
2. A well-organized referral mechanism that insures all the kinds, qualities, and quantities of the health services that patients need.
3. Numerous exit points also readily available to patients.

In addition to these elements, an ideal health services system should provide patients with uniform information as to their needs for health care upon entering the system and throughout the period during which they are receiving care. The latter is extremely important insofar as such judgments relate to conclusions that patients can no longer benefit from receiving more care—death and complete cure being but extreme cases in which such uniformity of judgment is often achieved.

Clearly, our health services system does not measure up to such standards. Critics are quick to point out such obvious departures from the ideal as shortages of personnel and services on the one hand, and enormous duplication of facilities and services on the other. Gaps exist in the referral mechanism, and professional barriers impede reorganization that would overcome some of these problems. If we were to start over without the weight of past history and tradition, it is doubtful that we would invent the current system as we know it now.

However, it should be recognized that few, if any, other activities of the magnitude and complexity of those that are involved in producing and distributing health services measure up to ideal standards that might be set forth. One only needs to consider our system of higher education and observe the disparity between existing accessibility, quality, and nonuniformity of results upon exiting from the system, as well as prevailing standards of education, to appreciate this fact. The fact that our higher education and health systems work well suggests that either there are deep-seated virtues to radical decentralization (as well might be the case), that the public is exceptionally ignorant, or that Americans are exceptionally tolerant.

One fact on which all who have studied the matter of health care delivery agree is that the process is extremely complex. No one can

[1]See James R. Jeffers, "Conflicting economic pressures in health care." *Hospital Administration*, Vol. 16, No. 3 (Summer 1971), pp. 22–23.

deny that the existing activities are highly organized and integrated. Most also would agree that the high degree of complexity that characterizes health delivery activities is a significant obstacle to understanding the system, and that it impedes our ability to discuss health policy issues intelligently. The systemic analytical perspective is a useful device for describing the myriad activities involved in health care delivery, and for analyzing organizational shortcomings. However, it fails to provide a viewpoint that is useful for analyzing issues of public policy that are not concerned with organizational alternatives.

The Industry Concept

An analytical perspective that is highly useful in many cases is that of an industry, a concept used by economists. An industry is a collection of production units called firms, all of which produce a similar product or service. While conceptually the term industry is rather precise, in practice the task of deciding which producers are to be included in the set of firms constituting an industry is often difficult. The difficulty lies in determining what goods and services or commodities are in fact similar. In general, the basis for making such a determination lies in ascertaining what needs the goods and services produced are intended to satisfy.

Obviously, the health services industry would consist of the firms producing goods and services designed to satisfy the desires of patients or consumers for an improved health status. However, the health services industry is by no means the sole factor influencing the health status of the population. Obviously, other factors impinge on health status, including hereditary traits, environmental factors, housing, and life style, to name a few. Therefore, the output of the health services industry should be regarded as health services and not health. The latter is the resultant of many influences in addition to the consumption of health services.

For analytical purposes, the health services industry may be viewed as the production processes centered around the activities of physicians, dentists, hospitals, and related health professionals and institutions. As in all service industries, it is difficult to separate the productive activity from the product that is produced, because the latter consists of rendering a service.

For our purposes these services may be defined to include services intended to improve health, alleviate suffering, increase comfort, enhance personal and financial security against illness, and aid in family planning. More specifically, these activities may be grouped into 11 broad categories:[2]

1. Professional and other services rendered to patients by physicians, dentists, nurses, chiropractors, podiatrists, veterinarians, religious healers, clinical psychologists, and others, together with assistants and capital employed. (To avoid double counting, this category excludes professional services rendered by employees of hospitals and other health services institutions.)

2. Professional and other services rendered to patients by the employees and capital in institutions, such as hospitals, mental hospitals, tuberculosis sanitariums, various nursing homes, and other extended care facilities.

3. Services rendered either to patients directly or to practitioners or to institutions by independent laboratories, consultants, transportation agencies, and other auxiliary agencies. For example, in many communities ambulance services are provided by local police and fire protection units.

4. The manufacture and distribution of consumable products, such as pharmaceuticals, eyeglasses, and hospital and medical supplies.

5. Public health activities not included above, such as environmental monitoring, control, and improvement; health screening; regulation of health services; accrediting; public education; consumer protection; and safety administration.

6. The operation of health insurance, income-protection insurance, fund raising, and other financial activities related to health and health services.

7. Formal education and training of health service personnel, professional and nonprofessional, including college and university training, proprietary school training, and continuing education. (Inservice training would be included in the other categories.)

8. Research related directly or indirectly to health services and conducted by government, universities, research institutions, private business, and others.

9. Patient and family time involved in using the health services system and in providing home care. This time factor must be included since it is a major ingredient in health care. For example, time spent waiting in a physician's office and in other health

[2]These categories are essentially the same as listed in Howard R. Bowen and James R. Jeffers, *The Economics of Health Services.* New York: General Learning Corporation, 1971, pp. 2-3.

facilities constitutes a significant expenditure of human resources that is seldom counted in reckoning the costs of health services.

10. Activities intended to modify the health services system; for example, efforts of professional associations (such as the American Medical Association) to influence public opinion and legislative action, efforts of specialized health organizations and other organizations to promote particular health activities, and activities of legislative bodies in the health services area.

11. Construction of buildings and other fixed capital employed in the health services system. (The capital item might more properly be handled as amortization—scheduled depreciation—of the structures and fixed equipment employed in the various parts of the system. However, in most discussions and statistics on expenditures and finance of health services, current construction is included as a separate item.)

Together, these varied activities may be regarded as an industry similar to the food or transportation industry, consisting of many specialized firms that employ various types of capital and labor, organize the production of many different services, and sell or otherwise dispense these services to consumers. Some of these services are complementary, for example, those of surgeons and hospitals or of dentists and dental technicians. Some are competing substitutes, like chiropractic and physical therapy, or self-administered proprietary drugs and physician's prescriptions. These services are seldom used in concert and often are viewed as alternatives.

The Concept of a Market

It is useful to think of a market for health services. In general, a market exists when suppliers and consumers exist and there is communication between them. In order to obtain a clear appreciation of the market concept, it is necessary to understand the basic concepts of supply and demand.

Supply. Supply is a multivariate functional relationship between the quantities of a particular commodity that suppliers plan to produce over a relevant time period and the factors that influence these plans. Among the factors that are important determinants of supply are the price of the commodities supplied, prices of alternative commodities that could be produced, the technology of production, and the costs of the inputs which when combined and organized appropriately enable the production of the commodity in question. The latter may be broadly viewed as labor (professional

Figure 1
Supply

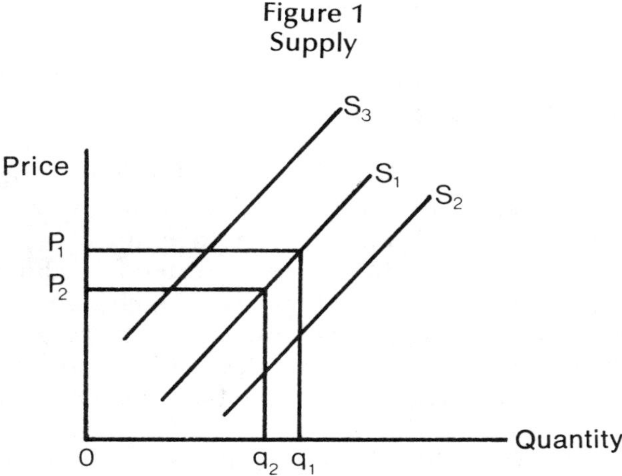

services); capital, including complex diagnostic and therapeutic equipment; and land, including building facilities; supplies, and so on.

Of considerable importance to economic analysis is the nature of the relationship between prices and the quantities of commodities produced. When graphed, this relationship is labeled a supply curve as reflected in Figure 1.

In Figure 1 the hypothetical supply curves S_1, S_2, and S_3 are all drawn as straight lines in the interests of simplicity. Actual supply curves may have a variety of shapes. However, the gradient or slopes of supply curves is usually upward, reflecting the fact that suppliers are willing to make a greater quantity of output available only if prices per unit of output are higher. This is the case because usually greater quantities of output can be produced only by incurring higher per unit costs.

A supply curve reflects the quantities of output of a particular commodity which suppliers will make available over a specified time interval at alternative prices assuming that the other determinants of supply, mentioned above, remain unchanged. That is, a given supply curve, such as S_1, exhibits a particular shape and position within the coordinate system according to given values of supply determinants other than price that are not explicitly incorporated in the diagram. Thus, focusing attention on S_1, at a hypothetical price, say P_1, the quantity that would be supplied is indicated by the quantity Q_1 on the horizontal axis. Assuming another hypothetical price, P_2, the associated quantity supplied is Q_2.

Because a single curve reflects supply under given conditions, changes in quantity associated with alternative prices are labeled changes in quantity supplied and not changes in supply. The latter is associated with a change in the entire relationship between price and quantity as reflected by a shift in the curve. Changes in the position and/or shape of the supply curve reflect net changes in one or more of the determinants of supply. For example, a technological advance often permits existing resources to produce a greater quantity of output with the same or lower costs of production. This development would be reflected by a shift or change in supply as illustrated by S_2 in Figure 1. The latter curve illustrates the consequence that a greater quantity of output would be made available at all alternative prices than was the case before the change in technology.

Then supply curve S_3 reflects a decrease in supply, indicating that some determinant of the quantity supplied other than the price of output changed adversely, say an increase in labor costs, thus making it possible to make quantities of output available only at higher prices as compared to the situation before the change as reflected by S_1.

Demand. The demand for commodities arises out of consumers' desires to satisfy psychologically formulated wants, or needs, for commodities as they perceive them. In a market economy, in order to satisfy wants for commodities that they cannot or choose not to produce for themselves, consumers seek out suppliers and offer money in exchange for those commodities that they desire. Since most consumers have limited financial resources, they cannot buy all the goods and services in the quantities that they desire. It may be assumed that, usually, consumers act rationally in allocating their limited financial resources among commodities that are available, purchasing that combination of goods and services which will provide them with the greatest satisfaction attainable in view of their financial constraints. Thus, the quantity of medical services that a given population will purchase over a given time interval depends on: 1) their collective wants or needs, as they perceive them, for those services as opposed to all goods and services; 2) prices of health services, and the prices of commodities other than health services that serve to satisfy alternative wants or perceived needs; 3) the size of the population; and 4) the financial resources extant in the population.

Demand is a multivariate functional relationship between the quantities of a particular commodity that consumers plan to purchase over a relevant time period and factors such as those mentioned above that impinge on those plans. As in the case of supply, it is important to focus on the relationship between price and

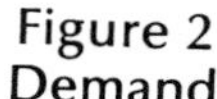

Figure 2
Demand

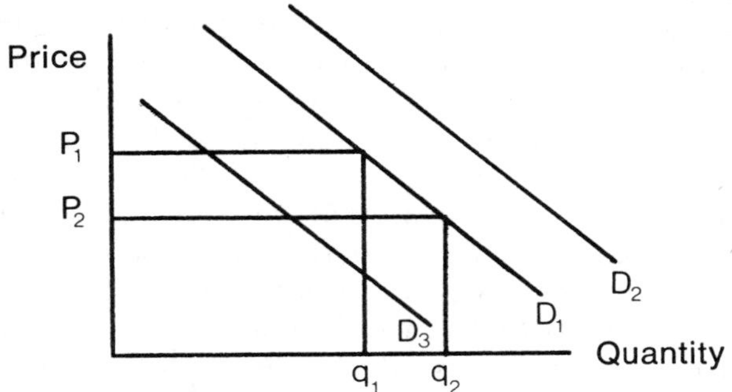

quantity. The relationship between price and quantity demand may be depicted geometrically as in Figure 2.

In Figure 2 the demand curves, like the supply curves of Figure 1, are drawn linearly in the interests of simplicity. However, demand curves are drawn so that they slope downward to reflect the usual case of demand, namely, that price and quantity demanded are inversely related. That is, assuming that all other determinants of demand remain invariant, including the prices of other desirable commodities, the quantity of health services demanded will increase in response to lower prices of health services. The reasoning supporting this proposition is as follows: It may be assumed that the population's collective financial resources do not permit everyone to buy all the goods and resources in the quantities necessary to satisfy all of their wants. Consumers are likely to strike some sort of compromise and consume less than desired quantities of all goods and services, including health services; the latter being the amount they would buy if prices of commodities were zero or if financial resources were unlimited. They will weigh the benefits of consuming various commodities against their costs as reflected by their respective prices. Assuming no change in potential consumption benefits, consumers reasonably may be expected to buy more of a particular commodity whose price diminishes relative to that of others. Since the demand curve of any particular commodity, in this case health services, is drawn under the assumption that prices of other goods and services remain constant, it is logical to imagine a greater quantity of health services being consumed as their prices diminish relative to prices of other commodities which are assumed to remain invariant.

Thus, focusing attention on D_1 in Figure 2, at a hypothetical price of P_1 the associated quantity demanded is Q_1 and at price P_2 the relevant quantity demanded is Q_2.

A single curve reflects demand under specified conditions. It is important to recognize that changes in quantity supplied reflecting the response of changes in quantity demanded to an assumed change in price should not be interpreted as changes in demand. The latter is associated with a change in the entire relationship between price and quantity demanded as reflected by a shift in the curve. Changes in the position and/or slope of the demand curve reflect net changes in one or more of the determinants of demand. For example, if the financial resources of the population were to increase, it is likely that demand would increase, i.e., greater quantities of health services would be demanded at all hypothetically relevant prices (see D_2) than was the case prior to the change as reflected by D_1. Similarly, if the population's financial resources were to decline, the demand would diminish as reflected by D_3 as compared to D_1.

Market Equilibrium. As stated at the beginning of this section, a market exists when suppliers and consumers exist and there exists communication between them. The market for health services may be represented by incorporating the demand for and supply of health services into the same diagram as is done in Figure 3.

Figure 3 characterizes the aggregate market for health services. In this view, the health services system is a large and highly complex industry producing a flow of goods and services used to improve health status. Demand flows from the public and, together with supply, determines prices and quantities exchanged. These are reflected in Figure 3 as Po and Qo respectively. Price and quantity exchanged change in response to changes in demand, supply, or both. These, in turn, change in response to changes in the nonprice determinants of demand and supply discussed earlier.

Admittedly, such a conceptualization is very abstract and artificial. No attempt has been made to define a unit of health services or to distinguish between types of services, even among broad categories such as therapeutic, preventive, and rehabilitative health care. No consideration has been made for alternative types of medical care organization, differences in quality of services, and so on. Obviously not all aspects, or even many, of existing health care delivery and consumption problems can be analyzed with such a simplified analytical framework. However, the simplicity of this way of characterizing health service activities has many strengths as well as these obvious weaknesses. It permits us to concentrate our thinking and analysis on considerations of enormous importance to public policy issues involving health care.

Figure 3
Market for Health Services

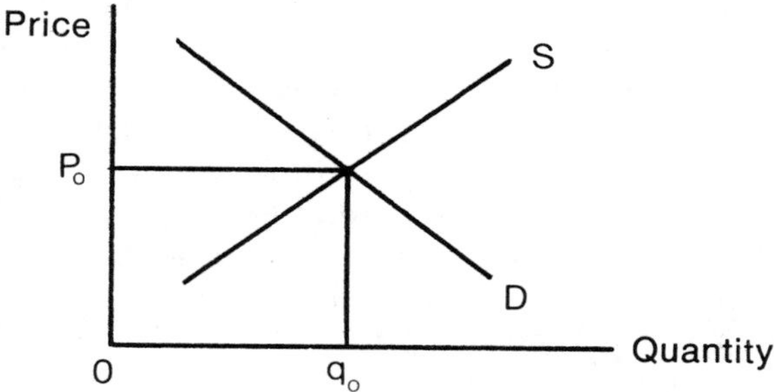

CHARACTERISTICS OF THE HEALTH SERVICES INDUSTRY

Frequently health professionals assert that "health is different" and, therefore, is immune from economic laws such as demand and supply. The implication is that economics has little to offer by way of assisting in the analysis of health delivery problems.

It is true that health services differ substantially from other commodities in the economy. However, these differences are differences in degree rather than in kind. As such, they in no way invalidate economic principles. However, the application of the latter must be modified to reflect the salient characteristics of health services as compared to those of other commodities. Several of these differences are discussed below.

Demand versus Need

Most would agree that consumers are more ignorant and uncertain in consuming health services than in consuming other goods and services. They are unaware of the quality of health services that they consume and are largely uninformed about the range of health care alternatives available for treating a given illness. Ethical standards adopted by the health professions preclude advertising. As a result, consumers are denied access to information concerning the comparative merits and costs of alternative procedures and care; however, admittedly, commercial advertising is not always a source of disinterested information. Also, health professionals are reluctant to discuss illness and therapy in nontechnical terms, thus keeping consumers ignorant of feasible alternatives. And, while in most cases individuals are free to choose their physician, physicians largely determine the kind, quality, and quantity of health services patients consume.

Physicians may be vaguely aware of an individual's economic circumstances, but there is little evidence that these considerations have significant influence over their prescribing patterns. As a result, therapeutic procedures tend to be heavily weighted by considerations of relative effectiveness, rather than by comparisons of potential marginal benefits relative to costs per unit of service. Even if a given therapy is twice as expensive as some alternative, it is likely to be prescribed even though its marginal effectiveness in improving health is only slightly greater than a lower cost alternative. Some have suggested that consumers often are prescribed Cadillac care when VW care would do and would cause less stress on their pocketbooks.

Consumers also often lack knowledge of their actual needs for health care. With the exception of obvious abnormalities such as pain, passing blood, and impaired function, consumers often do not recognize symptoms of illness or realize the consequences of failing to obtain early treatment of maladies that in later stages are extremely expensive to treat. While the incidence of illness can be predicted with fair accuracy for large groups of health consumers, illness for the individual is not nearly so predictable. Recovery from certain illnesses is almost as unpredictable as the incidence of the illness itself. Thus, the overall benefit of health services is highly uncertain from the point of view of consumers. Accordingly, demand for a sizable fraction of health services is based on judgments of health professionals who may or may not take into account the preferences of consumers and their financial capacities.

In summary, consumers are comparatively ignorant of standards of health, their own health status, and knowledge of what medical intervention can accomplish to improve their health status. Consumer wants for health services (needs as they perceive them) vary considerably from their needs as determined by health professionals. As a consequence, the quantities of health service consumers are likely to demand, even at zero prices, probably differs considerably from the quantities of health services that health professionals think consumers ought to consume to become as healthy as possible.

Given a difference between the maximum quantities of health services consumers want as reflected by demand at zero prices and needs as determined by health professionals, the discrepancy between the quantities of health services consumers demand at positive prices and quantities health professionals think that they need is undoubtedly even greater.

Supply

For the most part in other sectors of the economy, the supply of commodities is largely governed by the net return from producing them as compared to net returns derivable from the use of the same resources elsewhere. These net returns depend, in part, on the relative demands for goods and services. But the production of health services tends to be geared toward fulfilling needs rather than toward supply demand. A large segment of the industry, particularly voluntary hospitals, is, in principle, not profit motivated. Other health care units, including physicians and dentists, operate partially with an eleemosynary concern for supplying medical needs rather than for monetary demand. There is reason to believe that professional fees often are adjusted downward for consumers with lower than average incomes.

Capital does not flow freely into and out of the industry in response to market signals. Investment decisions are often made on estimates of need for new facilities (what health professionals feel is appropriate based on medical opinions) and not on economic grounds involving notions of the demand for services, profits, and efficiency. Charity, benevolence, and philanthropy underlie allocation of considerable resources in the health services industry. Many health facilities (not only coronary care units and facilities for open heart surgery) are overbuilt relative to expected utilization in order to obtain standby capacity sufficient to meet unpredictable emergencies. These facilities certainly provide a sense of security that contributes to the welfare of the community, but they are extremely expensive, and it is questionable whether or not members of a given community would pay for them if required to contribute directly to the costs of their acquisition and maintenance.

Many kinds of market imperfections exist in the health services industry. Monopolies over the education, certification, and licensing of health professionals have, as their objective, control over the quality of health services delivered. However, limited entry, licensing, and certification requirements serve to reduce the mobility of labor resources both within and among the producing units of the industry, causing prices of health services to increase to levels above those that would be expected to prevail in their absence.

Government Involvement

Another feature of health services is that often their benefits are comparatively indivisible. That is, once produced it is difficult and expensive to divide them into units and collect a price reflecting the value of each unit consumed. An example is medical research. Once knowledge is produced, it is largely available to all; it can be used over and over again; and its reproduction costs are trivial compared to costs of initial production. Similarly, many health programs provide improved sanitary conditions, pure water, fluoridated community water supplies, community hospitals (the entire community benefits from standby capacity), and so on. All these goods are public in nature, and many have appreciable externalities. For example, individuals benefit indirectly from the consumption of medical services on the part of others (such as immunization against communicable diseases or better health care resulting in higher national productivity).

Free enterprise market forces are not reliable for allocating resources used in producing public goods. In such cases, the sum of individual demands for units of service usually will fall short of the aggregate social benefit that these services yield. Collective action, possibly via governmental intervention, is necessary to achieve optimal outputs. Such action may take the form of subsidization, regulation, or nationalization of production. In fact, many medical services are subject to externalities in varying degree. As a result, the health services system is a mosaic of regulation and sponsorship activities by the health professions, by private industry, and by government.

The Role of Suppliers

Important economic decisions in the health services industry are usually made by the suppliers of health services. In the past, the answers to basic economic questions concerning how resources should be allocated have been supplied by health professionals. In cases where suppliers make all or most of the important decisions for consumers, technological imperatives, such as comparative effectiveness, tend to prevail over economic ones, such as comparisons of benefits relative to costs.

One way the health services industry differs from others is in its concern for maintaining the quality of health care and for otherwise protecting consumers. Many have suggested that health professionals view the health services industry as a quasi-public utility. Health professionals have assumed an enormous burden of public trust in attempting to decide what is best for the public in matters of health defense and health education. However, the burden of public trust, particularly when it involves decisions concerning the allocation of health services to consumers, makes health professionals who have little or no training in such matters distinctly uneasy.

Because of the genuine concern of health professionals for the plight of consumers who are randomly subjected to episodes of illness, the usual decision as to who should be permitted to consume the services has been that all should be permitted to consume the services that they need.

Herein, in large part, lies the basis for the familiar proposition that "health is a right, not a privilege." A similar posture is taken by professionals in other areas with respect to housing, education, defense, and, most recently, with respect to the right to legal counsel. By contrast, consider how ludicrous the public would regard a statement made by leaders of the auto industry (or those of some other industry producing similar goods) that "owning an automobile is a right, not a privilege."[3]

In summary, health is different in the sense that health services possess characteristics, each of which differs in degree from other commodities in the economy. However, many other commodities possess these same characteristics, but not all, education and defense services being but two examples. Such differences in no way render the analysis of health care problems immune from the laws of economics. Indeed, economics assists in sorting out certain differences implicit in the thinking of those advocating various public policy positions that are in conflict.

APPLICATION TO SELECTED PROBLEMS

The issues selected for investigation involve the general problem of determining the appropriate aggregate quantity of health services to produce. In analyzing this problem, care should be taken to distinguish between normative notions of desired levels of health care consumption from those notions that are economic in character.

Supply of Health Services

Elsewhere I have interpreted a given population's need for medical services as a normative professional judgment concerning the quantity of medical services that its members ought to consume

[3]The same point is made in Bowen and Jeffers, *Ibid.*, p. 10.

over some specified time period.[4] Clearly an accurate estimate of a population's health needs in this sense assumes that those making such an estimate have perfect knowledge of the health status of individual members of the population of concern, of what constitutes good health, and of what modern medicine can accomplish as the result of intervention. Obviously, perfect knowledge of these things does not exist; indeed, health professionals often violently disagree concerning such matters. Yet, every day health professionals make decisions concerning the health needs of individuals. In addition, health professionals who are members of various committees and commissions frequently make judgments as to the collective needs of people who are members of the population of states, regions, and nations.

It is important to recognize that assertions of needed quantities of health services consumption, be they based on professional judgments or on some other basis, are inherently normative in nature when they are not based on the preferences of consumers. As such they consist of value judgments as to what consumers ought to do in the interests of improving their welfare which are likely to differ from consumers' own perceptions as to what is best for them. I do not mean to imply there is anything wrong with being concerned with the best interests of others. However, I wish to stress that what consumers think is good for them likely differs from what others think is desirable. Such a distinction is extremely important to the problem of determining the quantities of health services to be produced and, as a consequence, has an enormous implication for optimal resource allocation throughout the economy in view of the magnitude of resources currently utilized in producing health services. The significance of these considerations is shown in Figure 4.

Figure 4 shows, hypothetically, aggregate demand on the part of consumers of health services (DD) interacting with the aggregate supply offered by suppliers of medical services (SS) so as to "clear the market" at a mutually satisfactory price and quantity of medical services exchanged equal to Po and OZ, respectively. If the market for health services were perfect, resources would be allocated optimally according to the collective tastes and preferences of consumers in all things, including health services; the distribution of income and wealth; the prices of other goods and services; the quantity and prices of resources available; and existing technology for combining them in production. Yet, even in the case of a perfect

[4]See James R. Jeffers, Mario F. Bognanno, and John C. Bartlett, "On the demand versus need for medical services and the concept of 'shortage.' " *American Journal of Public Health*, Vol. 61, No. 1 (January 1971), p. 46.

Figure 4
The Demand, Supply, and Need for Health Services

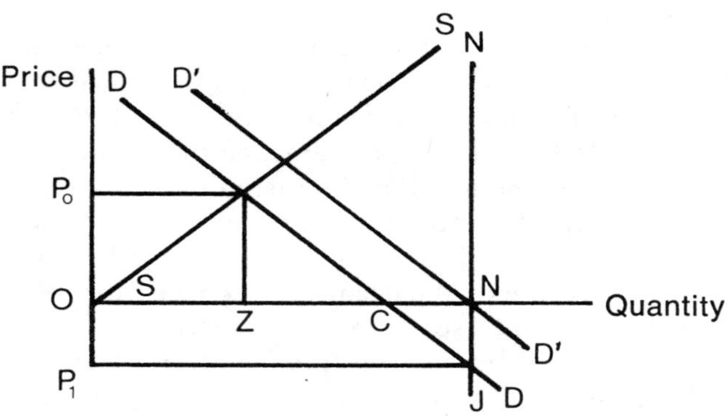

market, a shortage of health services may exist in the sense that consumption of health services falls short of what health professionals (or others) may feel is desirable. Figure 4 illustrates a shortage of this sort. The line NN represents the quantity of health services needed, in the sense that the quantity ON is the quantity of health services, independent of any economic considerations, which health professionals judge society ought to consume. Assuming that the market for health services is perfect, a declaration of the existence of a shortage equal to ON − OZ in the diagram is a normative value judgment and is not based on market criteria reflecting consumer preferences.[5]

Alternative Finance Schemes to Alleviate Shortages

Policies designed to increase the consumption of health services beyond current levels toward the quantity needed may be viewed

[5]However, in addition to the possibility of a normative shortage of the type just discussed, it is possible that a normative shortage exists in a different sense. The existence of perfect markets implies that resources are allocated optimally—that is, if every possible reallocation of goods among consumers results in the reduction of the satisfaction of at least one consumer and if every possible reallocation of inputs among firms results in the reduction of output of at least one firm. But there exists a particular optimum allocation of resources for every given distribution of income and wealth. While the diagram depicts the aggregate consumption of medical services, it does not reveal the distribution of the consumption of health services among consumers, which obviously depends on the distribution of income and wealth. Those with higher incomes and stocks, other things being equal, are no doubt consuming more health services than those not so well off. Thus, a normative shortage may exist according to notions of inequity in the distribution of the consumption of health services, stemming from inequalities in the distribution of income and wealth.

A reallocation of income and wealth very likely would result in a different optimum allocation of resources, and a consequent change in the distribution of the consumption of health services. The assertion that the existing distribution of income and wealth and consequent distribution of the consumption of health services as increasing demand, supply, or both. Such policies are being implemented at the present time. Current policies operating on the demand side of the market are too numerous to discuss in the space available; however, examples include Titles 18 (Medicare) and 19 (Medicaid), tax deductions for private health insurance, and proposals for compulsory national health insurance. Supply policies include a plethora of education assistance acts, facility construction subsidies, and special projects such as the establishment of neighborhood health centers. What are the consequences of these policies for the efficient use of limited resources?

Although it may not be obvious, almost all policies designed to increase the consumption of health services implicitly subsidize consumers of health services by drawing on resources that are currently being used to produce other goods and services, or which would have been used for that purpose in the future. Demand subsidies, such as Medicare, are rather explicit and therefore are obvious. Supply subsidies that increase the quantity of services supplied and, given the demand for them, result in lower prices to consumers, are more subtle, and thus are not so obvious. Yet, given a limited quantity of limited productive resources, any policy that results in an increase in the quantity of health services consumed implies that less resources are available for the production of other things.

In general, demand subsidies tend to result in higher market prices for all who consume health services not receiving the direct benefits of the subsidy, while supply subsidies tend to result in lower market prices for all those consuming health services. The fact that market prices tend to diminish or tend to rise less rapidly in the face of rising demand when supply is increased may explain why policies to increase supply in cases of a normative shortage are more popular than policies designed to increase demand. However, it must be emphasized that members of society lose the opportunity to consume other things when policies (demand, supply,

---

is inequitable is a value judgment implying that a normative shortage of the consumption of health services exists with respect to certain subpopulations of consumers. Thus, a normative shortage may exist in a distributional sense, as well as in the aggregate sense depicted in the diagram.

However, there is no doubt that the health services industry is far from perfect. The implication of all this is that demand and supply curves that actually prevail are something other than those corresponding to a perfect market and, consequently, resources are not even being allocated optimally, given the current distribution of income and wealth. Thus, the price and quantity of health services exchanged are not likely to be equilibrium values in the sense expressed in Figure 4. At any given price, it is likely that society is obtaining fewer health services than would be the case if the market were allocating resources efficiently.

or both) which are designed to increase the consumption of health services are implemented.

One point worth emphasizing in view of the prevailing apparent consensus that a greater quantity of health services ought to be consumed is that all members of society lose when too much of something is produced. This final point is illustrated in Figure 4.

Suppose that advocates of the notion that "health is a right, not a privilege" convince policy makers that health services ought to be produced in the quantities needed and sold at zero prices. This supply policy may be interpreted as making the supply curve for health services coincident with the needs line, NN, in Figure 4. Would people consume all the health services that they need? No, they would not, because at a zero price consumers would purchase a maximum quantity of health services equal to OC. Thus the quantity of resources committed to the health services industry necessary to produce a quantity of health services equal to ON − OC would remain idle, unless consumers were paid to consume medical services. That is, assuming no change in demand, only at a negative price of OP_1 would consumers be motivated to consume ON services as reflected by the intersection of the demand and needs curves at point J below the horizontal axis. To the extent that policy makers overestimate demand and it falls short of need at zero prices, society loses potential consumption through idle resources, the value of which, conceptually the real cost, is approximated by the area of the rectangle $ONJP_1$ in Figure 4. While the details of this may seem complex, the major thrust of it is that merely financing medical care will not necessarily mean meeting all health care needs.

SOME CONCLUDING COMMENTS

The concepts of demand, supply, the market, and industry are extremely useful tools for organizing analysis of resource allocation problems which underlie many health policy issues. Since health services are much different from those of other commodities, their production and distribution involves an expenditure of limited resources as in the case of any other commodity. Thus, economic principles and concepts are relevant and are essential to a fuller understanding of the consequences of most health policy issues.

REFERENCES

1. Arrow, K. J. Uncertainty and the welfare economics of medical care. *American Economic Review,* March 1963, 941-973.
2. Bailey, R. M. Philosophy, faith, facts, and fiction in the production of medical services. *Inquiry,* 1970, *VII,* 37-66.
3. Fein, R. *The doctor shortage: An economic diagnosis.* Washington, D. C.: The Brookings Institution, 1967.
4. Feldstein, M. S. *The rising cost of hospital care.* Washington, D. C.: Information Resources Press, 1971.
5. Feldstein, P. J. Research on the demand for health services. *Milbank Memorial Fund Quarterly,* 1966, *XLIV,* Part 2, 128-165.
6. Fuchs, V. R. The contribution of health services to the American economy. *Milbank Memorial Fund Quarterly,* 1966, *XLIV,* Part 2, 65-103.
7. Jeffers, J. R., Bognanno, M. F., and Bartlett, J. C. On the demand vs. need for medical services and the concept of "shortage." *American Journal of Public Health,* 1971, *61,* 46-63.
8. Klarman, H. Increase in the cost of physician and hospital services. *Inquiry,* 1970, *VII,* 22-36.
9. Pauly, M. V. Efficiency, incentives and reimbursement for health care. *Inquiry,* 1970, *VII,* 114–131.
10. Weisbrod, B. *Economics of public health.* Philadelphia: University of Pennsylvania Press, 1961.

8

Galloping Consumption: Consumer Participation in Health Programs

Rosalie A. Kane and Robert L. Kane

One of the more confusing contributions of the poverty programs that were begun in the 1960s has been their emphasis on consumer participation in the planning of public programs.* Health planners—some reluctantly and some with alacrity—have accepted the need for consumer involvement. The confusion has stemmed from the imprecise definitions of both *consumer* and *participation.*

Consumer participation in medical planning is a valuable principle and, as such, it is too important to be allowed to degenerate into a slogan which can be all things to all people, with precise meaning for none. Careful scrutiny of the concept demands an examination of the meaning of the term. What is consumer participation? Why is it useful in health planning? After definition and purpose have been considered, it is then possible to explore a host of secondary questions. Whom does consumer participation benefit? How should it be implemented? What are the potential problems? Should the goal and method of implementing consumer participation be identical across different programs and different population groups?

*A strong indictment of social programs and the consumers' misuse can be found in Daniel Moynihan's *Maximum feasible misunderstanding,* The Free Press, New York, 1969. Other accounts of the difficulties and misunderstandings involved in consumer affairs are compiled in the two-volume work, *Citizen participation in urban development* (NTL Institute for Applied Behavioral Science, Washington, D. C., 1968 and 1969), edited by Hans B. C. Spiegel.

WHAT DO WE MEAN BY "CONSUMER PARTICIPATION"?

Turning first to definition, one is confronted by a plethora of terms—consumer involvement, consumer representation, consumer participation—which are used almost interchangeably. The word *participate* is sufficiently vague to encompass a spectrum of involvement, ranging from attendance at meetings to the control of programs. The word *represent* implies a constituency to whom the representative refers. The various possibilities are discussed by Campbell who has outlined a hierarchy of levels at which consumers might be involved, ranging from the highest point of policy making through planning to the day-to-day operational level (1). Consumers may be given control or relegated to an advisory position, with no "clout" to implement advice. Some writers, such as Salber (2), have advocated a sharing of decision making by providers and consumers. In another, more pessimistic view, Jonas has predicted little possibility for consumers to occupy a genuine role in decision making on a local level whenever control of the health system rests in distant hands (3).

Meaningful consumer participation, however, must encompass some decision-making power. The consumers constitute the appropriate group to decide what the desired direction and outcome of services should be. On the other hand, technical plans and details should not be a consumer responsibility. A statement which gropes with defining the nature of the participation follows: Consumer participation is the process by which the recipients of care in a health program or community, through a representative mechanism, exercise some degree of authority in designating goals for health planning and share in the ongoing evaluation of the services designed to meet these goals.

The notion of *consumer* is also vague. A community does not have neat boundaries and arrows pointing to the appropriate health resources for given groups. Each geographic area, especially in the cities, is likely to contain a collection of overlapping communities, including the young and old, powerful and disadvantaged, white and black, established and transient, sick and well. The medical services available to these community groups reflect their haphazard and multiple origins by a confusion of eligibility standards, payment plans, and concentrations on specific disease entities. Given the diversity of the community and of its medical services, one who would define consumer participation is vexed by the question of who can best represent the sometimes amorphous community in question.

At the highest level of planning for national priorities in health delivery or environmental surveillance, everyone is a potential consumer. In an institution that serves a given geographical area (such as a state hospital for the mentally ill, a city hospital, a state medical school), one assumes that the interested consumers are narrowed to those within the designated region. Other programs are targeted for persons of certain incomes or with certain diseases, and the potential pool of consumers is thus delineated. But even in programs that serve a specified population the identification of consumers is not clear. Whom, for example, does a medical program for drug abuse or venereal disease serve? Certainly it serves the potential patient group but it is also designed to serve the needs of community members who are interested in suppression of the disease. The input of the primary consumers and the secondary consumers might be diametrically opposed when it comes to planning the nature of the program and its costs. Yet both are groups that should participate. Similarly, in a program for drug addiction, one set of concerned consumers would be the addicts who would want to insure that the treatment would be effective, not unpleasant, and not compromising to their legal status, while other consumers would include the residents of the area who might be more interested in the implications for crime control.

The medical profession has long recognized a dichotomy between the professional group and the laity. Community hospitals, for example, have always had lay representation on their boards. But the layman and the consumer are not always the same person. The consumer may be defined as an individual who is a direct or potential utilizer of services or who has a direct interest in a program. The meaningful group of consumers varies according to the purpose and power of the deliberating body. Within a nursing home, for example, the residents themselves may have a voice in day-to-day planning as they are the ones most involved. The institution, however, may have a board with consumer membership composed of potential users and other interested individuals; this board may well consider issues such as expansion of the facility or changes in direction of policy. At the level of regional health planning, the number of legitimately interested consumer groups proliferate and the size of the planning body can become unmanageable.

The issue of consumer selection is complicated when representation is required by law. Consumer representation was an inherent part of such federally funded activities as the Hill-Burton program, which supported the building of hospitals, and of the community mental health center movement. The Office of Economic

Opportunity's war on poverty went further by requiring a majority of consumers on boards. This principle was later adopted as a cardinal principle of the comprehensive health planning program which created the regional planning boards responsible for the coordination of all health activities in an area—preventive, environmental, and health services delivery.

With this change in policy the definition of consumer became critical. Even the distinction between professionals and the lay public sometimes became blurred as the consumer-dominated board became a more potent threat. Not infrequently such boards were filled with people generally thought of in association with providers—hospital executives, university faculty, voluntary health agency representatives, lawyers, and occasionally doctors' wives (4).

WHY SHOULD WE HAVE CONSUMER REPRESENTATION?

Anne Somers has stated that she sees no possibility of comprehensive health care for the individual without his understanding of and participation in the process (5). It can also be stated that there is no possibility of comprehensive health planning without the understanding and participation of the community.

Consumer participation responds to the real needs of both layman and professional in the medical system. From the planner's viewpoint, it offers a quicker and surer route to consumer acceptance of ultimate decisions. To health educators, consumer participation in the identification of a problem and the development of solutions implies that there will be a greater commitment to the solution, with less resistance to change (1), for participation in the problem-solving process is probably one of the best ways of understanding and accepting the necessity for change. For the citizen-consumer there is a need to feel that society's institutions are genuinely responsive to his requirements. In the health sphere, as in many others, participation can be an antidote to the sense of frustration and alienation so common in our rapidly changing communities. Like participants in participatory democracy in general, however, the health consumer is more likely to be conscious of his need to be involved when he feels alienated from the health system serving him.

Consumer participation also can fill needs which are peripheral to the business of health planning. For example, politicians may promote the involvement of consumers as a means of pacifying factions or putting key people into the picture. For some consumers, participation may represent a means to nonmedical ends, such as the development of a power base or a forum to express frustrations of a general nature. Moore has described the very conspicuous hostility and militancy among indigenous community health advisory groups (6). It is crucial that health planners remember the rationale for consumer participation as a response to mutual need, while remaining aware that the device can be subverted to respond to the tangential needs of both providers and consumers.

Consumer participation in health care has existed—in the form of hospital boards of trustees—even in prerevolutionary times (7). Such boards have traditionally been middle class institutions. Their generally harmonious functioning indicates that board members and hospital directors have understood the expectations of their roles and have not been threatened by the interaction. At first glance, the new demand for consumer involvement seems to be a lower class phenomenon. Middle class individuals, in general (with the transitory exception of students), rarely stand together to demand a greater voice in the institutions affecting them. They seem content with the belief that anonymous others are working in appropriate channels to draw attention to deficiencies for them. Especially in health planning, it has been difficult to involve middle class consumers in significant numbers (8).

The present impetus toward consumer participation, however, might more accurately be considered a have-not, rather than a lower class, phenomenon. The banding together may be prompted by individual insecurities and feelings of impotence, or by the conscious effort of the federal government to develop a sense of group identification among a segment of the population which is otherwise disorganized, apathetic, and voiceless. But some dissatisfaction with services is a necessary trigger to widespread concern about health in a given population.

Viewed in this way, agitation in ghetto or poverty neighborhoods for a voice in health planning can be seen as a logical response to services which are too expensive, inaccessible, or impersonal to meet the patients' needs. Middle class individuals have often become involved with planning around a specific disease entity, once personal or family experience has pointed up inadequacies in services. Women's liberation groups now are vociferously involved in a struggle to implement family planning and abortion services which meet their felt needs. Thousands of medically disadvantaged people who live in underprivileged urban neighborhoods feel victimized in all their experiences with health services. These groups can readily be mobilized and made to feel that consumer participation is important for them.

Because consumer representation serves legitimate purposes for both providers and recipients, it can be initiated either at the request of planners or at the demand of consumers. If planners are truly aware of the benefits of consumer input in devising a program that will best serve the felt needs of a community and for gaining its acceptance, they will not wait for the demands of citizen groups to set consumer participation in motion. A fearful, suspicious attitude towards consumers, or an oblivious disregard of their existence, or an elitist notion that consumers have nothing to add, are all mind sets which prevent providers from making the best use of consumer involvement. In Machiavellian terms, consumer participation is a tool which can be very skillfully wielded in the hands of the provider. Opposition can be disarmed and opponents brought together in an effort to solve mutual problems if providers carefully define their constituency and seek out their participation. Although such a policy may seem cynical, it is a realistic recognition of the important forces which make plans succeed or fail.

The consumers' role confusion is still more complex when one compares what he seeks to what others seek to make him. At a gross level, one need only contrast the consumer as policy formulator and decision maker with the figurehead role into which an inarticulate layman may be placed in an environment dominated by professionals speaking their own jargon. The voice of the community may thus be quite mute; or it may take on the militaristic overtones of a power broker demanding action with implied or overt threats and intimidation. This is no more consistent with the planner-partner collaborator role than is the silent, withdrawn figurehead. If the consumer representative is to fulfill his role, he must be supported by the other members of the board and encouraged to participate actively. Unfortunately, as Charlie Brown has observed, there is no greater burden than "a real potential."

WHAT IS A CONSUMER REPRESENTATIVE?

If consumer participation is to be useful for a particular program, some method of truly representing the target group must be developed. In many fields, there has been a continuous struggle to assure that representatives really represent their constituencies. Debates over methods of election or selection, appointment or self-appointment, have failed to resolve the issue. The poor's full-time struggle for survival has been reflected in their meager turnout for elections of consumer representatives (9). Often individuals present themselves as the representatives of a segment of the population, but the providers must establish the true criteria for this self-appointed representative. What confirmation is there for the size of his population base beyond his own claims, a show of forces, and veiled threats of intimidation or reprisal (10)?

Even when a representative's credentials clearly establish him as a genuine representative empowered to speak for a constituency, confusions of goal still exist. In reaching objectives for health services, planners need to tap the typical experiences of the consumers, not merely the experiences of a politicized or articulate elite. On the other hand, the qualities of leadership and the individual power base of the atypical consumer renders him an effective spokesman and advocate for health programs during their establishment phase. This is particularly true when the consumer group will need to place pressure on the centralized point of a hierarchical organization and appeal to congressional leaders for more funds.

A further problem remains: that is, how does one keep a representative representative after he serves for a time on a planning board? Prolonged association with providers may well render the consumer more like them and less like his constituency. Jargon, patterns of thought, sense of loyalty, perspective on problems may gradually realign and create a neoprovider. One only needs to look at labor union officials to note how closely they resemble managers and how little they seem to be of the laboring class.

As a way out of the dilemma of representation, a twofold relationship of consumers to health planning is necessary. First, there must be a method of achieving a broad base of typical consumers for the input of information and feelings necessary to plan objectives for and evaluate services. Serving on consumer boards are a group of representatives who are more politicized, more articulate, and by virtue of service on the boards, more sensitized to health care issues than the general public. As long as the board has continuous access to feedback from the larger community and some regular turnover of its membership, the specialized talents of its consumer-members should be an asset and not a threat to the purpose of the board.

ARE ALL CONSUMER GROUPS THE SAME?

Recent thrusts in federal health funding have been consistent—at least in their insistence upon some semblance of consumer participation. In some instances, we are urged to believe that a system of consumer representation that works in Harlem should also be applied in Appalachia or other rural areas. Yet clearly, there are important differences between rural and urban consumers, if not between urban consumers in various settings. Problems of sheer physical distance and travel present unique impediments in dealing with populations scattered over large areas. In such instances problems must be defined and dealt with at a local level, for even though total population density is low, the needs might be quite differently perceived in small clusters within the aggregate target.

Despite mass media, rural populations may be less well informed than are urban populations about the developments in health care and less willing to innovate and adapt to new systems of health care delivery. There would seem to be a totally different pace of life in which decisions are reached more slowly and communicated less directly. Cultural diversity, too, plays a part in the way consumers respond to health care; in groups which treat medical providers as impeccable authority figures, the model for consumer representation must be adapted to fit the cultural perceptions of the area.

Additionally, the history of decision making on other matters may play an important part in designing a model for how consumers should initially be involved in health care planning. In some urban ghettos, feelings of impotence have coalesced into a demand for representation, and perhaps control, in many spheres. Frustrations can lead quickly to violence. Rural dwellers may not express this same urgency to partake in planning, but may be content to leave decisions to elected or appointed officials. In fact, rural consumers must often be dragged unwillingly into the planning process. For health planners to expect an identical degree of consumer involvement in these contrasting examples could lead to either resentful noncooperation in the rural group or an unpleasant flare-up in the urban one.

The goal of consumer participation with all target groups is the same—the appropriate involvement of their representatives. Appropriate involvement suggests that the consumers have power over objectives and a share in evaluation. But the process of reaching this ideal mechanism will not always be the same.

WHAT ARE THE ADVANTAGES AND LIMITATIONS OF CONSUMERS?

Health planning and delivery has become such a technologically complex endeavor that many practitioners distrust the input of the consumer. They fear that, even with the best intentions and motivations, a consumer just could not have sufficient understanding to participate in decisions.

In this regard, the consumer of health services is somewhat like the novice at the art gallery who stares at the canvases and utters the much repeated cliché, "I don't know anything about art but I know what I like." The medical consumer may not know much about medical technology or computers or the complicated network of medical care delivery, but he probably knows what he likes. What a given community likes in medical care will differ according to the life style and culture of that group. Whatever the feeling of the consumer group about the quality of medical care available, these feelings must be treated as facts by planners who are challenged to design services which will be willingly and amicably utilized.

Consumer interest in medical care delivery is usually a response to dissatisfaction. Such discontent may be quickly focused on felt needs for more medical services. Attention centers on sins of omission, not commission; people tend to couch their initial demands in terms of more services rather than improved use of an old one. Consumers appointed to health boards, especially those most representative of the mythical average patient, will be vulnerable also to the quickly defined solution. When asked to enumerate a health problem, individuals often reply, "We need a new hospital," quite unconscious that they have really pointed up a solution instead. If meaningful dialogue is to be established, it must focus on problems and not become entrapped in a struggle over prematurely defined solutions.

One example is a small community in Kentucky which was about to lose its local hospital. The group turned to the regional medical school for assistance. State health planning officials were pessimistic about the potential for health developments in that area, claiming that the community was adamant in demanding a facility totally inappropriate to its small size. The medical school redefined the community's request for assistance by jointly exploring the kinds of health services the community wanted rather than discussing the feasibility of a single solution (the hospital). An appropriate pattern of service readily emerged as desirable to the consumers and feasible for the providers. The previous impasse had developed around conflicting definitions of *hospital* which to the patients had meant a facility to provide outpatient and emergency overnight accommodations plus an extended care facility. To health officials it had meant an inpatient facility devoted to acute care. When attention was directed away from a solution-oriented definition of the problem and onto a more specific delineation of the real problem, communication could take place. Then it became apparent that consumers knew what they needed but could not identify the precise techniques to meet their needs (11).

The object in reporting this incident is to illustrate that consumers and providers are not as far apart as it may first appear to both. Furthermore, the technological gap is not an important issue so long as consumers are not thrust into inappropriate tasks such as designing delivery systems. On the other hand, no amount of technical expertise can substitute for the consumer's expertise in the practical utility of a system for its users.

WHAT ARE THE POTENTIAL PROBLEMS IN CONSUMER REPRESENTATION?

A patient is expected to relate to the medical establishment in a dependent, trustful position during personal illness and as an informed critic when he serves as a representative of a policy-making group. Switching from patient to critic and back again calls for mental agility which may come at the expense of peace of mind. Medicine needs to be believed in to be maximally effective. This is as true of modern medicine as it was in the heyday of the general practitioner and the home visit. Experiments show that patients who feel confident about a procedure or regimen beforehand report the best alleviation of symptoms afterwards. It is not surprising that religion and medicine are closely linked in primitive cultures.

Medicine historically demanded confidence and cooperation from the patient and surrounded itself in a ritualism that inspired automatic belief. Providers sometimes fear that consumer participation in medical planning could shatter the patient's belief in the system. The mystique, however, is already cracking. The mass media have spread the word of advancing medical technology through newspaper facts and television fictions. Costs for modern medical miracles have soared to the point where officious money collectors or whole bureaucracies intervene between physician and patient. The time has probably passed for simple trust in mysterious medical functions. Patients must become informed consumers, and through knowledge gain confidence. This is especially true as new physicians' assistants and other kinds of personnel appear and begin to deal with patients. In place of trust built out of years of association and habit, the patient will need understanding and knowledge of how the new personnel can help him.

If the internal conflict between the role of consumer-patient and consumer-planner is largely illusory, a real conflict exists between providers and consumers when they serve together in health planning. Perhaps it is the providers who are most threatened by the need to adjust to the patient in two distinct roles. Professionals become alarmed at the thought that laymen are challenging their decision-making prerogatives. Hiding behind jargon and technical expertise, providers sometimes resist coming to terms with their own need to change (12). The physician, for instance, may need:

> . . . to be involved and challenged; to have his half-conscious needs for gratitude and subservience by his clients go unmet; to accept that clients have relevant skills, and that professionals are not the only (or primary) source of care (to recognize, for example, that most of the pediatric care in our society is given by sub-professionals called mothers, rather than by physicians); to have the Protestant ethic which often motivates him seemingly violated; and to surrender control (13).

The communications gap between providers and consumers may also be widened by the philosophy espoused by the experts. Richardson and Neuhauser distinguish two contradictory provider ideologies: assumption of public ignorance and assumption of public wisdom (14). Assumption of public wisdom not only belittles the usefulness of professionals' educations but also can lead to abrogation of professional responsibilities in the elucidation of a problem. On the other hand, assumption of public ignorance renders meaningful communication almost impossible. The provider must have some confidence that the public is capable of knowing its needs and of comprehending the possibilities and limitations of available technology upon adequate explanation.

A potential area of conflict or noncommunication between the provider and consumer group concerns the question of goal-setting. The providers can assume that the consumers are equally able to envisage long-term goals and lose sight of the need for immediate programs to meet immediately felt needs of the community. On the other hand, it is equally important that short-term goals not be the only ones realized, diverting attention and energy from long-term objectives.

A hazard lies in assuming either public ignorance or public wisdom, just as a hazard lies in assuming either professional wisdom or professional ignorance. An effective model must offer both the professional and the layman a distinctive role. Consumer participation should capitalize on the respective wisdom of each group and recognize that both consumer and provider have areas of ignorance which might be ameliorated by feedback from the other group.

RECOMMENDATIONS

With the above discussion in mind, it is now necessary to spell out the notion of consumer participation. Unlike technical advances, consumer participation is not a standard item to plug into health planning with a guarantee of better results. The present demand for consumer involvement reminds one of the enthusiasm for computers a few years ago. Belatedly, realization dawned—"garbage in, garbage out." The effectiveness of the computer depended on the input. Similarly, the effectiveness of consumer participation depends upon the establishment of a system which will permit the consumer to make a useful, informed, and appropriate contribution.

Ideally, a system of relationships must be developed which will maximize the potential contributions of both provider and consumer. In recognition of the strong tendency of consumers to define problems in terms of premature solutions, the model described here emphasizes process. It is an attempt to separate the roles of consumer and provider at various stages in the planning cycle.

For convenience in discussion, five steps may be distinguished, as shown in Figure 1.

1. *Identification of community health problems.* Consumers are in an ideal position to identify the problems and inadequacies in a delivery system which serves them. Emphasis should be placed on the types of services they feel they want and need. Consumers should describe how health services jibe with their life styles, for example, whether travel to health services takes them in or out of established and accustomed patterns. Opinions should be gathered over a broad population base with the recognition that feelings about health care are as important as facts. Providers, too, should have the opportunity to make their attitudes clear on the health care needs of the community. This information should be supplemented by relevant health data, including morbidity and mortality statistics, physical and personnel resources, and other pertinent information, such as trade and market patterns, and transportation and communication systems.

2. *Development of alternatives.* From the description of needs and resources, a series of alternative solutions or proposals should be generated by providers and outside experts. These models should include basic statements of benefits and costs and be described in terms of feasibility and potential impact, both positive and negative. At this stage, consumers should allow providers to

Figure 1

Steps in Collaborative Health Planning

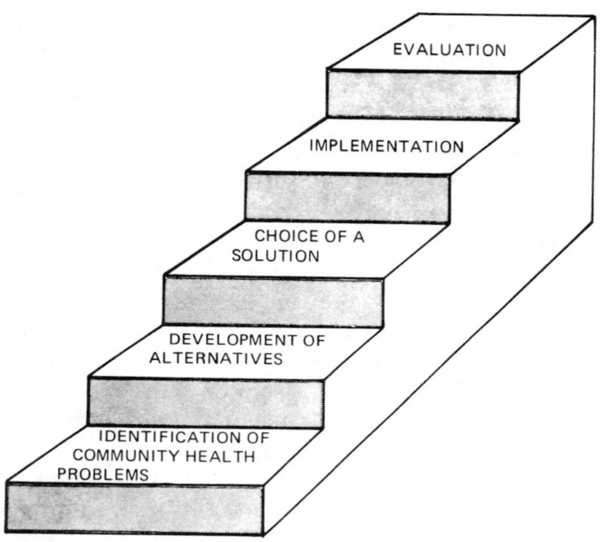

utilize technological expertise to provide the range of alternatives.

3. *Choice of a solution.* Together, the providers and consumers should then weigh the various costs and benefits of the alternative models and select the most appropriate proposal. It is also possible that the reviewers may reject all alternatives as inadequate and request additional models, or defer attack on that problem until better information is available. Given well-developed proposals, the consumers should exercise real power of selection or rejection.

4. *Implementation.* This task falls primarily to the providers who would be charged with the day-to-day administration of details. Opportunity for feedback from the consumers in terms of difficulties with the system in practice should be built in.

5. *Evaluation.* This step is best carried out by outside persons who can make use of both consumer and provider input to identify the overall effectiveness of the new approach in terms of impact on the population to be served. In addition, measurements should be made of consumer satisfaction, provider satisfaction, and financial solvency of the newly established program. This evaluatory material then becomes part of the data in the repetition of Step 1, Identification of community health problems, and a new cycle starts.

This model does not address itself to how much of the community should be involved at each stage. Clearly, decision making cannot be effectively achieved in mass meetings. Smaller groups of provider and consumer representatives must thrash out the details of the various alternative proposals. When the issue is important enough or arouses enough general concern, community choice through plebescite may be justified. In any event, a major sector of the community can and should be involved in the first step of problem identification and the final step of evaluation. Whether through probability sample surveys or community-based meetings, every attempt should be made to reach all sectors of the community to solicit their input.

Community surveys serve two important functions. Properly designed and appropriately administered to focus on problems, rather than solutions, they provide a rich source of data. But perhaps even more vitally, they offer a means of involving a substantial segment of the population. Carried out amidst adequate publicity about their purpose, they represent a means of reaching the nonvocal segment of the population which might otherwise be mutely carried along with the more vociferous elements. A necessary step in this involvement process is to report back to the community. The survey findings then represent the collective sum of individual opinions rather than the sway of a single powerful voice. While it may be argued that in many instances the data derived can be predicted, given adequate social and demographic information, involvement cannot be so readily duplicated.

Effecting such a model requires a catalyst. In those areas where health professional schools are not embroiled in political skirmishes with the community, they might fill this difficult role. Unobtrusively, the catalyst must identify and nurture potential leadership. It must help both consumers and providers to define problems and avoid premature solutions. It articulates unvoiced concerns and sustains relationships during the period of data gathering in spite of the inevitable testing and conflict. Yet as a catalyst, it must remain out of the equation, without ambitions of its own.

This five-step model of consumer participation is by no means simple to apply. At each stage, its implementation implies more trust than is presently enjoyed between provider and consumer groups. The consumers must trust that the providers present alternatives honestly. The providers must trust that the consumers are capable of judging these alternatives intelligently. The hope is that by identifying more distinct and appropriate roles for both consumer and provider, each group may drop some of its defensiveness and develop a trust in the other's good faith. Without this, there can be no joint problem solving.

REFERENCES

1. Campbell, J. Working relationships between providers and consumers in a neighborhood health center. *Amer. J. Pub. Hlth.*, 1971, *61*, 97-103.
2. Salber, E. J. Community participation in neighborhood health centers. *New England J. Med.*, 1970, *282*, 515-518.
3. Jonas, S. A theoretical approach to the question of "community control" of health services facilities. *Amer. J. Pub. Hlth.*, 1971, *61*, 916-921.
4. Lewis, C. E. The thermodynamics of regional planning. *Amer. J. Pub. Hlth.*, 1969, *59*, 773-777.
5. Somers, A. R. Comprehensive care and the consumer. *J. Med. Educ.*, 1970, *45*, 467-472.
6. Moore, M. L. The role of hostility and militancy in indigenous community health advisory groups. *Amer. J. Pub. Hlth.*, 1971, *61*, 922-930.
7. Notkin, H., and Notkin, M. S. Community participation in health services. *Med. Care Rev.*, 1970, *27*, 1178-1201.
8. Schwartz, J. L. *Medical plans and health care: Consumer participation in policy making.* Springfield, Illinois: Charles C Thomas, 1968.
9. Geiger, H. J. Community control—or community conflict. *Bull. Nat. Tuberc. and Resp. Dis. Assoc.*, 1969, *55*, 4-10.
10. Wolfe, T. *Radical chic and mau-mauing the flak-catchers.* New York: Farrar, Straus, 1970.
11. Kane, R. Determination of health care priorities and expectations among rural consumers. *Hlth. Serv. Res.*, 1969, *4*, 142-151.
12. Freidson, E. *Professional dominance: The social structure of medical care.* New York: Atherton Press, 1970.
13. Geiger, H. J. Of the poor, by the poor, or for the poor: The mental health implications of social control of poverty programs. *Psych. Res. Rep.*, 1967, *21*, 55-65.
14. Richardson, W. C., and Neuhauser, D. First question in health planning: Does the public know what it wants, or not? *Mod. Hosp.*, 1968, *110*, 115 passim.

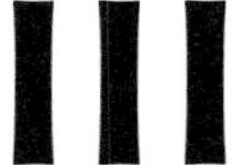

Evaluation of Health Care and Its Programs

Evaluation is an ever-present and increasingly important aspect of any community program. Accountability seems to have become the watchword of the day at both the individual and program level. Increasingly, the medical profession has been asked, if not required, to justify its actions, particularly its actions in regard to the expenditure of the growing amounts of this nation's gross national product being spent on medical care. As the government and private third-party payers become the purchasers of major segments of medical care, they want to know what they are buying. The kinds of questions raised by practitioners in the various disciplines represented in community medicine and the methodologies used to seek the answers have important implications for these evaluative efforts.

A focus on the population served provides a means of assessing the outcomes of medical care efforts. In Chapter 9, Brook summarizes the state of the art in quality of care assessment and indicates many areas in which further research is needed. Chapter 10 discusses program evaluation and moves the reader toward the larger perspective of collective responsibility for outcomes.

9

Critical Issues in the Assessment of Quality of Care

Robert H. Brook

One of the most important issues to be confronted in resolving what many believe to be a health crisis in this country is the complex problem of assessing and assuring the quality of medical care. Though quality assurance is central to current debate concerning future government programs and funding, techniques for measuring quality of care are still in their infancy. Most of the studies in this area have demonstrated that the American medical care system has many deficiencies in the care it provides.

It is the purpose of this paper to examine the relevant components of the quality of care issue especially as they pertain to the medical care received by enrollees of prepaid group practices. The specific objectives are: (a) to discuss problems with the definition and use of the words "quality of care," (b) to present the different methods of assessing quality of care and to illustrate their weaknesses and strengths, (c) to summarize the available literature concerning the quality of medical care received by people enrolled in prepaid group practices, and (d) to suggest possibilities for future research and development in this field.

This chapter is adapted from the original article by Brook, "Critical Issues in the Assessment of Quality of Care and Their Relationship to HMOs," which appeared in the *Journal of Medical Education*, Volume 48, No. 4, April 1973, Part 2. It is reproduced with the kind permission of the author and the journal.

The study reported here was supported in part by grants 5R01HS00110 and 5T01HS00112 from the National Center for Health Services Research and Development, by contract HEW-05-71-171 from the Department of Health, Education and Welfare and Georgetown University, and by the Carnegie Corporation and Commonwealth Fund.

DEFINITION AND USE

The phrase, quality of care, is vague and has acquired various emotional overlays. Some people use these words to be synonymous with quality of life. This means that ideals such as liberty, happiness, and individual autonomy become components of quality of care; consequently, any valid measurement of quality of care must take into account these different ideals. Others assume that almost any proxy measurement in the health field which shows improvement implies that quality of care has improved. They argue, for example, that if the number of doctors in a population previously underserved is increased or if a comprehensive health center is built, the quality of medical care improves since more services are provided.

This paper will take a middle position, which is based upon two concepts. The first, as stated by H. Blum (personal communication), concerns the relationship of health to the medical care system. He defines four major influences on health: (a) the medical care system, (b) genetics, (c) the environment, and (d) patient behavior. For the purposes of this paper, only measures of that component of health which can be altered by the medical care system will be considered as indicators of quality of care. Quality of care then, differs from quality of life.

The second concept is defined by Scheff (1) by means of the following two equations (which at first glance appear rather complicated):

$$E_T = P_S V_S^S + (1 - P_S)\, V_H^S$$
$$E_N = P_S V_S^H + (1 - P_S)\, V_H^H$$

In these equations, P equals probability, a superscript refers to the way the patient is treated, a subscript refers to his actual conditions, S signifies sick, H signifies health, V is equal to value or cost of (non) treatment, E_T is equal to the expected value of treatment, and E_N is equal to the expected value of nontreatment. Translated, these two equations read:

1. The expected value of treatment is equal to the probability that a patient is sick times the value of treating a sick patient as sick plus the probability that a patient is healthy times the cost of treating a healthy patient as sick.

2. The value of nontreatment is equal to the probability that a patient is sick times the cost of treating a sick patient as healthy plus the probability that the patient is healthy times the value of

treating a healthy patient as healthy. These two equations illustrate that, when a patient visits a physician, two of the four possible results are unlikely to be of any benefit to him and may indeed be harmful. (He may be healthy and be labeled sick or may be sick and treated as healthy.)

It has been virtually impossible to measure and assign weights to all four terms in the above equations; nevertheless, the usefulness of them is illustrated in the work of Bergman and Stamm (2) when they examined school children with cardiac disease in Seattle, Washington. The schools' medical records on all 20,500 junior high school students were reviewed. In 110 records a note was found indicating that the student had a heart condition. Ninety-three of these students were then examined by a member of the research team. Of the 93, only 18 still had evidence of heart disease; the other 75 were probably misdiagnosed. Of these 75 healthy children, with or without innocent heart murmurs, 30 were either psychologically or physically restricted. The authors concluded that the disability from cardiac nondisease (healthy person being treated as sick) was greater than the disability due to actual heart disease (sick person being treated as sick). It is also possible to conclude that the services which were established to diagnose heart disease in children in this community produced more harm than good.

This paper will analyze the quality of care issue in light of the above concepts of Blum and Scheff. Only that part of a patient's health for which the medical care system is responsible will be used as a final indicator for measuring quality of care. In arriving at a value judgment concerning the level of quality of care rendered, either some improvement in an individual's health must be demonstrated or a strong causal relationship based on epidemiological data must be shown to exist between the indicators used to measure quality of care and health. Finally, the implications of the four terms in Scheff's equations will be included in the analyses.

METHODS OF ASSESSMENT

Two fundamental questions which must be answered when comparing the validity and reliability of methods for assessing quality of care are: (a) what type of data should be collected upon which an assessment of quality of care can be based and (b) who should be responsible after examining this information for developing a value judgment as to whether quality of care is good or bad? The emphasis in this paper will be placed on the former question for two reasons: (a) most of the research in the quality assessment field is concerned with it and (b) this writer believes and will subsequently show (at least for one institution) that decisions based on the first question are far more likely to influence the results of the quality assessment than decisions based on the second question.

Types of Data

In order to analyze and classify different types of data for assessing quality of care, three different frameworks have been devised. Donabedian (3) suggests three different ways of assessing quality: (a) structure assessment, which includes input measurements, such as the number of health facilities available or the ratio of physicians to the population served; (b) process assessment, which includes the physician's technical and socio-economic management of health and illness as well as aspects of the patient-doctor relationship; and (c) outcome assessment, which includes what happens to the patient in terms of his symptom level, major activity level, whether he is still living, and how he functions in his community.

DeGeyndt (4) has extended Donabedian's system by dividing it into five different ways of assessing quality of care. The assessment of structure remains the same, but the assessment of process is divided into an assessment of content (which studies the physician-patient interaction with major emphasis on what the physician does for the patient) and an assessment of process which describes how the physician and the "whole patient" relate to and use other members of the health team in arriving at solutions to health problems. Donabedian's outcome assessment is divided into an assessment of outcome which examines the health status of the patient and into an assessment of impact which emphasizes the social and emotional well-being of the patient and how he functions in relationship to family and community responsibilities.

Roemer (5) has proposed his own six levels of assessment: Level 1—assessment of health status outcomes; Level 2—estimated quality of service; Level 3—the quantity of services provided; Level 4—attitudes of recipients; Level 5—resources made available; and Level 6—costs of the program. Level 1 corresponds to Donabedian's outcome assessment; Level 5 corresponds to structure assessment and the other levels combine to form the process assessment. Roemer considers one of the major advantages of his system to be its natural hierarchical arrangement. In general, it is preferable to assess the highest possible level (Level 1 rather than Level 3, etc.).

For the purposes of this paper, Donabedian's classification

scheme of structure, process, and outcome will be followed. It is a simpler scheme and, in general, the research undertaken in this field can be more readily classified by this terminology. It must be remembered, however, that usage of this categorization is arbitrary, and there are likely to be instances when what this writer designates as a structural measurement, for instance, would by others be considered a process measurement and what is considered a process measurement may by others be called an outcome measurement.

Deciding what types of data to collect is only the first step in assessing quality of care. The second, and equally important, step is the development of criteria to place value judgments on these data such as acceptable or unacceptable. Both the data collection and criteria problems vary with the method (structure, process, or outcome) used.

Structure Assessment

When one considers two variables such as structure and quality of care, between which exist many intervening variables, the first legitimate question is why attempt any assessment of quality of care based on structural information. The answer to this question is relatively straightforward. Structural information is relatively easy to collect and categorize. Items such as the specialty board certification status of physicians, the physical condition of the health facility, or the number of meetings attended by staff physicians can usually be assessed by use of simple, routine questionnaires. Since this information is largely objective, establishing criteria based on these data is a relatively simple task.

The problem of how to use this information in evaluating quality of care is quite different. The relationship of criteria based upon structural measurements to health and, therefore, to quality of care is largely unknown. Studies which have attempted to examine this relationship have usually found either unpredictable or weak correlations. Examination of the data from the major studies in this area may help illustrate this point.

In his classic study of North Carolina general practitioners, Peterson (6) examined many structural variables, such as place of medical training, number of journals received, number of hours spent in postgraduate training, place of practice, board certification, membership in the local medical society, and number of months in various residency training programs. He rated the quality of care provided by these practitioners independently through direct observational measurements and then attempted to correlate these variables. The only structural variable which he found to correlate substantially with the physician's observed practice habit was the number of months the physician had spent in an internal medicine training program.

Using virtually the same methods as Peterson, Clute (7) could not find any significant relationship between the observed quality of care and membership in the Canadian College of General Practice. In one of the studies in the 1950s sponsored by the American College of Physicians, Blankenhorn (8) could not find any significant relationship between the quality of care as judged either by a record review or by structural variables, such as: (a) the presence of a full time pathologist or radiologist on the hospital staff, (b) autopsy percentage, (c) number of scientific meetings held by the staff during the past year, and (d) the percentage of members of the staff who were certified by their respective boards. Morehead (9), in examining the care received by a sample of the teamsters' population in New York City, correlated an assessment of quality of care based on a chart review with structural variables such as board certification and the type of hospital in which the physician practiced. In general, she found that the place in which the physician practices was far more important than whether he was board-certified or not. Patients admitted to university teaching hospitals and city hospitals received the best care.

Perhaps the most detailed study attempting to relate structural variables to physician performance has been conducted over the last 20 years by Price and Taylor (10,11). They have selected various samples of Utah physicians and have attempted to examine relationships between 80 independent variables, such as average number of society meetings attended annually, number of refresher courses taken during career, grade-point average in first two years of medical school, grade-point average in last two years of medical school, gross income from medical practice, and the confidential rating of the physician's performance as obtained from different professionals working with these physicians. Results indicated that the prediction of physician performance is extremely complex. No simple, concise series of factors were identified to explain physician performance. Variables such as performance in either premedical education or medical school were independent of performance as a physician. These studies emphasize the tremendous complexity of determining physician performance from structural data. It may be virtually impossible to predict physician behavior for different types of physicians by means of a statistical technique designed to handle a large number of structural variables. These authors demonstrate that this is unlike the situation in professional football where there is a very high correlation between the round in which the player is drafted and his later success as a professional football player.

These studies suggest at best an unpredictable relationship between structural variables and quality of care and, at worst, an unexpected relationship. The question can then be asked: why should structural data be collected? For use in the assessment of quality of care it can perhaps only be justified as a fraud control mechanism. For instance, if a given health facility is only open two hours per day, if the building is in disrepair, or if rodents are running around in the operating room, this information could be used to infer a low level of quality of care. Collected by an unannounced, ad hoc sampling technique, structural data may be relatively inexpensive and successful in controlling against overt fraud.

Process Assessment

The complexities of both data collection and criteria-setting are greatly increased when process data are used. Process data may be based upon subjective interpretations and, consequently, are more difficult to categorize than structural data; however, analysis of process data is one step closer to directly measuring changes in health. The distance between improving the process of medical care and improving the health of a person, however, is still large enough that the question of what is the relationship between an assessment of medical care process and health must be answered if process assessment is to be used as a measure of quality of care.

Before attempting to answer this question, it is important to describe the state of the art of process assessment and comment about its reliability and validity. Donabedian (12), perhaps the leading advocate of process assessment as a basis for evaluating quality of care, emphasizes the assessment of process for, apparently, three reasons: (a) many outcomes can be considered processes for further ultimate outcomes, (b) knowledge and agreement among experts concerning expected outcomes are not highly developed, and (c) assessment of process provides feedback concerning the performance of the system. An abbreviated version of Donabedian's outline of medical care processes which indicates the variety of processes which could be used to assess quality of care is contained in Exhibit 1. It is interesting to note that the usual process assessment reported in most studies is confined to components I-A-1, 2, and possibly 3, of this outline.

In order for the assessment of quality of care based on process data to be valid, it must meet certain standards: (a) the procedures for collecting the information must produce valid and reliable results; (b) the criteria which are established must also be valid and reliable; and (c) there must be a previously established positive relationship between a high score on the process assessment and health.

Most process assessments are based upon a review of the medical record to determine whether certain information is present or absent and, if present, normal or abnormal. Most of the information felt necessary in order to judge care, however, may not be recorded in a chart. For instance, a doctor may examine the eyegrounds and/or urine of a patient with high blood pressure and not record that information in the chart because the examination was negative. Another doctor may not do these procedures at all, and he, likewise, would have no information recorded in his patient's chart. If these two procedures, eye examination and urine examination, are required as indicators of good quality of care, should both of these doctors be judged as providing low quality of care? Certainly, a chart review would produce results indicative of low care for both. Some experts would state categorically that if results are not re-

EXHIBIT 1
Donabedian's Outline of Medical Care Process

I. Physician Behavior
   A. Technical Management of Health and Illness
      1. Adequacy of diagnosis
      2. Adequacy of therapy
      3. Parsimony or minimum redundancy in diagnostic and therapeutic procedures
      4. Full exploitation of medical technology
      5. Full exploitation of professional and functional differentiation
   B. Socio-Economic Management of Health and Illness
      1. Attention to social and environmental factors
      2. Use of larger social units as the units of care whenever appropriate
      3. Use of community resources on behalf of the patient
      4. Attention to broader community interests
   C. Psychological Management of Health and Illness
   D. Integrated Management of Health and Illness
   E. Continuity and Coordination in the Management of Health and Illness
II. Client-Provider Relationship
   A. Some formal attributes of the client-provider relationship
   B. Some attributes of the content of the client-provider relationship

corded, procedures should be considered not done, since the results cannot be recalled reliably for future use in treating the patient. Other experts may argue that the routine recording of negative information just to fulfill requirements of a quality assessment program is time-consuming and expensive.

The problems of process assessment based upon a routine medical record review can be illustrated with some data from various studies.

1. In studying the quality of care provided in the offices of internists, all members of the American Society of Internal Medicine, Kroeger found that only 67 percent of the physicians kept records which the physician-reviewers considered adequate on the basis of legibility and completeness for nonphysicians to review (13).

2. In assessing the quality of care provided for a group of patients with gastrointestinal illness in a university hospital, Brook found that only 25 percent of the records were available in the first week of the study; most of the rest were temporarily lost (14).

3. Brook also reported that in a public hospital only 20 percent of the results of the laboratory tests done for a group of ambulatory patients were recorded in the patient's chart (15).

4. Fitzpatrick et al., examining the appropriateness of length of stay for a group of patients hospitalized in Michigan, showed that their judgment varied in 10 percent of the cases, depending upon whether the information was derived from the medical record or from an interview with the physician taking care of the patient (16).

Perhaps the major implication of these data is that the routine use of detailed process data (especially those relating to the recording of negative physical findings and normal objective laboratory tests for assessing quality of care) may produce major artifactual relationships based on the amount of data recorded, which is unpredictable and varies from institution to institution and from physician to physician. One may only be examining the quality of the medical record and not the quality of the medical process.

There is a second major limitation in assessing quality of care by process measurement. Recalling Exhibit I, most of the comments made in the above paragraphs pertained to parts I-A-1, 2, and 3 of the outline. This is what Donabedian calls the technical management of health and illness. Why have sections IB and II been left out in this discussion? Although books have been written on the importance of this aspect of medical care process, a sound conceptual framework leading to a series of valid and reliable measurements which can be obtained routinely is lacking.

Once the data collection problems are overcome, the next level of problems involves setting and selecting criteria for assessing care. There are two different approaches to solving these problems. The first, or implicit approach, is to present to a physician or some other competent judge a medical chart or an abstract of a medical chart and ask him to rate the care received by the patient.

The second approach is to develop a list of explicit criteria and then to audit the chart to determine whether or not the criteria are fulfilled. An example of how these two methods differ in assessing quality of care for patients with high blood pressure is as follows: In the first method, a physician would be given the chart and told to use some reasonable standard for good care and determine whether this patient received adequate or inadequate medical care. In the second method a previously agreed upon set of criteria would be applied to the case. A nonprofessional could audit the chart for whether or not the patient had a repeat blood pressure reading, a cardiogram, a chest x-ray, and/or had blood pressure medications prescribed. A scoring system based upon a series of relative weights would then be constructed. Each case would receive a score reflecting the adequacy of the medical care process. The trade-offs between the two systems are that the criteria approach will tend to be more rigid and reliable and can be done by non-physicians, but the chart review approach is less rigid, possibly more valid, and less reliable and would require personnel with better qualifications to perform it.

The principal exponents of the explicit criteria approach have been Payne and his group in Michigan (17). They have developed, using a nonrandomly selected sample of physicians both in Michigan and Hawaii, lists of criteria, mostly for inpatient care, for over 75 conditions. These criteria are somewhat weighted towards justification for admission and appropriateness of length of stay. Brook (15) has also developed a list of criteria for hypertension, urinary tract infections, and an ulcerated lesion in the somach or duodenum, using two different groups of physicians from the Baltimore area. These criteria lists emphasize follow-up care and therapy for the ambulatory component of these diseases. Barnoon* is developing explicit criteria for hypertension, diabetes, urinary tract infections, and the routine adult physical examination by using a sample of physicians in a few selected states who belong to the American Society of Internal Medicine. Richardson (18), working with the New York state government, has also been developing

*Barnoon, S. Medical Care Appraisal and Quality Assurance in the Office Practice of Internal Medicine. Progress Report III. San Francisco, American Society of Internal Medicine, 1971 (mimeographed).

explicit criteria mainly for biliary tract surgery, diarrhea in children under two years of age, and obstetrical complications. Other groups, such as the San Joaquin Foundation in San Joaquin, California, and the Hospital Utilization Project of Western Pennsylvania in Pittsburgh, are also using criteria lists to evaluate care.

Studies comparing the explicit criteria approach to the implicit approach in evaluating the process of medical care have been done by Richardson (not yet published), Taylor et al. (19), and Brook (15). In a series of studies on biliary tract surgery, DeRouville (20) and Richardson attempted first to judge quality of care using the implicit technique (no specific criteria supplied). In these studies, 394 cases were reviewed by a consultant over a six-month period. Four percent of the first 50 cases were judged to have received unsatisfactory quality care, while 40 percent of the last 50 cases received the same judgment ($p < 0.001$). This variation was attributed to the consultant's unintentional exposure during the review period to attempts to develop criteria for biliary tract surgery. Other studies using different judges have indicated that some judges lost interest in their job and changed their response pattern in order to accomplish the task more quickly. On the basis of this variability, Richardson has rejected the implicit approach in favor of a series of weighted, objective binary variables. An estimation of quality of care for patients undergoing biliary tract surgery can be obtained by checking the chart for the presence or absence of information on 26 indicators. A mathematical model utilizing regression techniques and these indicators as independent variables can produce a 0.9 correlation with a judgment of quality of care derived from an implicit process review by a consultant to the Bureau of Medical Review in the New York state government.

Payne and his group have conducted many studies using explicit criteria. The two major methodologic studies are reported here. In the first study (16), using a sample of Michigan general hospitals, the data obtained from the medical chart using explicit criteria were compared with data obtained from an interview with the physician caring for the patient. Data were collected regarding: (a) appropriateness of admission, (b) appropriateness of procedures done while hospitalized, and (c) appropriateness of length of stay. Roughly 87 percent of the cases were found to have been appropriately admitted, 68 percent had the appropriate number of procedures (30 percent did not have enough), and length of stay was appropriate for 75 percent of the cases, with 9 percent of the patients having overstays. In general, the agreement between the methods used was excellent, with differences being less than 10 percent.

The second study (19), performed at four Michigan general hospitals, compared the assessment of quality of care based on three different techniques: (a) review of the medical record alone; (b) review of the medical record in presence of the explicit criteria developed in the Payne's *Hospital Utilization Review Manual;* and (c) a combination of the medical record review, the criteria list, and a case abstract prepared by a nonprofessional. Cases of uterine fibromyoma, urinary tract infection, and heart disease were included in the study. Each of the 90 cases was reviewed three times by each of the three methods for a total of nine times. The following results were obtained:

1. Using majority opinion (at least five of the nine judges rating the care as adequate), 13 percent of the cases of uterine fibromyoma (four of 30), 17 percent of the cases with urinary tract infection (five of 30), and 70 percent of the heart disease cases (12 of 30) were judged adequate.
2. For only six of the 90 cases were all nine judges in agreement, indicating a striking lack of consensus.
3. For only two of the 90 cases did the method utilized for review significantly change the judgment of adequacy of care. This implies that when explicit criteria were made available as an aid to judging the medical record they were ignored by the physician judges and not used to increase the reliability or validity of their judgments. By examining the proportion of adequate responses among total responses, 58 percent of the cases judged by the medical record alone (157 of 270) and 48 percent judged by the medical record and criteria (130 of 270) were judged adequate.
4. Further analysis suggested that physicians were rating adequacy of care on the basis of minor variables instead of the major ones included in the explicit criteria lists.

Brook's recently completed methodologic study evaluating the quality of care received at a city hospital by 296 patients with either a urinary tract infection, hypertension, or an ulcerated lesion in the stomach or duodenum compared four different methods of assessing quality of care using two different groups of physicians. Only the results of the evaluation of the medical care process will be discussed in this section of the paper.

Adequacy of process was assessed in two different ways. First, a detailed case abstract was presented to the reviewing physician with instructions to rate the adequacy of the medical care process using the following general definition: for medical care process to be rated adequate, interventions or investigations likely to be important in altering the patient outcome must be included, while those likely to be harmful without substantially altering the patient outcome must be excluded. Each case was read independently by three different judges. There were 296 total cases and each judge read 88 or 89. At least two out of three judges rated process of care adequate for 69 (23.3 percent) of the 296 cases. For 66.8 percent of the cases the judges were in perfect agreement (all three rated the case adequate or all three inadequate). Significant variation was found among the different judges with one judge rating 39 (44 percent) of 88 cases as having adequate medical care process while another judge only rated 6 (6.7 percent) of the 89 cases as adequate. In order to test intra-physician variability, a sample of the same cases was reread after an elapsed time interval. A change in the process judgment occurred in 24 (15 percent) of the 160 cases reread. This percentage varied with whether or not there was perfect agreement among the three judges on the initial reading. Only eight (seven percent) of the 113 cases on which there was perfect agreement initially had an opinion changed on rereading, while 16 (34 percent) of 47 cases on which there was initial disagreement had an opinion changed on rereading by one of the initial three judges.

The second method of assessing the adequacy of the process in this study was the use of objective explicit criteria developed by two different teams of physicians, both chosen from a defined statistical sampling frame. One team, selected from the Johns Hopkins Hospital, consisted of a group of specialists for each condition studied, and the other team consisted of internists from the city hospital from which the cases were selected. Criteria for judging care were developed using the same definition of adequacy of care as stated above. Results from these methods showed that four of the 296 cases met all of the required criteria of the generalists, and six met all those of the specialists. There was no statistical difference in a judgment of care based upon the criteria of either team of physicians.

From this long discussion of medical care process assessment, several conclusions can be drawn:

1. Neither the implicit approach nor the explicit criteria approach for assessing quality of medical care process has sufficient validity or reliability to permit the accurate assessment of care provided to an individual patient. Either method, however, can be used in judging a large number of similar cases. For example, quality of the process of care can be rated with reasonable reliability by either method for 100 or more patients with a given disease. This may mean that it is impossible to rate a single physician but possible to judge groups of physicians.

2. Results from an evaluation based on explicit criteria are likely

to differ significantly from results of one based on the implicit chart review approach.

3. An extremely tentative examination of criteria lists developed by physicians in different areas of the country suggests that, when they are applied to actual cases, little difference in the assessment will be found. Results of Brook's study (15) show no significant differences between a criteria list developed independently by a group of general internists and by a group of internists who are specialists in the conditions under study. Barnoon's study also has tentative results suggesting no significant differences in criteria lists developed by groups of internists in Washington or Colorado. A national set of criteria lists may then be feasible; however, the acceptability of such a list to practicing physicians is unknown and difficult to predict.

Consideration of the problems intrinsic to assessing the process of medical care does not answer the question raised initially in this section: what is the relationship of medical care process to the health of a patient? If one's desire is to regulate or educate physicians on the basis of assessment of the medical care process, then certainly a strong causal relationship between medical care process and patient outcome must have been demonstrated, hopefully by well-documented, experimentally controlled clinical trials. Summarizing the entire literature on the efficacy of the process of medical care is beyond the scope of this paper; however, some examples may help to illustrate the major gaps which exist in this area.

In terms of medical problems which physicians feel are important (importance was defined as the frequency of a condition times the ability of medical care either to prevent or to treat mental or physical disability), especially in an urban population, conditions such as hypertension, obesity, malnutrition, alcoholism, trauma (especially from industrial and automobile accidents), unwanted pregnancies, and mental illness predominate. For all of these conditions except hypertension, it would be extremely difficult to arrive at standards for efficacious care based on any data from the literature. If one examines hypertension, the medical condition for which the best controlled clinical studies were done, slightly less discouraging results are obtained. The two controlled studies (21,22) which show that blood pressure control is advantageous for the subsequent reduction in morbidity were done on male, middle-aged veterans. Only those veterans whose diastolic blood pressures after hospitalization for a few days were greater than 104 (relatively high) were included in the study population. The tendency is to generalize this study to the entire United States population and to patients with less severe levels of hypertension. It is difficult to know whether or not this is justifiable. Over a long time period different levels of blood pressure severity may have different effects. Drug therapy designed to reduce the risk of a stroke 20 to 30 years in the future may result for some hypertensive patients in immediate chemical changes in the blood which may lead to a heart attack at an earlier date. In terms of biological response to high blood pressure, women and men behave differently, as do blacks and whites. Even after two excellent experimental studies have been done, it is still unknown what is an adequate medical care process for many hypertensive patients.

Examination of data for five other conditions (ulcerated lesion in the stomach or duodenum, urinary tract infections, diabetes, cancer of the cervix, and cancer of the breast) produces similar discouraging results. Considerable information is known about the various components of these diseases, but it is doubtful that enough is known to accept detailed process criteria as a mechanism to judge adequacy of medical care. For an ulcerated lesion in the stomach or duodenum, valid questions remain: Do antacids promote healing? Is any good done by operating on patients with cancer of the stomach? Do diet and/or drugs promote healing of the ulcer? Or is the attitude and warmth of the physician the most important component in managing these patients? For urinary tract infections, questions to be answered are: Is it necessary to repeat a urine culture after a defined period of time to determine if the patient is still infected? Is this likely to alter the patient's health? For diabetes the major question is whether or not mild diabetes should be controlled with oral drugs that reduce the level of the blood sugar. After a costly 10-year study (23) which was designed in part to answer that question and which demonstrated greater morbidity in patients on these drugs than in those on the placebo, major changes in physician behavior have not occurred. Depending upon one's bias, this may be viewed as due either to errors in the design of the study, which implies that the conclusions are unwarranted, or an unwillingness of physicians to change their behavior and stop prescribing these drugs. Questions also remain for patients with cancer of the cervix: Has the reduction in the death rate from cervical cancer been due to the Pap smear and subsequent therapy or to changes in habits such as sexual behavior? How often is it necessary to repeat a Pap smear? The major question for cancer of the breast, still unanswered after 50 years of controversy, is whether a radical mastectomy or a simple mastectomy is the procedure of choice for removal of the cancer. This question is not a trivial one because some patients following radical mastectomy have life-long swelling of their arm which produces disability due to limitation of arm movement. If there is no difference in survival rates between these two procedures, then radical mastectomy must be considered a mutilating procedure. Finally, for the common conditions such as headache, fatigue, and weakness with which patients present to doctors in primary practice, no reasonable process criteria have been developed. The important component of physician care in handling these patients may be a feeling gained by clinical experience in deciding whether simply to reassure the patient or to do an extensive diagnostic evaluation. There is little doubt that this feeling can be defined; but, when defined, it is doubtful that it can be objectively measured from examination of a patient's chart.

In considering the use of process judgment in assessing quality of care, one would like to point to studies which have judged process as, for instance, adequate or inadequate and have shown that there is a high correlation between this process judgment and the patient's functional capacity in terms of symptoms, major activity level, or an abnormal physiological measurement after a defined period of time. The judgment of medical care process would then serve as a tool for identifying patients with an increased likelihood of having preventable impairment.

A literature review attempting to find such correlations produces disappointing results. Fessel (24) developed a scale for judging the quality of care received by patients with appendicitis or heart attacks by means of a record review. He applied this method at three different hospitals and found no correlation between this process judgment and the impairment present at follow-up. Brook and Stevenson (14,25) found no correlation between the process judgment of patients presenting to two different emergency rooms with subacute or chronic gastrointestinal complaints and their symptoms and/or activity level at follow-up. In another study, Brook (15) found only a mild correlation between judgment of medical care process (even though the judges were specifically asked to judge the process of care only on the basis of those processes likely to alter the impairment level of the patient at follow-up) and impairment produced by either hypertension or urinary tract infections and found no correlation between process judgment and impairment produced by ulcer disease. The mild postive correlations found were between blood pressure control at follow-up and process judgment and between the presence of a positive urine culture at follow-up and the process judgment. For other important parameters of impairment, such as symptom level and how well a patient was performing his major activity or job, there was either no significant correlation or even an occasional negative one. The explanation for these phenomena seems to be the severity with which the process of medical care was judged. The judges' rating of the process of care seems largely to be based on components of the medical care process for which there has been no available evidence to suggest that inclusion of these procedures would alter impairment levels. Their judgments were thus based on conventional wisdom which may be inaccurate; their severe judgments eliminated the expected relationship between process judgment and follow-up impairment.

The assessment of quality of care based on process data must be dependent on physician judgment in terms of either establishing a list of process criteria, reading the medical record, or reading a case abstract. In terms of the studies noted above, this judgment is likely to include many tests and procedures whose benefit in preventing future impairment is questionable. The end product of a system assessing process is likely to be higher medical care costs without major improvement in the health of the population.

Many more studies on how physicians arrive at judgments are necessary if this opinion is to be verified. An analogy, however, can be drawn from the biomedical literature. Many procedures are accepted ethically and morally as indicators of good practice. For instance, hypertensive patients should have a standardized evaluation, a Pap smear should be done every year even on women unlikely to develop cancer of the cervix, and a radical mastectomy is better than a simple mastectomy. Once a medical procedure has passed into this stage of conventional wisdom without being experimentally tested, it is difficult and at times ethically and morally impossible to test whether or not such a procedure is efficacious. Perhaps because of this sequence of events, much of the medical care which is delivered today is not efficacious but merely costly. It would be regrettable if the outcome of a movement desiring to measure and improve quality of care would accelerate this process.

Outcome Information—Based Assessment

Just as Donabedian is the leading advocate for assessing quality of care from medical care process, Williamson et al. (26,27) are the primary proponents of measuring quality of care on the basis of outcome data alone. They have defined their method as follows: The first step is the identification of the high priority health problems in a defined population using judgments obtained from local experts. This team is asked to list in descending order of importance 10 to 15 conditions for which the frequency of disease times the preventable impairment not being prevented by the medical care system is maximal. The second step is to have a different team of experts estimate for groups of patients with an important condition various impairment levels that would result after a defined period of time. These estimations are made after the patients have been divided into homogeneous clusters based upon prognostic characteristics. The impairment levels are then estimated given the possibility of no therapy, present therapy, or adequate therapy. Possible impairments to be estimated for high blood pressure, for example, are: (a) the percentage of patients who would have died by the end of one year; (b) the percentage of patients whose blood pressure is not below 140/90 a year after initially being seen; and (c) the percentage of patients who have lost their jobs or who are unable to perform their major activity. In the third step the physician teams place a value judgment on their estimations by establishing criteria for the maximum acceptable outcome impairment. Step four involves the collection of outcome data; if observed impairment exceeds the maximum acceptable outcome impairment level, medical care process is examined to determine how to improve care. Subsequent steps involve the repetition of this cycle.

In addition to sharing some of the problems inherent in using process data to evaluate care, using outcome data presents other problems.

1. The success of this method depends upon knowledge of the natural history of the illness. Such information, if known, is usually reported in terms of death; information concerning other outcome parameters such as symptoms or activity level measured after a defined follow-up period is generally unavailable.

2. Physicians have not been trained to think in terms of group prognostic terms, that is, given a group of black, male, elderly hypertensives with an average blood pressure of 220/130, to predict the percentage of patients who will die after one year if the patients receive no therapy. The ability to think in these terms, however, is crucial to Williamson's method.

3. Outcome data are not recorded routinely in a patient's chart; this information must usually be obtained from a patient interview.

4. When nonphysiologic outcome parameters are measured, such as symptom level or activity level, at least two major method's questions are encountered: the way symptoms affect a patient's life style depends upon social and economic factors as well as purely medical ones. For instance, the level of impairment resulting from

an amputated arm in terms of loss of work will differ between a group of businessmen and a group of carpenters. The expression of symptoms varies with ethnic origin and other factors; this also makes comparison of data difficult.

5. Evaluation cannot depend upon long-term outcome measurements, such as death from hypertensive disease, but instead must depend upon less certain, short-term outcomes such as blood pressure control. This is self-evident because by the time one has finished collecting the long-term outcome data, the institution one is evaluating is likely either to have disappeared or to have changed remarkably and the purpose of the evaluation is no longer apparent.

Williamson et al. have reported studies in which estimations of certain impairment measures fall within 10 to 20 percent of the known values. Brook attempted to apply this method by using it to estimate quality of care. Patients with either hypertension, urinary tract infection, or an ulcerated lesion of the stomach or duodenum were divided into prognostic groups, and estimations were obtained for several outcome parameters (symptom level, major activity level, death, appropriate blood pressure control, or presence of a positive urine culture). In general, estimates for the nonphysiologic outcome parameters were significantly different from those actually observed. Estimates of the more specific measurements (blood pressure control and positive urine culture at follow-up) were significantly different from the results obtained from the other methods, both process and outcome, used to assess medical care quality.

A judgment of the quality of care based on outcome data can be obtained in an entirely different way. Outcome parameters can be measured after a defined time interval and individual cases examined to determine whether outcome could or could not have been improved. If this method (case-by-case outcome) is chosen, both outcome and process data must be collected simultaneously. It makes no sense, for instance, to state that after a year had elapsed a patient with hypertension had died of a stroke and to ask the physician to judge whether or not this outcome could have been avoided. If, however, the additional information is given that this patient's high blood pressure was not being treated and he had not received any care in the follow-up period, the physician could probably state that the outcome obtained by this patient could have been improved if the medical care process were better. Using this method in the same study as previously reported, Brook found that for 109 (36.8 percent) of the 296 cases, outcome was judged improvable by at least two of the three judges reading the case. The three judges were in perfect agreement for 211 of the 296 cases (71.3 percent). This agreement is slightly but not significantly better than that obtained for the process judgment. Intra-physician variability was similar to the variability reported for the process judgment.

The value obtained from assessing quality of care varies with the method chosen to measure it. It is this investigator's opinion that the "true value" lies somewhere between the value obtained from the implicit process method (23 percent acceptable) and the case-by-case outcome method (63 percent acceptable). The first method tends to underestimate quality of care because physicians require more tests and procedures than are actually necessary to improve health. The second method overestimates quality because for almost every disease a proportion of patients will recover without medical care, but this does not necessarily mean that they should not have received any care.

PREPAID GROUP PRACTICE CARE

It can be concluded from the preceding discussion that little is known about quality of medical care in general, let alone about care received by enrollees of a prepaid group. A review of the annotated bibliographies on the subject of quality of care revealed that nearly every study published demonstrates large deficiencies in the quality of care generally provided Americans. For instance: (a) in examining a group of new patients in a general medical clinic using specific criteria, Huntley (28) found that only 15 percent of required routine laboratory tests were performed and 39 percent of the abnormal laboratory tests were not followed up; (b) Brook found that, of 296 consecutive patients presenting to a city hospital with either hypertension, urinary tract infection, or ulcerated lesion of the stomach or duodenum, only 27.1 percent had a level of quality of care judged acceptable by the staff at the institution; (c) a study of the quality of care provided by various groups of the Health Insurance Plan of New York demonstrated that care provided by five of the 26 groups fell into the lowest level indicating that inadequate histories and physicals were being performed (29); (d) a record review of selected cases at four different hospitals indicated that the care received by 50 percent of the cases in two teaching hospitals was judged fair or poor and 75 percent were so judged in the two nonteaching hospitals (30); and (e) in Peterson's classic study of care provided by general practitioners, 39 of the 88 physicians were placed in the lowest two categories on a scale of five which indicated, at best, mediocre care.

It is not only difficult but impossible to provide a direct answer to the question of whether or not people enrolled in prepaid group practices or variants of it receive better or worse care than that provided to the rest of the population. Information on this subject is meager, and much of it may not be in the public domain. Nevertheless, an attempt will be made to summarize the major studies that exist.

Perhaps the three best studies in the area were conducted at the Health Insurance Plan of New York (HIP). The first study compared the perinatal mortality and prematurity rates of HIP subscribers with those of patients treated by private physicians. Patients were matched for race, age of mother, and ethnic characteristics. HIP patients had significantly lower rates for prematurity and perinatal mortality than the controls in almost all comparison groups including poor blacks (31). Even though the perinatal mortality rate of blacks was lower in HIP, it was still higher than the rate for a matched population of white patients. This suggests that even though outcome was improved by an organizational change in medical care, further steps are necessary if equal perinatal mortality rates are to be achieved.

The second study was a comparison made of mortality patterns of two groups of patients on old age assistance. The first group used HIP and the second used the welfare medical care system. After the first year in which the mortality rate was the same in both groups, mortality became statistically lower in the HIP group (32).

The third study (33) examined mortality following discharge from a hospital for patients having suffered a heart attack. Members of the lower socio-economic classes tended to have a higher death rate.

These studies, performed in one type of prepaid group system, tend to indicate at first glance that the outcome of care can be favorably modified by organizational changes in the system of American medicine; however, major questions must be resolved if this statement is to be accepted at face value. Over 20 years ago Makover examined the quality of care provided by different physician groups in the HIP plan. He found a number of them extremely deficient. Questions as to what has happened in the intervening 20 years must be raised. Has a similar study been repeated? If so, why has the information in it not been made public? If another study has not been done, why not? Is a partial explanation of the poorer outcome of care received by patients in the lower socio-economic classes the result of a differential in quality of care being provided, or is it a result of social and/or economic variables beyond control of the medical care system?

In the book, *Welfare Medical Care* (34), which describes an experiment in organization of the welfare medical care system, a comparison was made of the care received by patients enrolled in a comprehensive medical clinic at Cornell and by a control group using traditional medical care services. The findings are generally mixed. No differences in perinatal mortality rates or overall mortality rates were observed. Some differences in problem solving for patients with urinary tract infection were described with the experimental group having the better results. In general, the quality of care provided by the comprehensive medical clinic was not appreciably different from that provided by traditional medical services.

One maternal and infant program at the New York Medical College has been examined using outcome data collected during the 10 months before initiation of the program and after one year of operation. Results indicated a 29 percent drop in prematurity and a 43 percent reduction in early infant mortality, which the article suggests are the result of better medical care (35). A more comprehensive study of maternal and infant projects conducted by Hebel et al. is in preparation. It is difficult to make definitive statements at this time, but perhaps it is fair to state that prematurity and perinatal mortality rates have dropped in the areas served by maternity and infant programs, but this has also occurred in the areas in which no program has been established. Except for perhaps a few rural counties, the data cannot support a cause-and-effect relationship between establishment of a maternal and infant program and reduction in perinatal mortality.

Evaluation of the quality of care in neighborhood health centers has been conducted largely by Morehead et al. (36) at the Health Evaluation Center at Albert Einstein College. A questionnaire for ascertaining selected items of medical care processes considered necessary for good medical care was developed. Charts were reviewed to determine whether these items were included. A second clinical audit was conducted by a clinical surveyor-physician who rated care as good, fair, or poor using broad guidelines, such as justification for diagnosis. Both audits were done from a record review. No data are available from the clinical audit. Major problems uncovered in the baseline audit were the lack of performance of routine hemoglobin and urinalysis in children and, in obstetrics, the failure to record sufficient information about the delivery period and method of contraception.

In further study by Morehead, the quality of care was assessed at 35 Office of Economic Opportunity (OEO) neighborhood health centers, 10 medical school affiliated hospital outpatient departments, 7 private group practices, 5 health department well-baby clinics, 6 maternal and infant care projects (M and I), and 4 children and youth projects (C and Y). A total of 3,040 records were reviewed and abstracted. Using the arbitrary standard of 100 for the overall average of care, the following results were obtained: (a) overall rating: OEO centers, 107; group practices, 103; (b) obstetrics rating: outpatient departments, 124; OEO center, 121; group practice, 122; M and I, 138; (c) pediatric rating: outpatient department, 83; OEO center, 90; group practice, 84; well-baby clinic, 93; C and Y, 133; and (d) medical rating: outpatient department, 94; OEO center, 112; group practice, 102. It should be emphasized that these measurements are based on short-term processes, on an audit system whose components and weighing values are not fully published, and on an unclear sampling system. Despite these limitations, these data are useful for preliminary comparisons between programs and tend to indicate that quality of care was not significantly better in an OEO health center than in a hospital outpatient department.

Another major federal program providing health care to the poor is the Children and Youth Program which is being studied by the Systems Development Project (37). Each C and Y program is required to submit a quarterly report to the national headquarters. From this report the following data are abstracted: (a) relative change in the most frequent episodic diagnostic conditions before and after initial health examination, (b) relative change in the frequency of diagnosis found at the initial health examination and at the recall examination, and (c) hospital days per registrant. Data were collected from about 20 centers during their first two years of operation. Results showed a decrease in episodic dental conditions, a 50 percent increase in the number of examinations ending with a well-child label, a decrease in children needing eye refraction, and a 47.5 percent decrease in hospital utilization.

A more detailed examination of one C and Y program produced less positive results (38). Records were audited to identify all patients with a hemoglobin lower than 10 grams percent (anemic). Patients were then interviewed at the end of the follow-up period and their charts reviewed to determine whether or not the cause of their anemia had been established and appropriate therapy begun. Results indicated that 45 percent of these patients did not have their low hemoglobin recognized. Twenty-two patients had therapy instituted but eight did not complete this therapy. At the end of the follow-up period, at least 26 of the 53 patients still had a hemoglobin below 10 grams percent.

In a recent study completed under the sponsorship of the Hawaii

Medical Association, Payne used his physician performance index (PPI) to measure the quality of the process of medical care provided by physicians in different organizational settings. Separate sample frames were designed to study the hospital and ambulatory components of medical care. For the hospital component of the study the average patient received a score of 72 percent of the weighted optional criteria indicative of good care. The physicians practicing in the prepaid practice setting had a PPI of 79 percent, while the value for physicians in multiple specialty group practices was 74 percent and for those in solo practice 69 percent. When these data are controlled for the care being rendered by the model specialist (the doctor who typically cares for the diagnosis studied), the differences between the organizational settings disappear. Thus, as Payne concludes, the value of the prepaid group setting appears to be to direct the patient with a specific diagnosis to the appropriate specialist. There is no evidence that the quality of care rendered by individual physicians is increased by practicing in the prepaid group setting. Furthermore, whatever differences there are among levels of practice in different settings, they appear insignificant when compared with the deviation of the level of practice from optimal behavior in all of the organizational settings.

The ambulatory component of the Payne study confirms the above findings. In this component, however, the average PPI value was much lower, 41 percent. The difference between the prepaid group setting and solo setting and multiple specialty group was 3.9 percent. These slight differences were both in the direction of the prepaid group setting but in both instances are of minor importance when compared with the overall inadequate level of care.

Finally, Donabedian (39) in his article summarizing what is known about the performance of prepaid group practice makes the following points: (a) about 10 percent of all subscribers to a prepaid group plan are dissatisfied with most aspects of the plan; (b) perhaps as many as 30 to 40 percent of subscribers in a few groups may not consider the plan doctor to be their family or regular doctor; and (c) unjustified surgery, especially appendectomy, hemorroidectomy, operations on the female genital tract, and tonsillectomy and adenoidectomy, is significantly lower in prepaid group practices.

In summary, there is no convincing body of evidence to suggest that care provided to enrollees of a prepaid group practice is, on the average, substantially better than that provided in other organizational settings. This may mean that: (a) the care provided is similar, (b) the proper instruments to measure quality of care have not been employed, or (c) the proper comparative studies have not been done. Part of the answer to the question of what the value of the health maintenance organization movement is to American society may lie in the solution of the above dilemma.

CONCLUSIONS

As the health maintenance organization movement in the United States matures, it must contend with a statement attributed to Colton in the 1820s: "We ought not to be over-anxious to encourage innovation in cases of doubtful improvement, for an old system must ever have two advantages over a new one: it is established, and it is understood" (40). If the major and only significant advantage of prepaid group practices over fee-for-service practices is to reduce hospital utilization for a few selected surgical conditions, then the question must be raised whether or not this is sufficient justification for such a dramatic change in the medical system. Certainly there are other perhaps better ways to control cost. However, if it can be shown that prepaid group practices provide better quality of care at reasonable costs which in turn lead to improved health status, then considerably more justification for the change exists.

If appropriate documentation of the quality of care is to occur, new and more appropriate methods for assessment of quality of care must be developed. This will almost certainly necessitate the inclusion of the many different professionals working at academic medical centers. Close cooperation between academicians and practitioners in health maintenance organizations could lead to objective studies which would eventually demonstrate the belief of many organizers of prepaid group practices that they indeed provide high quality medical care.

Much of the research at academic medical centers has been concerned with exotic diseases at the frontier of medical knowledge. As indicated previously, large gaps exist in our knowledge concerning the accurate diagnosis and treatment of common important medical conditions. Except for a few diseases, the knowledge of what procedures or therapies are effective for many common conditions is quite rudimentary. There are at least two current forces which should lead academic medical centers into major research endeavors which will attempt to relate a variety of health services variables of common conditions to outcome. The first is their desire to produce well-trained doctors. In an era of rapidly multiplying laboratory tests and procedures, how can a doctor be appropriately trained if the basic knowledge concerning the natural history of disease and the effectiveness of a variety of procedures and services is missing? How can appropriate textbooks of medicine be written in the absence of this knowledge? The second is the desire of government to control costs of medical care. It would be invaluable to the health of some people if cost containment were based upon knowledge concerning effectiveness of services as opposed to arbitrary standards. It almost appears that academic medical centers have a responsibility to society to gather such data and help reduce the chance of adoption of arbitrary standards.

If this is to occur, academic medical centers must begin to form better relationships with prepaid group practices. Studies of the above type cannot be performed on the select referral population existent in most academic medical centers. The facilitation of such studies seems at least partially dependent upon the ability of the academic medical center to be operationally tied to a geographically defined population which exists in many prepaid group practices.

This paper has attempted to present a frank and open discussion of the problems of quality assessment and their relationship to the health maintenance organization movement. At times it has indicated that serious gaps in knowledge exist in these fields. This fact could be used as a basis to justify total inaction, especially in academic medical centers. It is hoped that this will not be the outcome of this paper. Even though the perfect system for assessment and assurance of quality of care may not yet exist, innumerable simple efforts can be made to improve quality of care. If applied in a systematic manner, many are likely to be successful. Similarly the enormous discrepancy which exists between the quality of care rendered to hospitalized patients versus that given to ambulatory patients is obvious. Almost any effort to change this situation seems warranted. As these changes occur, it is hoped that academic medical centers, aware of their tradition of teaching and research, will carefully study these natural experiments in order to produce useful information to correctly direct further change.

REFERENCES

1. Scheff, T. J. Decision Rules, Types of Error, and Their Consequences in Medical Diagnosis. *Behav. Science, 8*:97-105, 1963.
2. Bergman, A. B., and Stamm, S. J. The Morbidity of Cardiac Nondisease in School Children. *N. Engl. J. Med. 276:* 1008-1013, 1967.
3. Donabedian, A. Evaluating the Quality of Medical Care. *Milbank Mem. Fund Quart., 44,* Part 2:166–206, 1966.
4. DeGeyndt, W. Five Approaches for Assessing the Quality of Care. *Hosp. Admin., 15:*21-42, 1970.
5. Roemer, M. I. Evaluation of Health Service Programs and Levels of Measurement. *HSMHA Health Rep., 86:*839-848, 1971.
6. Peterson, O. L., Andrews, L. P., Spain, R.S., et al. An Analytical Study of North Carolina General Practice 1953–1954. *J. Med. Educ., 31,* Part 2,1–165, 1956.
7. Clute, K. F. The Quality of General Practice. *The General Practitioner.* Toronto: University of Toronto Press, 1963, pp. 262–340.
8. Blankenhorn, M. A. Standards of Practice of Internal Medicine and Methods of Assessing the Quality of Practice in Hospitals. *Ann. Inter. Med., 47:*367-374, 1957.
9. Morehead, M. A., Donaldson, R. S., et al. *A Study of the Quality of Hospital Care Secured by a Sample of Teamster Family Members in New York City.* New York: Columbia University School of Public Health and Administrative Medicine, 1964.
10. Price, P. B., Taylor, C. W., Nelson, D. E., et al. *Measurement and Predictions of Physician Performance, Two Decades of Intermittently Sustained Research.* Salt Lake City: Lynn Loyd Reid Press, 1971.
11. Richards, J. M., Jr., Taylor, C. W., Price, P. B., et al. An Investigation of the Criterion Problem for One Group of Medical Specialists. *J. Applied Psych., 48:*79-90, 1965.
12. Donabedian, A. Promoting Quality Through Evaluating the Process of Patient Care. *Med. Care, 6:* 181-202, 1968.
13. Kroeger, H. H., Altman, I., Clark, D. A., et al. The Office Practice of Internists, 1. The Feasibility of Evaluating Quality of Care. *J.A.M.A., 193:*371-376, 1965.
14. Brook, R. H., Berg, M., and Schecter, P. Effectiveness of Non-Emergency Room Care Via Emergency Room: A Study of 116 Patients with Gastrointestinal Symptoms. *Ann. of Inter. Med., 78:* 333–339, 1973.
15. Brook, R. H. *Quality of Care Assessment: A Comparison of Five Methods of Peer Review.* Rockville, Maryland: National Center for Health Services Research and Development, 1973, DHEW Publication No. HRA-74-3100.
16. Fitzpatrick, T. B., Riedel, D. C., and Payne, B. C. Character and Effectiveness of Hospital Use, Project 2, Hospital and Medical Economics. McNerney, W. J. (ed.). Chicago: Chicago Hospital Research and Educational Trust, 1962, pp. 361-592.

17. Payne, B. C. *Hospital Utilization Review Manual*. Ann Arbor: University of Michigan Press, 1966.
18. Richardson, F. MacD. Peer Review of Medical Care. *Med. Care. 10:*29–39, 1972.
19. Taylor, F. C., Payne, B. C., Mann, F. C., et al. *The Use of Hospital Utilization Review Manual.* Criteria and Record Abstracts for Medical Record Review in a Hospital Committee Setting. Ann Arbor, Michigan: Center for Research on Utilization of Scientific Knowledge, Institute for Social Research, University of Michigan, 1970.
20. DeRouville, W. H. Peer Review in Biliary Tract Surgery. *N. Y. State J. Med., 71:*1544-1548, 1971
21. Veterans Administration Cooperative Study Group on Antihypertensive Agents. Effects of Treatment on Morbidity in Hypertension. *J.A.M.A., 202:*1028-1033, 1967.
22. Veterans Administration Cooperative Study Group on Antihypertensive Agents. Effects of Treatment on Morbidity in Hypertension: II. Results in Patients with Diastolic Blood Pressure Averaging 90 Through 114 mm Hg. *J.A.M.A., 213:* 1143-1152, 1970.
23. A Study of the Effects of Hypoglycemic Agents on Vascular Complications in Patients with Adult Onset Diabetes: II. Mortality Results. University Group Diabetes Program. *Diabetes, 19:* (Suppl. 2), 789-830, 1970.
24. Fessel, W. J., and Van Brunt, E. E. Quality of Care and Medical Record. *New Engl. J. Med., 283:*134-138, 1972.
25. Brook, R. H., and Stevenson, R. L. Effectiveness of Patient Care in an Emergency Room. *New Engl. J. Med., 283:*904-907, 1970.
26. Williamson, J. W., Alexander, M., and Miller, G. E. Continuing Education and Patient Care Research. *J.A.M.A., 201:*938-942, 1967.
27. Williamson, J. W., Alexander, M., and Miller, G. E. Priorities in Patient-Care Research and Continuing Medical Education. *J.A.M.A., 204:*303-308, 1968.
28. Huntley, R. R., Steinhauser, R., White, K. L., et al. The Quality of Medical Care: Techniques and Investigation in the Outpatient Clinic. *J. Chronic Dis., 14:*630-642, 1961.
29. Makover, H. B. The Quality of Medical Care. Methodology of Survey of the Medical Groups Associated with the Health Insurance Plan of New York. *Amer. J. Public Health, 41:*824-832, 1951.
30. Rosenfeld, L. S. Quality of Medical Care in Hospitals. *Amer. J. Public Health, 47:*856-865, 1957.
31. Shapiro, S., Weiner, L., and Densen, P. Comparison of Prematurity and Perinatal Mortality in a General Population and in a Population of a Prepaid Medical Care Plan. *Amer. J. Public Health, 48:*170-185, 1958.
32. Shapiro, S., Williams, J. J., Yerby, A. S., et al. Patterns of Medical Use by the Indigent Aged under Two Systems of Medical Care. *Amer. J. Public Health, 57:*784-790, 1967.
33. Shapiro, S. Social Factors in the Prognosis of Men Following First Myocardial Infarction. *Milbank Mem. Fund Quart., 48:*37-50, 1970.

34. Goodrich, C. H., Olendzki, M. C., and Reader, G. C. *Welfare Medical Care: An Experiment.* Cambridge: Harvard University Press, 1970.
35. Gold, E.M., Stone, M. L., and Rich, H. Total Maternal and Infant Care: An Evaluation. *Amer. J. Public Health, 59:*1851-1856, 1969.
36. Morehead, M. A., Donaldson, R. S., and Seravalli, M. R. Comparisons Between OEO Neighborhood Health Center and Other Health Care Providers of Ratings of the Quality of Health Care. *Amer. J. Public Health, 61:*1294-1306, 1971.
37. DeGeyndt, W. *Quality of Care: End Results Based on a Performance Reporting System.* Minneapolis: Systems Development Project, Minnesota Systems Research, Inc., 1971.
38. Starfield, B., and Schef, D. Effectiveness of Pediatric Care: The Relationship Between Processes and Outcome. *Pediatrics, 49:*547-552, 1972.
39. Donabedian, A. An Evaluation of Prepaid Group Practice. *Inquiry, 6:*3-27, 1969.
40. Colton, C. A Selected Public Health Bibliography with Annotations. Wylie, C. M. (ed.). *Amer. J. Public Health, 62:* 116, 1972.

10

Program Evaluation: Is It Worth It?

Robert L. Kane, Ruth Henson, and O. Lynn Deniston

From the perspective of community medicine, evaluation must extend beyond an examination of the patient care process to review the impact of a total program. Perhaps no other area is so burdened with confusion and misunderstanding. Political pressures, the need for continued funding, community concern, and individual ambitions combine to influence the conclusions reached as one attempts to evaluate a situation.

By definition evaluation is value laden. It requires a clarity of thought in planning that is difficult to achieve and more difficult to maintain during administration, particularly under the multiple stresses of normal operation. To be meaningful, evaluation must include the selection and measurement of certain choices and a rigorous application of these in terms of the underlying conception of the project (1). The necessity for differentiating between various approaches to evaluation is illustrated in this excerpt on mental health services (2).

> . . . Some mental health professionals argue that formal evaluation studies are inappropriate to the mental health field and that program decisions are better based on professional intuition than on such studies. We contend that, although program decisions must ultimately be based on judgment regardless of whether evaluation is conducted, good evaluation can provide information that can contribute to the decision making process.

Let us underline and expand this statement. Evaluative judgments are always made, whether consciously or subconsciously, objectively or subjectively, and with varying degrees of completeness. As this is so, a valuable component in any program will be the inclusion of plans for meaningful evaluation. The choice, therefore, is what to evaluate, when to evaluate, and how to evaluate—not whether to evaluate.

Before program evaluation can be seriously considered, however, agreement must be reached about what constitutes a program. The word is commonly used in many different ways. For our purposes, a *program* is any enterprise organized to eliminate or reduce one or more problems. This enterprise will have one or more objectives to be accomplished by the performance of one or more activities, which are supported by a detailed expenditure of resources (3). Any size enterprise or response could then constitute a program. Therefore, program evaluation should focus on the stated objectives (achievements, results, goals) in terms of their appropriateness, adequacy, effectiveness, efficiency, and side effects.

In pursuing clarity of thought in all stages of program design, it is mandatory to state standards in precise terms. Unfortunately, not only do evaluative standards vary in meaning among laymen, professionals also become confused by the clouds of ambiguity. Many words have too broad an application and take on a spectrum of value-laden meanings, not necessarily consistent from user to user. In view of this inherent difficulty in semantics, a few basic definitions are in order.

Appropriateness is directly related to value—the good-bad continuum. In considering appropriateness, the question at issue concerns the desirableness of the objectives. The answer naturally depends on who answers the question. Most people agree on certain values—peace is good, murder is bad—but considerable disagreement exists about other values: for example, U.S. involvement in Vietnam, registration of guns, keeping people biologically alive through heroic medical manipulations. The dimension of appropriateness may be viewed in several ways. First, is the proposed program intrinsically desirable or undesirable? More difficult to decide is the degree of desirability, or priority, of the program in relation to other programs. Even if an objective is desirable, it must be located on a scale of relative values with other possible objectives. Ambiguity, either in stating the objective(s) or determining its appropriateness, will severely handicap any subsequent attempt at evaluation.

Effectiveness and adequacy of the program are closely related. They should be separated more for psychological than logical reasons. *Adequacy* is concerned with the degree to which the whole problem has been prevented or eliminated. *Effectiveness* is a measure of the actual accomplishment of the program compared with the amount intended or planned which may be less than total eradication or prevention. Thus a program to reduce the incidence of lung cancer by 50 percent, which attained that level, would be 100 percent effective but only 50 percent adequate, since half of the problem still remained. Objectives should specify both what is to be attained (the valued condition) and the amount of proposed attainment. Many programs either propose the eradication of an existing disease problem or its reduction by an unspecified amount. Eradication is usually unrealistic—few people really expect it, and it is only rarely possible. Unqualified reduction is an inadequate goal because it provides neither a basis for planning nor a standard for comparison.

Efficiency is a measure of the cost in resources that is incurred in attaining the objectives. An accurate appraisal of effectiveness is therefore prerequisite to a consideration of efficiency, since one must first know what was attained before estimating the cost of that effect.

Thus, four criteria (appropriateness, adequacy, effectiveness, and efficiency) focus on the program objective. A frequently neglected aspect is the side effects. We can never be sure that only the goals intended will result. Side effects, either good or bad, nearly always occur. The thalidomide experience is one of the more familiar examples of undesirable side effects. The recent discovery of a highly selective and effective raticide made while testing cancer drugs is an example of a good side effect.

Five questions should be asked both before a program begins and after it is in operation. Asked early, the questions are guideposts in the planning process. When applied to a program in progress, they constitute an evaluation of performance. These questions focus on: 1) whether the program has in fact been directed toward important problems; 2) how much of the total problem has been controlled; 3) the extent to which the predetermined program objectives have been attained; 4) the actual costs of attaining objectives; and 5) the effects of the program other than those intended.

Others have found it useful to view evaluation in different terms. *Definitive* (an evaluation of results or outcomes) and *presumptive* (an evaluation of the process) are key terms in another approach (4). Definitive evaluation utilizes direct information about the condition of interest, usually a program objective or goal. To evaluate a food protection program, definitive evaluation would examine the food if the objective were stated in terms of food composition or contamination, or would study the people who consume it if the objective were stated in terms of incidence of food-borne illness.

Presumptive judgments are based on data concerning the resources and activities of a program rather than its objectives. Administrators often presume that if the budget is of a particular size, if the personnel involved possess certain credentials, and if certain activities are performed, the program will automatically have some degree of effectiveness.

Some criteria commonly used are objectivity, reliability, and validity. These apply in all evaluative approaches. In many cases, different conclusions are reached because of variations in the objectivity with which measures are applied. *Objectivity* refers to the precision with which the measurement procedures are specified. Stanley (4) has suggested the terms impressionistic and proven to describe two different evaluation methods; we believe they represent the ends of a continuum of objectivity. Measuring fever by placing a hand on the forehead tends toward the impressionistic, or subjective, end of the scale; when fever is measured by a certified thermometer, the proven, or objective, end is approached.

A related component is the *reliability*, or repeatability, of information. For example, to evaluate a program designed to achieve high quality water in a river, would a second measure of the water yield the same results as the first (assuming water quality had not changed)? The validity of the data must also be assured. *Validity* is the degree to which the data actually assess the nature of the phenomenon of interest. Our ability to ascertain validity depends upon the results of a comparison of the test measure to an established standard. The degree to which these independent measures correspond is the extent of the validity of the test measure. Thus the choice and precise identification of a standard is critical and may, in some instances, lead to great difficulties if the standard is ill chosen.

Other characteristics of measures include preciseness, completeness, and coverage. *Preciseness* means the extent to which a measurement technique discriminates between differences in magnitude. The ends of this continuum are crude or precise (e.g., an adult weight scale would not be precise in measuring weight increases in infants). *Completeness* implies the degree to which the entire problem is assessed. For example, air pollution is a complex condition made up of many contributing factors, a few of which are SO_2, hydrocarbons, particulate matter, and the nitrogen oxides. If all components were assessed, one would have a complete measure of air pollution; to the extent that only certain components, often termed indices, are measured, the appraisal is incomplete. *Coverage* defines the extent to which measures are applied to each instance of the phenomenon of interest. Are all, or only a representative sample, of air pollution sources analyzed in a given area? Problems with coverage usually center on making too few measures or on bias resulting from measuring a nonrepresentative sample.

Every program has one or more program objectives. These represent the desired result. Each objective implies one, or more, necessary conditions, termed sub-objectives, which must be accomplished in order that the program objective may be accomplished. Activities are performed to achieve each sub-objective and consequently the program objectives. Resources are expended to support the performance of activities. A sharp distinction is made between activities, which imply the performance of work, and objectives, which refer to the conditions of people or of the environment that are deemed desirable.[1] Every program plan, whether explicit or not, makes three assumptions: 1) that the expenditure of resources as planned will result in the performance of the planned activity; 2) that each activity, if properly performed, will result in the attainment of the sub-objective with which it is linked; and 3) that each sub-objective must necessarily be accomplished before the next one can be achieved and, if all sub-objectives are attained, the program objective will be attained.

OBJECTIVES

In evaluating program effectiveness, specific measures of accomplishment for each sub-objective and program objective are set up; data on each are collected systematically, using accepted principles of research design. In addition, data are collected on the degree to which each activity has been performed as planned and on the amount of resources used. The results are then used to strengthen subsequent program planning.

Considerable attention to program objectives is necessary because rarely are the objectives explicitly stated. Another hazard in program evaluation that often occurs when objectives have not been spelled out in detail prior to operation is a shift in emphasis with the passage of time. This may be due to an umbrella-like, all-encompassing objective; or the original objective may have

[1]For a more complete treatment of this distinction see Deniston, O. L., and Rosenstock, I. M. Evaluation health programs. *Public Health Reports*, 1970, *85*, 835-840; Deniston, O. L., Rosenstock, I. M., Welch, W., and Getting, V. A. Evaluation of program efficiency. *Public Health Reports*, 1968, *83*, 603-610; Deniston, O. L., Rosentock, I. M., and Getting, V. A. Evaluation of program effectiveness. *Public Health Reports*, 1968, *83*, 323-335.

proven so difficult to implement that other more practical projects have been expediently substituted. But, valuable as these consequences may be, they are not what was originally sought.

The importance of establishing specific objectives and the difficulty of carrying out effective evaluation without them can be appreciated by a review of the history of the Neighborhood Health Center programs, established by the Office of Economic Opportunity (OEO) in the 1960s. These centers were originally funded as pilot programs to test what approaches and methods are most effective in bringing health care to people who have not been reached. Their implied goal was thus to improve the health of indigent persons by providing health care and related services. Implied subobjectives were increased accessibility and availability of health services to these populations. These distinctions become increasingly important as one examines their implications, for we have very little evidence to support the contention that providing medical services to populations, particularly populations suffering from a number of social ills, will have any profound effect on their health in the absence of other changes in their social and physical environment. Nor can we immediately conclude that making services available will necessarily guarantee that the services will be utilized.

Clearly, some of these problems were recognized by the OEO. They have begun to talk in terms of people enrolled in health care programs, utilization rates, and other measures of increased accessibility. They carefully avoid the issue of improved health status. Unfortunately, as the cost of providing this kind of care grew (in part caused by the extensive outreach system mounted to increase utilization), more people began asking for demonstrations of results. As the OEO fell back on measures of comparative quality of care between the services delivered in their Neighborhood Health Center and other comparable institutions such as medical schools and private practices, signs of new or altered objectives began to appear. The Neighborhood Health Centers were now referred to as instruments for health and social action whereby the participation of residents in the decision-making process was emphasized above the effects on the health of the population. The numbers of indigenous persons hired for new careers on the health ladder was emphasized as playing a major role "in bolstering community and individual self-respect, trust, and comfort." The Neighborhood Health Center was now talked about as "a health institution, a social institution, a training and employment agency, a financing mechanism, a political institution, and many other things" (5).

Thus, we see that it is very difficult to evaluate the success of such a program until one can be specific in delineating the objectives which the developers had intended to achieve. Perhaps the shifting objectives have not been altogether accidental. Our political system has a strange habit of demanding far stricter standards of evaluation for programs designed to aid the poor than it does in other areas of endeavor. It may indeed be totally unfair to expect the Neighborhood Health Center to defend its actions on the grounds of improving the health status of a population when indeed the rest of the medical care system can make no such claims. The Office of Economic Opportunity has taken refuge in the claim that "some of the Center's most valuable assets and outputs do not easily fit into the ledger. They deal with the human condition and who can measure self-respect, independence, and hope?" (5). It would seem that if we are to make any progress and have any assurance that we are going in a positive direction, we must find ways to measure these traits since it is no longer practicable to measure the original goals.

Selznick describes some consequences of this lack of predetermined objectives (6):

> Once an organization becomes a "going concern," with many forces working to keep it alive, the people who run it can readily escape the task of defining its purposes. This evasion stems partly from the hard intellectual labor involved, a labor that often seems but to increase the burden of already onerous daily operations. In part, there is the wish to avoid conflicts with those in and out of the organization who would be threatened by a sharp definition of purpose, with its attendant claims and responsibilities.

The threat engendered by making program objectives explicit becomes intensified when one seriously proposes to measure achievement (4,7,8). There is just no easy way to eliminate all threatening factors, but threats may be lessened if the benefits can be perceived as outweighing the costs.

Another difficulty exists in some programs when the objectives for individual participants of the target population are different. This is particularly likely to occur in mental health and home care programs. In these situations, it would be more appropriate to state a separate objective (and sub-objectives) for each person served. The health professional establishes a unique objective for each patient, e.g., by the end of a certain time period, Mr. A will return to work; Mr. B will bathe and dress himself. The program objective can then be summarized as: all, or some proportion of, program clientele will attain their unique objectives within specified periods.[2]

STEPS IN SYSTEMATIC EVALUATION

But how does the individual project director, or program evaluator, go about doing a more systematic evaluation? For the most part, it is a frame of mind, an attitude. Evaluation of program effectiveness involves three steps, the first of which is to accurately and completely describe the project. This description may simply consist of the program title and a list specifying the objective(s), sub-objectives, activities, and resources. If these things have already been described in the planning phase, this step is relatively simple and may require only copying the items from the program plan. However, it is rare in current practice to find program plans with the objectives spelled out in sufficient detail and precision to permit substantial evaluation of program effectiveness.

The program objective may or may not be an ultimate objective. The program may cover the entire spectrum of a problem, or portion of it. Nevertheless, the program objective is an arbitrary point on a continuum of desired goods that is expected to culminate in an ultimate good. In this way a specific program might contribute to rather than be an ultimate goal.

An evaluation of effectiveness must include measurements of the condition that is specified in the program objective. In addition, it should include as many measurements of sub-objectives as time and resources permit. Generally, it is useful to measure several sub-objectives in order to locate sources of trouble when a program proves less effective than expected. If an administrator wants to evaluate the effectiveness of several programs but has limited resources for evaluation, he may prefer to measure only the objectives for all programs, returning to measure sub-objectives in those programs where trouble was indicated.

In step two all program activities are listed, and each one is linked to the objective or sub-objective it is intended to accomplish. Making activities explicit can serve as a check on the adequacy and completeness of the objectives. If a planned or continuing activity cannot be linked to an objective or sub-objective, either a

[2]Kiresuh and Shuman have described a model for implementing this general idea in their discussion, Goal attainment scaling. *Community Mental Health Journal*, 1968, *4*, 443-453.

necessary objective or sub-objective has been omitted, or the activity is unnecessary. Conversely, if a stated objective or sub-objective has no activity linked to it, either an essential activity is not being planned or performed, or the stated objective or sub-objective is not necessary to the program. Another reason for including activities in the program description is to determine the extent to which they were performed. For this reason, each activity must be carefully specified—what was done, by whom, and when and where.

If an objective or sub-objective has not been accomplished, either an activity was not performed as planned or the assumption linking the activity and the objective was not valid. Of course, if the activity was not performed or performed improperly, the linking assumption must remain untested.

The final task, specification of program resources, determines whether resources were used as planned. Obviously, if projected activities were not performed, knowledge of whether resources were used will allow determination of the validity of assumptions linking resources and activities made earlier.

In summary, the first step in evaluating program effectiveness requires 1) a clear statement of the program objectives and sub-objectives, 2) specification of program activities, and 3) a description of program resources.

PROBLEMS IN MEASUREMENT

A complete treatment of the details involved in measurement and statistical determinations is not possible here. This material is readily available in standard texts which cover the field in detail (9,10,11,12). In addition, consultation with experts, such as statisticians and behavioral scientists, will often be helpful in completing these steps. These procedures require identification of the kinds of data needed to determine the status of an objective. Of course, valid and reliable measures of program accomplishments are required.

Validity and reliability are important because test scores do not always measure consistently what they are intended to measure. Suppose a series of measures are obtained on a group of persons, or restaurants, or samples of water. A range of scores will be obtained. Differences in scores may reflect true differences in the characteristic being measured, but these scores may reflect other factors as well. If the measure is of people suffering from headaches, responses may not only reflect the complaint being measured but also such transitory factors as mood or fatigue. In measures of the physical environment, variations in the administration of a test and the care with which instruments are read will also directly affect scores.

A variation in scores is always possible when such complex concepts as health status, morbidity, or cleanliness are measured. These concepts are composed of many factors. For example, good health might be defined to include an almost infinite number of measurements of the functions of various organ systems. It is unlikely that any one test could measure all functions. A test of two or three functions, an incomplete index, applied to a group of people might show that some are healthier than others without recognizing the fact that other tests would have yielded other conclusions.

Because test scores vary not only by true differences in what is being measured but also for other reasons, it is never completely safe to accept a test score at face value. When possible, evidence should be assessed to determine whether the test is valid and whether it is reliable.

The selection of an adequate measure of accomplishment may prove the most taxing part of the evaluation process. Where reliable and valid methods are not immediately available, the literature may yield relevant procedures. Failure to locate acceptable standards may necessitate developing a unique one which satisfies the basic criteria of measuring instruments. The lack of an adequate measure for certain objectives may mean omitting some data from the evaluation, thus reducing the resultant amount of information bearing on the success of a program.

Ideally, the timespan in which accomplishment should take place is laid out initially. This planning would indicate critical times for appraisal and program readjustments. Indeed, evaluation will be most valuable if it is considered as a more nearly continuous process, rather than a one-time procedure.

In deciding how to make the needed measurements, two problems are particularly important: how to avoid bias and how to select a representative sample. Bias is a systematic overperception of that which one desires to see. The possibility of bias is great if one evaluates his own work; it is especially great if subjective rather than physical measures are used. Laboratory tests that detail blood counts, changes in blood pressure, and other such data are less apt to be biased than subjective estimates of whether a patient is better, unchanged, or worse. Bias could be reduced by using objective measures when possible; or, if observation or judgment is necessary, by having several independent judges and using a standardized rating form. Blind therapeutic trials (where the patient does not know whether he has received the treatment or a placebo) and double blind studies (where neither patient nor observer know) are common ways to minimize bias.

Sampling procedures are often used in evaluating a program because it is rarely feasible to measure the attainment of objectives for everyone involved. In such cases, a probability sample which accurately represents the total population must be selected. The size of the sample required depends on such technical considerations as variance in the distribution of the parameter being measured, the amount of change expected as a result of program activity, and the level of certainty desired when inferring that what is true of the sample is also true of the population from which it was drawn.

ANALYZING EFFECTIVENESS

When evaluating effectiveness, the investigator asks not merely whether the program objectives were accomplished but to what extent achievement of the objective can be attributed to the activities of the program. That is, would the changes have occurred without the program? Or, would the situation have worsened without intervention? These questions may also appropriately be asked during planning. Would other factors have led to the same results? Control groups are a particularly valuable source of information for answers to these queries.

Analysis of program effectiveness can be simplified by using a set of ratios involving the three program variables—resources, activities, and objectives. Simplest is the ratio of actual resources to planned use of resources, AR:PR. Slightly more complicated is the ratio of actual program activities performed to planned activities, AA:PA.

The ratio that indicates accomplishment is still more complex: AO:PO. AO is the net attainment of the objective attributable to program activity and PO is the attainment desired less the amount that would have existed in the absence of the program. It might be thought that the proper comparison would be between the actual status of the objective at the time of evaluation and the desired status. However, such a comparison is not valid because it does not take into account the effect on the program objectives of activities and events outside it. Evaluation should assess the extent to which achievement of the objective can be directly related to activities performed in the program. Therefore, it is necessary to find a way to compare the net accomplishment attributable to the program with the accomplishment intended for the program. One way is to determine the status of the objective at the time of evaluation and then to subtract from it an estimate of what the status would have been had the program not been undertaken. For example, if a program operator finds that 90 percent of a group of children are immune to measles after an immunization program, he cannot properly take credit for all 90 percent, but only for those who would not be immune had his program not been undertaken.

What is true for the actual status of the objective, the numerator, is also true for planned attainment, the denominator. One must subtract from planned attainment that portion of the desired goal that would have occurred in the absence of the program. Suppose it was hoped that 90 percent of the children be immune to measles. Evaluation shows that 80 percent actually became immune but that half, 40 percent, became immune through activity outside the program (visits to outside or nonprogram physicians and so forth). Program effectiveness would than be 80-40:90-40 = 40:50 = 80 percent.

CONTROL GROUPS

How is it possible to estimate the status of the objective in the absence of the program? The most certain way is to use a control or comparison group similar to the one exposed to the program. The control group procedure maximizes confidence in judging the results that may be properly attributed to the program.

It is not always feasible to use control groups in evaluating health programs, but they could be employed more often than they currently are. For example, when a new program cannot be initiated throughout an area, it may be possible to begin in a few places at random and to use the remaining areas as controls. Alternate procedures might be tested in different sections of the target area. This is frequently done in clinical field trials to test whether one procedure is superior to another.

However, if a strict control group is not available, a possible control group can be approximated by comparing community status before and after the program with information about similar nearby communities that were not exposed to the program. While this is not an ideal procedure, it may provide guidance as to the impact of the program.

A major danger in using such natural groups for comparison or controls is that an available group, within or outside the community, may not actually be similar to the study group in crucial respects. The laboratory practice for minimizing this danger is to assign subjects randomly to both treatment and control procedures. While this practice can sometimes be used in health programs, it will often be impossible to withhold treatment for ethical reasons. A notorious example is the recent disclosure of the extended U.S. Public Health Service study of the long-range effects of untreated syphilis. In 1932, when the project was started, treatment for the disease was indeed risky. While the more than four hundred persons with latent (noncommunicable) cases who did not get treated received significant benefits in other ways for their participation in the program, they never received treatment for syphilis, even after the discovery of penicillin and its effectiveness. Anyone who considers the use of such an evaluative control group should review the furor caused in this one instance.

When random assignments to experimental and control groups cannot be made, baseline information is helpful. Careful planning should include basic data about the target population and potential comparative situations. Such data can help in making reasonably accurate predictions as to accomplishment of the objectives. In this way, even without a classic control group, during planning various methods for comparison will have been weighed. If baseline data show that the program and comparison groups are similar at the beginning of the program, one may be more confident that the status of the comparison group at evaluation will represent what would probably have occurred in the program group without the program. If the groups differ at the beginning, one should be much less confident.

When no comparison group can be devised, it may still be possible to obtain information on the probable impact of program activity on the objective. One can formulate alternative explanations for the outcome of the program and check whether available facts support such alternatives. Suppose one wishes to determine whether a decline in the incidence of tuberculosis in a community can properly be attributed to an ongoing tuberculosis control program. Improved nutrition and housing are possible alternatives. If neither improved substantially, the director could attribute the reduced incidence of tuberculosis to his program with greater confidence. If one or both alternative explanations were borne out by evidence, he could not claim all the improvement. At this point he could, however, use cross-tabulation analysis to study the interrelationships among the alternative explanations and thus throw more light on the relative contribution of each explanation to the program objectives that were attained (12).

The conclusion that program activities caused program outcomes requires a judgment that can never be made with absolute certainty. With the use of control groups and/or tests of alternative hypotheses, however, it is possible to make a more confident judgment than would be legitimate without the use of such procedures. Work is underway to determine the conditions under which various approaches to isolating the effects of program activity can be relied upon (13).

A PRACTICAL EXAMPLE

A practical example of an evaluation problem can be seen in the study of an Israeli community health center which had been established for the purpose of integrating the then existing multiple services so as to make them both more efficient and economical (14). In reviewing the alternative methods by which the work of the health center could be evaluated, the investigators recognized that before-and-after comparisons would not be possible because of inadequate preplanning for an evaluation and lack of baseline data. They considered comparing the neighborhood served with a similar one that had a different type of health service. Unfortunately, no demographically comparable area with reliable statistics could be identified. A matched sample could not be extracted from national figures due to lack of suitable data. Therefore, the investigators compared the local statistics with national ones on a one-shot basis as well as using the latter as a moving indicator.

Having checked the comparability of their local population to the nation as a whole in terms of such factors as age distribution, sex, country of birth, family size, size of dwelling units, and members receiving social welfare aid, they then compared the two populations in terms of mortality, morbidity, and hospitalization rates. Mortality data showed similar perinatal mortality rates and similar proportional mortality. However, the study area had significantly lower infant mortality rates and lower standardized mortality rates. Morbidity data for selected specific conditions showed identical figures for typhoid, but a significantly lower incidence of diphtheria, tuberculosis, and anemia during pregnancy, and a significantly higher incidence of bacillary dysentery in the study area. The number of hospitalized patients was significantly lower and the average stay in the hospital per patient was significantly shorter among those in the study area.

Community response to this information was reflected in a

number of projects, as well as in attendance at mass radiography tuberculosis screening programs where attendance rates exceeded those experienced in other areas. Calculations for cost indicated that the study's per capita expenditure was in the same range as that dispensed in other parts of the country.

To provide a closer causal link between the parameters observed and the activities in the local community, the evaluators suggested using national rates as a moving indicator against which to contrast the rate of change in local areas. In this way, the rate of change in parameters, such as infant mortality rates, could be graphically displayed for the national and the local area with the hope that local changes would be moving at a faster pace than national ones toward a theoretically irreducible minimal level. This approach, while focusing on disease reduction rather than health improvement, illustrates how available data sources can be creatively utilized to address basic objectives of a health delivery unit.

ANALYSIS OF EFFICIENCY

Most program evaluations will reveal imperfect success in accomplishing objectives and sub-objectives. Evaluation does more, however, than demonstrate the amount of achievement. It pinpoints areas where problems exist. This model for evaluation of effectiveness assumes that programs have been planned to expend resources to promote activities—these activities, in turn, are designed to accomplish the program objective.

If the attainment of objectives were valued regardless of cost and if unlimited resources were available, efficiency would not be of great concern. Since neither of these conditions exists within the realm of political reality, efficiency must be a primary concern in all program operations. Efficiency represents the cost in resources necessary to accomplish the program's objectives, or the ratio between an output (net attainment of program objectives) and an input (program resources expended): AO:AR. The inverse of this ratio, which would be AR:AO, yields a measure of average cost. Clearly it matters little whether one examines efficiency or average costs, since the same relationship will emerge. However, it is sometimes more meaningful to look at one than the other. For example, it is easier to understand that it costs $10,000 to locate and cure one case of tuberculosis than to understand that 1:10,000 of a case was located and cured for $1.00.

Efficiency studies may answer questions about the relationship between the degree of accomplishment and the resources expended, between the degree of attainment and the number and kind of activities conducted, and between the number and kind of activities conducted and the resources expended.

Knowledge of how effective and efficient a program is will permit decisions on whether its results are worth the cost and reveal opportunities for expansion. The addition of a multiple-antigen immunization program to a functioning program could be made with little additional cost. Other embellishments could prove cumbersome.

Evaluation always entails comparison with a standard. In evaluations of effectiveness, the standard for comparison most frequently selected is the attainment level that had been planned before program implementation began. A similar standard may be used for determining efficiency. One may ask whether the actual level of efficiency or the average costs are similar to what had been planned.

Frequently, no sound basis for estimating planned efficiency is available. For example, there are situations in which little or no data can be obtained about the resources required to support an activity, or the number and kinds of activities that will be required to attain an objective. In this situation, where quantitative estimates are not available from the program plan, another standard for comparison needs to be selected. A frequently used but dangerous standard for comparison is the operation of the same program in an earlier year. The fact that a program is cheaper to operate one year than the next need not necessarily imply greater success. Costs and circumstances may vary so from year to year that conclusions drawn from efficiency ratios obtained in two different years may be invalid. Nevertheless, a knowledge of local circumstances and of the costs of living may enable a person to estimate from data obtained periodically whether efficiency is increasing or decreasing. The important point is that a comparison of the actual operation of a program with a reasonable standard permits a judgment as to whether the efficiency attained is satisfactory or unsatisfactory.

QUALITY VERSUS QUANTITY

Since each program variable includes quantitative and qualitative components, measures of the variables must reflect both dimensions. In most instances, quantitative measures alone do not provide a sufficient basis for judging how adequately a program component has been implemented.

Generally, an assessment of quality as well as of quantity is desirable. When resources are described in terms of a given number of "qualified" physicians, nurses, or sanitarians or a given number of "adequate" clinic facilities, the nature of the resources themselves needs to be described and quantified. What factors determine the qualifications of the personnel? What is meant by "adequate"? How "good" were the physicians, nurses, sanitarians, or clinics provided? When activities are described in terms of numbers of nursing visits, santitation inspections, physical examinations, or educational efforts, the qualitative as well as the quantitative aspects must be specified and subsequently measured. The evaluator needs to measure not only the number of activities, but also the way in which each was performed and at what level of expertness.

At present, few ready procedures are available for developing and applying qualitative measures; we can only point out that more qualitative measures are needed. Considerable work has been and is being done on development of measures of the quality of medical care. As we examine these efforts, we must keep in mind that two quite different kinds of studies are conducted under the general rubric of quality. To some quality means (as we do here) the extent to which physicians, nurses, and others are carrying out the correct activities in diagnosis, treatment, and so on. To others, quality care is that which cures; it is really a test of an activity-objective assumption. It is desirable to bear in mind that effectiveness and efficiency may be influenced as much or more by the quality of resources and activities as by their quantity.

WHO SHOULD EVALUATE?

One important consideration has been tangentially mentioned but never directly considered. This is the problem of deciding who should conduct the evaluation. As with other problems discussed here there is no ready answer. An outside agency is often most able to be objective and unbiased. It is particularly difficult to refrain from "reading in" those things one wants to find and from "ruling out" those factors which detract from one's plans. In addition, the desire to insure the survival of projects and personnel cannot help but influence such a reading. It is hard to believe that many administrators would rate themselves and their programs poorly if their job security depends on effective performance. Balanced against these hazards are the opportunities to adjust quickly any defects as they arise and to incorporate the findings into meaningful program changes which will substantially alter the course of events. The most effective evaluation, and perhaps the most efficient as well, will generally be some combination of outside people working with program management. The evaluators will need access to personnel and management data as well as cooperation from staff. Management can provide background information and gain ready feedback before the final report.

Application of the methods described here to real program situations will be fairly simple in those programs for which resources, activities, and accomplishments can be readily quantified in reasonably meaningful terms and in which the concept that represents success is clear enough to be shared by all. While conceptual clarity is a prerequisite to meaningful quantification, it does not follow that all things which are conceptually clear can be readily measured. For example, the goal of achieving the regular use of a seat belt is conceptually clear, although ascertaining actual accomplishment might require considerable ingenuity.

Such simple situations, however, are not common; more often program objectives are lacking in conceptual clarity. When a program director thinks in terms of raising the level of health in a group, he is dealing with ideas that may have no common meaning even among a group of experts. One director or physician may think of the absence of certain symptoms, a second of certain physical signs, a third of emotional stability, a fourth of physical vigor, and a fifth of individual productivity. Others will think in combinations of several or all of these ideas. Before the program director can prepare an index of accomplishment, he has to define the objective(s) he is going to try to measure. This task frequently proves to be the most difficult part of the evaluation process. Similarly, in many settings, the conceptual meaning of the performance of planned activity is unclear. What is really meant by a "nursing visit" or an "inspection"? When a person's role is termed "education," what precisely is meant by education? Until one can specify, first in terms of concepts and then in terms of measures of quantity and quality, how the professional should behave in a particular situation, evaluation cannot be comprehensive, and programs cannot be systematically improved.

The tools described for evaluating effectiveness and efficiency are most useful for programs in which: a) the objectives have been specified qualitatively and quantitatively and have been fixed in time to particular geographic areas and to particular target audiences; b) the programs are described in sufficient detail to permit reliable observations of performance of planned activity; and c) all the resources that are directed toward program activity are identified.

Thus, the first step in evaluating effectiveness and efficiency appears to be to attain conceptual clarity about what the program is and what it contains. Then evaluation becomes straightforward.

SUMMARY

A program is an organized response to eliminate or reduce one or more problems where the response includes one or more objectives, performance of one or more activities, and expenditure of resources.

Five foci have been identified for evaluation of the program. For appropriateness, were the proper values used to select the problem? For effectiveness, to what extent were objectives attained? For adequacy, how much of the total problem was eliminated? For efficiency, at what costs were the objectives attained? And for side effects, what outcomes occurred that were not central to the objectives of the program?

Programs are always evaluated, but the evaluations vary as to whether the measures are presumptive or direct and the degree to which the measures are impressionistic or objective. Valid and objective measures of program goals make it possible to assess a program systematically. Ideally, we should compare the actual status at the time of the evaluation with the status that would have existed had there been no program.

In the process of setting objectives, one should not only specify the desired amount of change but also the absolute level expected. If both estimates are specified when the program is being planned, subsequent evaluation can reveal both the extent to which an intended amount of change has occurred and also the accuracy of the planning estimates. When the findings are fed back into the planning process they should have the effect of increasing both the effectiveness of the program and the accuracy of planning.

Whatever mechanisms or approaches are used in planning a program, the administrator needs to make three major kinds of decisions after specifying the problem toward which the program is to be directed. These decisions comprise: a) a determination of the program objectives and sub-objectives deemed necessary and sufficient for attaining the program objective; b) a selection of one or more activities believed to have a high probability of resulting in attainment of each sub-objective; and c) a determination of the kind and amount of resources needed to support the performance of the planned activities. In attempting to implement a program plan, an ideal plan will frequently have to be modified on the basis of extant constraints. Resources may not be sufficient to support all desired activities, or limitations of personnel may make it impossible to undertake certain desired activities. In such instances, modifications must be introduced to restrict the level of activities and perhaps the scope or breadth of the program objective. The logic of program operation is to expend resources wisely to support the performance of activities and thereby to attain sub-objectives and the program objective.

REFERENCES

1. Weckworth, V. On evaluation: A tool or a tyranny. Paper presented at an annual meeting of the American Public Health Association, Philadelphia, November 12, 1969.
2. Fox, P. D., and Rappaport, M. Some approaches to evaluating community mental health services. *Archives of General Psychiatry*, 1972, *26*, 172-178.
3. Deniston, O. L., Rosenstock, I. M., and Getting, V. A. Evaluation of program effectiveness. *Public Health Reports*, 1968, *83*, 323-335.
4. Stanley, D. T. Excellence in the public service: How do you really know. *Public Administration Review*, 1964, *24*, 170-174.
5. Bryant, T. E. Goals and potential of the neighborhood health centers. *Medical Care*, 1970, *8*, 93-94.
6. Selznick, P. *Leadership in administration*. New York: Row, Peterson and Company, 1957.
7. Bergen, B. J. Professional communities and the evaluation of demonstration projects in community mental health. *American Journal of Public Health*, 1965, *55*, 1057-1066.
8. Herzog, E. *Some guidelines for evaluative research*. Children's Bureau Publication, No. 378, U.S. Department of Health, Education and Welfare, 1959.
9. Selltiz, C., Jahoda, M., Deutsch, M., and Cook, S. *Research methods in social relations*. New York: Henry Holt and Company, 1960.
10. Cronbach, L. J. *Essentials of psychological testing*, 2nd ed. New York: Harper and Row Publishers, 1960.
11. Kerlinger, F. N. *Foundations of behavioral research*. New York: Holt, Rinehart and Winston, Inc., 1966.
12. Hyman, H. *Survey design and analysis*. New York: The Free Press, 1955.
13. Deniston, O. L., and Rosenstock, I. M. The validity of nonexperimental designs for evaluating health service. *Health Services Reports*, 1973, *88*, 153-164.
14. Medalie, J. H., and Mann, K. J. Evaluation of medical care: Methodological problems in a 6-year follow up of a family and community health center. *Journal of Chronic Diseases*, 1966, *19*, 17-33.

IV
Environmental and Social Factors

The environment in which we live is an arena of major concern and current controversy. We seem to be suffering from toxic pollution created by an industrial society, with no alleviation in sight, although this pollution may have serious deleterious effects on our health. Equally serious may be the effects of stress produced by our life style in such a society. People themselves may become a type of pollution as the resources of the planet are being depleted to satisfy a rapidly growing population. If the facts are confusing, at least the confusion may be brought into perspective by the following chapters. King outlines the social and philosophical dilemmas that interfere with the interpretation of the various sets of data available on environmental pollution, and with decision making in regard to taking action. Peters examines the areas of high dosage and job-related exposures, and offers some practical suggestions on how to detect and deal with them.

Cassel reviews a relatively new area of epidemiologic concern —the effects of stress in producing a wide variety of disease states. If such factors can be detected and alleviated, we may be able to alter the susceptibility of human hosts on a scale equal to that achieved by immunization in the area of infectious diseases.

With our gradually increasing awareness that our behavior is a major factor in maintaining our own health, the function of the behavioral sciences in studying and influencing health care becomes even more vital. Coe outlines some of the roles behavioral scientists can and do play in community medicine.

Population is not only the denominator for a community problem; it may be the source of that problem as well. Growing concern over the population explosion makes it important to review some basic demographic concepts in the hope of understanding why certain things are happening and what might be done to alter the course of events. Weisbuch gives us such a review in Chapter 15, entitled "Population, Politics, and Public Health."

11

Environmental Health: Effluence, Affluence, and Influence

Thomas C. King

A major problem in dealing with the influence of the environment on health is that we know so little about what causes good health. Throughout recent history and probably throughout the history of the medical profession, there has been a preoccupation with disease. The causes of disease have been studied in great detail, but rarely have concerted, thoughtful studies of what contributes to good health been made. As a result, a great deal is known about the diseases which plague mankind, but little is known about the causes of good health in man. We deal with that dilemma by making inferences about health from our study of disease. The World Health Organization's proclamation to the contrary, we operationally define health as the absence of disease.

Environmental health experts have been struggling to improve health by eradicating disease and during the first seven decades of this century they have been amazingly successful. Prior to World War I, one out of every ten births resulted in the death either of the child or the mother. Twenty-five percent of all deaths occurred before the thirtieth year of life; and the life expectancy of man was approximately 43 years (1). An English Renaissance scholar described himself at age 43 as having "fallen into the winter of my life" (2). An English poet of the time, without any significant personal jeopardy, praised "the autumnal face" of a 39-year-old woman (3). It would be interesting to see him try such a description now, for at the present time more than half of all deaths occur after the seventieth year of life (4). Note that life expectancy at that time was influenced predominantly by deaths occurring in the first two years of life. For most of those surviving childhood, life expectancy has probably not increased beyond the biblical entitlement of "three score years and ten" (5).

A closer analysis of the changing pattern of illness over the past 70 years is intriguing. Before the First World War, the leading causes of death in this country were influenza and pneumonia —then at 202 per 100,000, now 30 per 100,000, most of which occur in elderly people in whom pneumonia is the terminal episode of a chronic debilitating disease. Tuberculosis has dropped from 195 per 100,000 to 3 per 100,000. Gastroenteritides, which occupied third place as a cause of death in the first decade of this century, has dropped from 143 per 100,000 to 1.1 per 100,000. Throughout most of recorded history, people lived in constant dread that some fulminating, infectious disease would carry off one or more of their children. Contagious diseases accounted for most health worries. In the last 20 years these diseases have become so rare that it is difficult for us to recall the horror and morbid fear with which many mothers contemplated each febrile illness in a child. While this dramatic success in eradicating those major causes of death is generally attributed to recent progress in medical science, scrutiny of the data suggests an alternative hypothesis. René Dubos in his challenging book *Mirage of Health* (6) questioned the influence of medical intervention on the eradication of these diseases. It is not unlikely that the same results might have occurred simply as a result of the nonmedical activities of epidemiologists, public health officers, and sanitation engineers who have identified the vectors of diseases and systematically eradicated them.

For whatever reasons, dramatic results have led society to believe that medical men are miracle workers. The medical profession perpetrated that illusion by advertising its miracles and promising solutions—if only society would invest enough money. The tremendous burst of public investment in medical research which occurred in the 1950s and 1960s was an expression of the people's faith in their miracle workers. Unfortunately, that faith was largely misplaced, for the medical practitioner continues as he has always done to deal with the end stages of disease. Encouraging society to "expect a miracle" resulted first in rising expectations and, more recently, in increasing disenchantment.

In the pre-twentieth-century world most men had a fatalistic attitude toward disease. When serious illness struck, they cursed their fate, the will of God, or the forces of nature. They accepted the fact that the cause of their trouble was external to man; realistic expectation for its correction was meager, and driving out demons or appeasing gods was the therapeutic objective. Mankind was caught up in the grip of apathy, fatalism, and superstition regarding disease, its causes and consequences. But as mankind began to control and correct the cause of some diseases, the grip of apathy was broken. Rising aspirations led to a growing faith in man's ability to deliver his fellowmen from the influences of external forces. Now man curses himself, his employer, the political party in power, or his doctor, but he has come to believe that men can correct the problems leading to disease. The medical profession has fed our hopes for a health utopia as they have lobbied legislatures for appropriations and philanthropies for contributions with which to cure the ills of men. Their promises, however, are based on invalid assumptions about the nature of illness and the nature of society.

The structure of human society has been profoundly altered by the eradication or control of diseases which, in the past, have dominated man. Throughout history, populations have been controlled by recurring plague, famine, and epidemic diseases. Whenever population pressures became excessive, crowding increased the risk of contagion as the disposition of wastes became more difficult. By periodically decimating the ranks of the older generation, disease also provided unexpected opportunities for the young. Such opportunities are now rare because of a troublesome shift that has occurred in the dependency ratio. As more people live beyond retirement age, that segment of the population which is both absolutely and relatively beyond their productive years increases. The greater technological demands of our society have extended the educational period which precedes entrance into a productive life. As the years of training crowd through the third decade of life, and as the number of people living into the seventh, eighth, and ninth decades of life increase, the average individual may have only 30 or 35 years of productive employment during his 70 to 80 years of life. Thus, man spends more than half of his life in a dependency status.

CHANGING PATTERNS OF DISEASE

The eradication of infectious disease as a predominant killer; the shift in the dependency ratio; and the consequences of the nonagrarian urban society with its smog, slums, speed, and stress have led to important changes in the nature of the diseases with which man must deal. Previously, the diseases which preoccupied man and characterized his medical training, and around which the health care system was organized, were diseases typified by acute onset and acute recovery. Generally, people were healthy and fully employable until suddenly stricken by disease. If they survived, they usually recovered completely and returned to full employment. The diseases were generally of a single biological cause; the bacterial, unitarian concept of disease determined our style of inquiry into disease processes. The single cause was generally biological and the vectors of the biological causes were identifiable and usually manageable. The rats, lice, or vermin that carried the dangerous organism could be identified, studied, and understood.

What are the new patterns of disease which have evolved to replace those earlier concerns? At the present time the leading causes of death and morbidity are characterized by gradual onset and indefinite recovery. Most are diseases of aging and, while specific catastrophic episodes may punctuate the progress of the disease, they tend to develop gradually. Any acute exacerbation which leads to medical intervention rarely allows an expectation of permanent cure. The aim of medical intervention has shifted from cure to palliation; from relieving men of disease to teaching them how to live with it. No longer unitarian in concept, the major diseases are made up of multiple risk elements such as chronic long exposure, genetic predisposition, and the complex interactions of many other factors including automobile and highway design, food processing, poverty, and nutritional problems (both undernutrition and overnutrition). How fast a man drives, what he drives, where he drives; how much he eats, what he eats; what he smokes; and his life style now become determinants in debilitating chronic illness. Rats, lice, and vermin were the vectors of disease in an earlier age; similarly, the vectors of vascular diseases, cancer, and accidents can be identified and understood. These vectors are predominately nonbiological, multiple, and generally man-made; they relate to the environmental setting in which man lives. In an earlier day, increasing longevity by eradicating disease could be expected to increase man's productivity and to decrease his morbidity; in the diseases with which we are now confronted, increasing longevity results in increasing morbidity. When a man recovers from the acute phase of his chronic illness, impaired social function remains.

Our present pattern of premedical and medical education is built on assumptions about disease derived from that earlier pattern of causes and consequences. It is built on a premise of biological origins which predicates individual intervention as an appropriate therapy. Preclinical education focuses on biology, chemistry, and microbiology, with little emphasis on those etiological causes of contemporary diseases which stem from human behavior and man's manipulation of his environment. Hospital-based medical education perpetuates the illusion that sickness has a beginning and an end. As a consequence, we too often train our physicians to play an insignificant role in maintaining health; they are left to deal with terminal stages of chronic diseases or to help patients adjust to the failures of a system which has not effectively managed the environmental causes of man's developing disabilities.

A probable consequence of this historic preoccupation with disease is the interesting paradox that the esteem with which medical education and society in general have held various medical disciplines during recent decades is inversely proportional to the impact those disciplines have had on health. In the more prestigious specialty fields (e.g., cardiovascular surgery, neurosurgery), the major effort of the practitioner is focused on the terminal stages of individual illness; his successful interventions, when they occur, have minimal impact on the overall health of society. In a society which has failed to attend to the ordering of its health priorities, an extraordinary disproportion of its economic commitment to health has been diverted to these areas. Our purpose here is to shift the focus and deal briefly with some of the problems which have resulted from this disordered priority.

Because environmental health can be viewed as a field that involves everything related to man's well-being, it includes far more than can be reasonably reviewed here. But we can identify some of the problems which confound priorities, decision making, and policy setting for human health, and discuss some of the perceptions that extend our concerns beyond the relatively simple matters of water and sewage disposal, which historically have characterized the field.

MAN'S EFFECT ON THE ECOLOGY OF THE EARTH

A decade ago, Buckminster Fuller conceived a new model for analyzing the earth's destiny and the ecologic consequences of man's action—the planet is a spaceship and man its passenger (7). The earth, at its launching, was outfitted with provisions in a finite quantity; when depleted, there are no replacements. The basic resources of fossil fuels and inorganic materials must be conserved and reused or they will run out. As resources cannot be added, wastes cannot be jettisoned. There is no method for their permanent disposal. Whatever is discarded accumulates, unless it is discarded in a form which allows it to reenter the pool of resources. If waste materials are not recycled, not only will raw materials be trapped, but the planet will eventually be filled with garbage. Thus, every act of man, particularly industrialized man, must be analyzed for unexpected or undesired effects on the health of man. Furthermore, each generation should be obliged to neither detract from the resources available to the next, nor to add to the waste load it must carry. That we have not yet fully defined the health consequences of the accumulating oxides, isotopes, dirt, and junk should not permit us to ignore the fact that there may be some.

Accepting the finite limits of resources and space makes implicit the fallacy in the concept of "free goods." Until now man has viewed his world as one of unlimited frontiers. He could always move on to find air, water, and the other necessities at no cost beyond the cost of moving. Exploitation was acceptable because it could be afforded; it cannot be tolerated in light of our new perceptions. Usable space, air, and water now require some expenditure from man in either effort or inconvenience. It is urgent that we identify the cost and avoid further loss of resources.

Our spaceship does have one continuing external input. Solar energy is the original and ultimate source of energy and when existing storage cells are depleted, man will need to tap solar sources to solve his food, fuel, and other energy problems. Even this external resource has an important side effect on human health. The effect of actinic rays on the skin provides one of the clearest examples of a direct, deleterious consequence of the environment on man's health. The carcinogenic effects of actinic rays on human epidermis have been clearly demonstrated.

The growing list of environmental problems deserves our attention, for environmental health encompasses far more than can reasonably be reviewed here. Consequently, the extremely important problems of accident prevention, ionizing radiation, thermal injury, war, psychological consequences of crowding, and noise are among relevant topics that will not be discussed. A recent monograph (8) edited by P. W. Purdom provides a useful review of these subjects for the interested reader. The remainder of this chapter will consider two of the major environmental issues which have a significant impact on the health of man—air and water.

Effects of Air Pollution on Health

> . . . this most excellent canopy, the air, . . . this brave o'erhanging firmament, this majestical roof fretted with golden fire, why, it appears no other thing to me than a foul and pestilent congregation of vapours. (*Hamlet* II, ii, line 311)

The present state of our knowledge allows only some very tentative hypotheses regarding the way in which the gases, chemicals, and particulates that man inhales each day influence his health and well-being. The number of interacting variables make this a complex problem. There are some intriguing correlations of various types of air pollution with the aggravation, at least, of certain acute and chronic diseases, such that the assumption of a relationship can be reasonably made. The exact nature of that relationship and the factors which contribute to it are poorly understood. The tradition of medical inquiry focusing on single causes for specific diseases has encouraged attempts to relate specific air pollutants, such as sulfur dioxide, to a specific disease. Such efforts have failed. It is probable that the SO_2 in the air must occur in a particular concentration and in certain combinations of humidity, temperature, and particulate size if it is to reach the vulnerable level of the respiratory tract. It may be that even then an adverse effect would only occur when the pulmonary field was already prepared for the insult by underlying disease or genetic predisposition. Measuring the level of oxides of sulfur in the ambient air and correlating that with any specific disease yields inconclusive findings. In spite of the nonspecific nature of these correlations, the association of sulfur dioxide and particulate pollution with serious increases in mortality and morbidity in a few specific disasters seems inescapable.

Our information about the constituents of air contamination is obtained largely by measuring those substances for which analytic methods have been developed. Because we know how to measure the oxides of sulfur, carbon, and nitrogen, we struggle to correlate disease incidence with those gases. Future technology may allow us to measure many other inert or noxious gases, or trace metals, which could prove to be far more significant than those substances we now strive to indict. We are in a sufficiently primitive and inferential stage in the science of exploring the complex relationships between environment and health that specific attention must be afforded the alternative hypotheses which could explain findings. In the discussion which follows, some simplifying generalizations have been made in order to clarify the problems and facilitate an analysis of the relationship between air pollution and human health, but the reader is urged to remember that the serious methodological problems, and the complex interplay between the atmospheric variables and the pathophysiological variables, vitiate the confidence with which these generalizations can be applied.

For descriptive purposes, air pollutants can be divided into at least four general groups. What is ordinarily referred to as Type I pollution (9) constitutes the primary air contaminants—carbon monoxide, the hydrocarbons, the oxides of sulfur and nitrogen, and the particulates (soot, fly ash, other industrial emissions, and volcanic debris). Figure 1 indicates the approximate percentage by weight distribution of these pollutants as they are found at various sampling stations throughout the United States (10). Sources of pollutants are also shown. Carbon monoxide comes almost totally from internal combustion engines, predominately the automobile. The hydrocarbons are largely residue from incompletely burned gasoline. In most communities the automobile is the major hydrocarbon source, though in and around refineries and volatile solvent plants, other sources become significant. As depicted in Figure 2, fossil fuel combustion in stationary sources, principally power plants, contributes 73 percent of the SO_2; 23 percent of the SO_2 comes from a variety of industrial sources, including smelters and refineries. Of the particulates, 32 percent are emitted from stationary fuel combustion sites, 27 percent from various industrial processes, 23 percent from forest fires, 4 percent from solid waste disposal combustion sites, 4 percent from transportation, and 10 percent from miscellaneous smaller sources (11).

This breakdown of the particulates refers only to the lower atmosphere. Particulates in the upper atmosphere may have another effect on man's health and well-being, for they have the potential of significantly changing the heat balance of the earth as they disrupt incoming and outgoing patterns of radiation. This stratospheric (> 40,000 feet) particulate contamination comes largely from natural sources, predominately in the form of volcanic dust. Some concern has been expressed about the consequences of supersonic jet travel at the 65,000 foot elevation where wind currents are minimal and particulates deposited may remain one to three years. Carbon dioxide is the most abundant combustion product of the SST and that molecule remains in the stratosphere from three to thirty years before passing into the biosphere (12). Water vapor, another significant residue of SST exhaust, remains an average of 18 months (13). These data have serious implications for long-range weather and earth surface temperature modification.

Type II pollutants are secondary pollutants which result from the chemical reactions of Type I pollutants in the atmosphere. These reactions are largely due to the catalytic effect of the sun and, where they occur, they peak during midday. Aldehydes, ozone oxidants, conjunctival irritants, and plant toxicants are produced. These secondary pollutants occur primarily where the predominant Type I atmospheric contaminants are the hydrocarbons and nitrogen oxides. As a consequence, they are characteristic of urban

Figure 1

AIR POLLUTION EMISSION IN THE UNITED STATES, 1968
Percentage by weight

What They Are

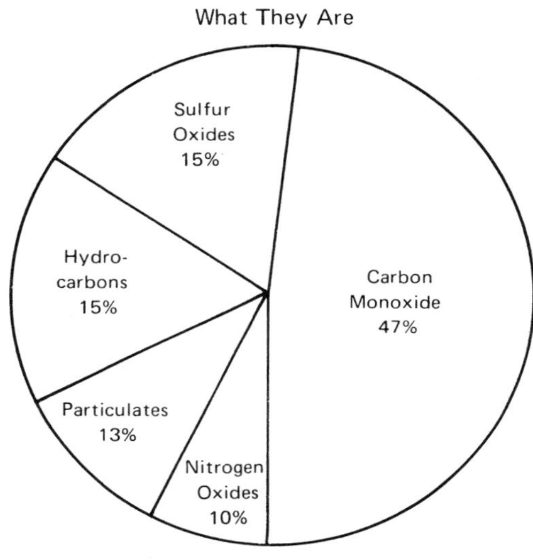

Where They Come From

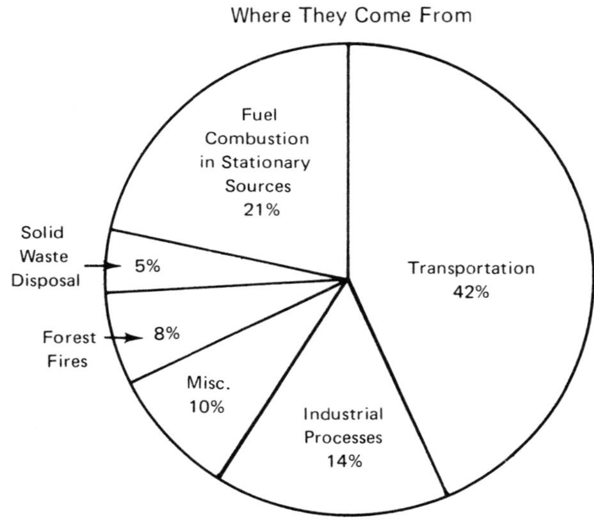

From: *Environmental quality: First annual report of the Council on Environmental Quality*. Washington, D.C.: U.S. Government Printing Office, August 1970.

Figure 2

SULFUR OXIDES AND PARTICULATES EMITTED INTO THE U. S. ATMOSPHERE

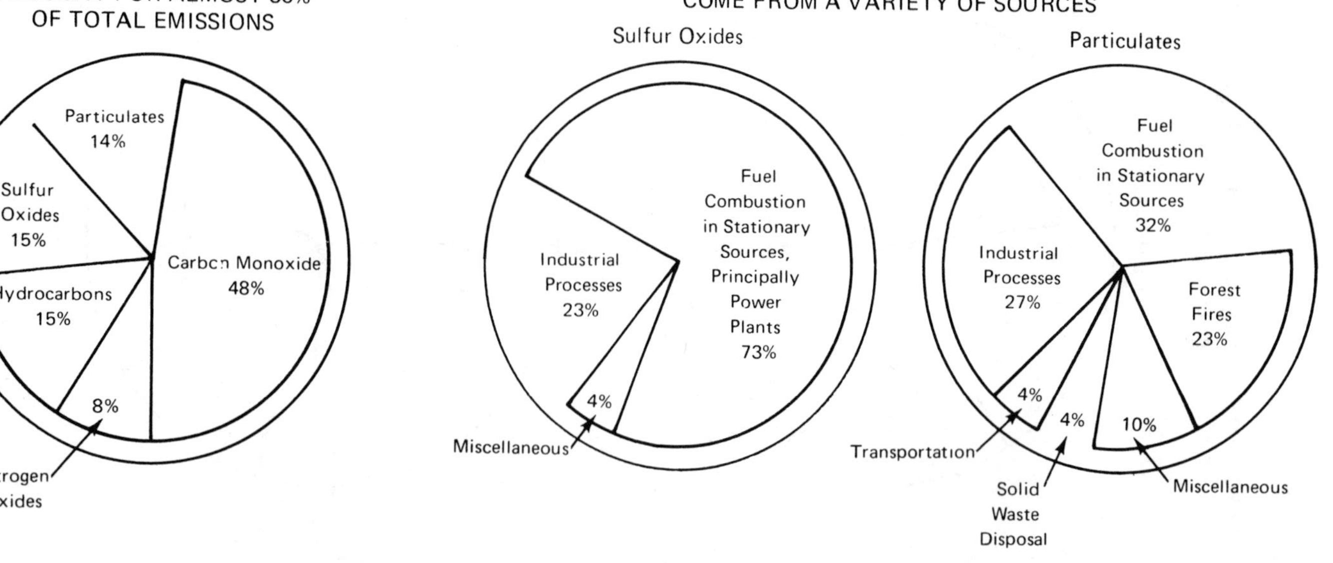

From: Danger in the Air: Sulfur Oxides and Particulates, May 1970. U.S. Department of Health, Education, and Welfare, National Air Pollution Control Administration, Publication No. 1. Washington, D.C.: U.S. Government Printing Office, 1971.

centers whose primary source of pollution is the internal combustion engine and where the atmospheric conditions allow stagnation of the air mass and enough sunlight to act upon the pollutants. Los Angeles smog is typical of this type.

Situational air pollution, the third type, is both the best studied and the least studied. This includes occupational and domestic air hazards. Occupational air pollution, about which there is considerable information, has been dealt with elsewhere in this book. It is an interesting paradox that domestic air pollution, which is similar in many ways to occupational pollution, has received so little attention. The fumes from cooking and heating, from hair and deodorant aerosols, and from other volatile chemicals used around the home provide potential risks about which comparatively little is known. Among Mexican-born women living in Los Angeles and working in the home, the death rate due to lung cancer significantly exceeds that for their male counterparts (14). In most populations that have been studied, the frequency with which lung cancer occurs is markedly higher in men than in women (15). In populations of U.S.-born women of Mexican descent, this increased frequency of occurrence of lung cancer is not seen (16). The only other population in which this sex ratio reversal seems to appear is in rural and nonmetropolitan nonsmokers (15), suggesting that domestic pollution may be a factor among nonsmoking rural Americans. There are many alternative hypotheses which might explain these differences, but situational air contaminants in rural homes remain an intriguing possibility.

A fourth type of air pollutant which may have health consequences and about which very little is known is the group of trace elements, e.g., cadmium, lead, arsenic, beryllium, vanadium, and fluorine, which are accumulating in the atmosphere or are contained in the ambient air. Ordinarily, an individual inhales 30 pounds of air a day. The possibility exists that significant amounts of trace elements might accumulate within the body over an extended period. The size of the particle on which the trace element may be carried, the level of the pulmonary tree which that particle reaches, the halflife of the trace element within the body, are relevant issues. With the wide use of gasoline containing tetraethyl lead, the quantity of lead accumulating from atmospheric sources could influence body-lead levels, particularly in infants and children who may be exposed to lead from other sources.

Particulates may have other effects as well. Winkelstein has noted increased rates of cirrhosis of the liver (17), stomach cancer (18), and prostatic cancer (19) in those parts of Erie County, New

York, where particulate contamination is high. Certainly this observation warrants further study.

In assessing the health consequences of pollution, several issues should be reemphasized. The various organ systems or cell types of the body may respond in a nonspecific way to a wide variety of insults. Genetic predisposition, preexisting disease or chronic cellular irritation from allergic or incidental occupational influences, fatigue, dietary or smoking indiscretions, stress, or age may establish a tissue receptivity which greatly enhances the likelihood that inhaled agents will precipitate disease. These varied host factors then interact with a confusing interplay of environmental circumstances which influence the magnitude of insult from general community pollution. Patterns of home heating, humidity, particle size, temperature and range of temperatures, wind patterns, situational and atmospheric "sinks" of stagnant air all may be relevant. Each or any of these may be necessary in some exact relationship with several other factors before they produce a significant health consequence in a given individual. The search for causal relationships is exceedingly complex.

With the exception of certain of the industrial and occupational pneumonoconioses, the presence in the air of specific chemical pollutants will ordinarily not increase the health hazard. Statistical analyses of health patterns in relation to specific pollutants are extremely confusing. The contrary problem also adds to confusion in the literature; that is, the confusion of statistical correlation with causation. Most of the epidemiological data which have been accumulated are based upon the correlation of disease incidence, hospitalization frequencies, morbidity, and excess mortality, as these are associated with specific changes in air pollution patterns. The temptation to draw causal conclusions from these correlative studies continues to plague researchers and we must continually force ourselves to look for alternative hypotheses as we attempt to unravel these intriguing correlations. Frost on the window does not cause the winter.

Having identified the major types of air pollution which commonly occur and may contribute to ill health, it is worth discussing those patterns of disease response which correlate with air pollution.

1. *Acute episodes of aggravated pulmonary disease.* While there are a number of historical episodes which seem to implicate air stagnation-pollution with increased deaths from pulmonary disease, the first clear correlation occurred in the Meuse Valley of Belgium in 1930 (20). Since that time a number of increasingly

well-documented episodes have taken place. Perhaps the most dramatic was December of 1952 in London where, beginning on the ninth of December, a temperature inversion over London combined with an intense seasonal fog. There was virtually no air movement. The resultant stagnation of the trapped air with the progressively accumulating levels of sulfur dioxide, hydrocarbons, particulates, and carbon monoxide was associated with a dramatic increase in hospitalizations for pulmonary complications throughout the London area. The increased death rate for the period accounted for 4000 additional deaths (11). Most of these deaths occurred in the very young or the very old and in people with preexistent chronic pulmonary disease. Other episodes of significance occurred in Donora, Pennsylvania, in 1948; in Poza Rica, Mexico, in 1950; in New York in 1953. An intriguing worldwide episode occurred between November 27 and December 10, 1962 (9). First in Washington, Philadelphia, New York, and Cincinnati, a sharp rise in the pollution levels was noted. Over the next ten days to two weeks, sweeping rapidly from West to East, this pollution belt moved across Europe and Asia to Osaka, Japan. In London the sulfur dioxide levels exceeded those of the 1952 episode, although the particulate level remained somewhat lower. In Rotterdam there was a fivefold increase in the normal level. In Hamburg a similar fivefold increase was noted and by the tenth of December this sharp increase was measured in Osaka. In each of these cities, sufficiently accurate health studies were made to verify a significant increase in both deaths and morbidity. Significant increases in pollution levels were also noted in Paris, Frankfurt, Prague, and a number of other cities, but concomitant health studies correlating these pollution peaks with morbidity or mortality were not made. It is interesting to note that this West to East pattern did not seem to extend beyond Japan, for no increases were noted in other parts of the world where air pollution monitoring is done, Australia and the West Coast of the United States, for example.

Infants and children comprise a population particularly susceptible to air pollution hazards (21). The increased incidence of lower respiratory infections whenever average annual SO_2 concentrations are above 0.06 ppm (22) or the oxides of nitrogen exceed that concentration (23) seems to be reasonably well demonstrated, although Colley and Reid (24) have concluded that socioeconomic factors may account for some of the demonstrated difference, at least in the 9-11 age group.

2. *Chronic respiratory disease.* The incidence of chronic respiratory diseases has been undergoing a dramatic increase in the

U.S. in recent decades. Efforts have been made to attribute these increases to air pollution, but the evidence is ambiguous. The many variables involved are such that the precise role played by air pollution can be identified only with great difficulty, if at all. Additional studies will be required on large populations over a period of many years. Epidemiological evidence, particularly in the United Kingdom, does allow some tentative conclusions that, although air pollution is probably not the major precipitating cause of chronic lung disease, it is certainly an aggravating factor. A number of studies reviewed by Bates have suggested that whenever annual average sulfur dioxide levels exceed 0.08 ppm, accompanied by particulate pollution of more than 150 μg per cubic meter as an annual average, the morbidity from chronic bronchitis is increased (25).

Lave and Seskin have discussed the evidence which relates air pollution and human health and concluded that a relationship has been established, particularly for bronchitis and urban air pollution (26, 27). In his 1971 James Waring Memorial Lecture, David V. Bates came to the same conclusion (25). On the other hand, extensive studies in Los Angeles over the past two decades have failed to identify any clear data which would implicate community air pollution as having a direct causal relationship to emphysema or to bronchitis, particularly for nonsmokers, though it does seem to increase both cough and sputum production in older workers who smoke (28). In this same Los Angeles population there is some slight suggestion that pollution might increase coronary disease but such influence is difficult to establish. Evidence supports the supposition that for selected asthmatics and those with chronic lung disorders, community air pollution may have an adverse effect (29). Although personal air pollution from cigarette smoking has been established as a cause of lung cancer, there is no evidence to implicate community air pollution. The incidence of lung cancer in urban dwellers who smoke is somewhat higher than for their counterparts in rural areas (30), but these associations may be related to the factors of migration and urban life, rather than air pollution per se. The intriguing reversal of male-female lung cancer ratios which occurs in Mexican-born women is worth mentioning again (14,16) as possibly implicating domestic air pollution.

3. *General well-being.* Occult changes may prove to be significant even though substantive evidence is lacking at present. Pulmonary function may be temporarily impaired during and after severe episodes of pollution but little clear evidence has been developed to implicate chronic community pollution.

There is a variety of more obvious impediments to general well-being that result from air pollution. Irritation of the conjunctiva results from secondary pollution when aldehydes and ozones are formed. Bad odors, impaired visibility, corrosive property damage, damage to vegetation, and the psychological depression that accompanies dismal, gloomy, overcast, polluted days are sufficiently obvious and disturbing to be a focus of public clamor to clean up the air. Many of these concerns relate more to aesthetics than primary health, but their effect on health and general well-being should not be discounted for this reason.

Nearly half of the air pollution presently encountered in the United States is carbon monoxide (Figure 1). Because it diffuses more easily across the alveolar membranes than oxygen to form carboxyhemoglobin, carbon monoxide in even small amounts is important. At one part CO per million, 0.16 percent carboxyhemoglobin is formed (31). Whenever the carboxyhemoglobin levels reach 20 ppm, studies done by Shulte (32) and others have demonstrated clear-cut impairment of psychomotor functions. Because levels of about 20 ppm are frequently reached in tunnel or congested urban traffic environments (33), the implication of carboxyhemoglobin and consequent oxygen deficits in automobile accidents should be analyzed more carefully. Recent studies have shown that in certain urban office buildings and apartments near high traffic volume freeways and tunnels, carbon monoxide levels exceed federal health standards from one-fifth to one-half of the time. These potentially toxic levels of the invisible odorless gas existed up to the thirty-second floor of buildings in New York during the 1973 heating season (34).

Since 1962 half of all American deaths have been caused by diseases of the heart and blood vessels. In the 16-to-45 age group, accidents, predominantly automobile accidents, are the leading cause of death. Cancer of the lung presently kills more Americans than all other cancers combined. Since the early 1950s, emphysema has been rapidly increasing in the United States, with incidence doubling every five years (35). Although air pollution cannot be shown directly to cause any of these diseases, it has been implicated in most of them. Aggressive research efforts must continue in order to build the data base upon which rational decisions can be made regarding society's priorities for cleaning up the air.

Water Pollution

The fish died and the river stank, and the Egyptians could not drink water from the Nile. (Exodus 7:21)

It is likely that man's first recognition of the consequences of fouling his nest occurred with the contamination of his water supplies by raw sewage. Throughout history, man has been ravaged by the plague and other epidemic diseases. Wars were lost and nations destroyed when the population increased to the point where its sewage exceeded its capability of protecting the water supply. Major advances in urbanization and civilization have been correlated with specific technological advances in man's ability to obtain clean water for growing populations (36). Until the middle of the nineteenth century, however, most of these advances were built around inventive ways of transporting water to the populations and seemed to be founded on assumptions that the rivers, lakes, and oceans had an infinite capacity to absorb waste. The terrible typhoid epidemics in London in the early nineteenth century finally precipitated extensive organized efforts to control the pollution of man's water. The technological progress in sanitary engineering can probably claim major credit for the substantial eradication of infectious epidemic diseases which has occurred throughout the developed nations of the world.

The old problems of contaminated drinking water still recur occasionally during times of natural, or man-made, disruption of sewage disposal and water protection mechanisms. There are other special circumstances under which water supplies may become contaminated and cause special health problems; for example, during periods of heavy rain in urban centers where most of the soil has been covered by concrete, an engineering blunder arises to haunt us. In virtually all American cities, sewage and domestic waste are intermingled with runoff water in drainage systems. This mixture of clean and dirty water places extraordinary and unnecessary loads on treatment facilities; during heavy rain and rapid snow melt the overload becomes more than treatment plants can handle and untreated overflow occurs. Additionally, low-grade intestinal infestations still occur frequently among travelers who ingest endemic organisms; these organisms are nonpathogenic to the native population who have developed effective immunological defenses but are capable of ruining the vacation of the unprotected visitor. Occasionally specific microorganismal contaminants flare up in some interesting ways. The recently reported outbreaks of intestinal infestation of giardiasis after visits to Leningrad (37) or Aspen, Colorado (38), are well-documented examples of such episodes. In spite of these exceptions, waterborne epidemics are largely things of the past and the procedural mechanisms for tracing down and controlling the occasional offender are well established. Because of this, most attention to water pollution in this country has shifted to the problems of availability, aesthetics, recreation, and economy.

There are, however, a number of concerns which, while primarily related to one of these other issues, may have health consequences which should not be ignored. One concern is simply that we are facing the possibility of running out of clean water. With the rapid increase in population which has occurred during this century, there has also been a sharp per capita rise in water consumption. In 1900 a typical American used an average of 100 gallons a day. That average has now risen to 200 gallons per day (39). The earth's supply of fresh water has not only not increased, it is decreasing. At the present time only 0.325 percent of the earth's water supply can be classified as fresh water, and of that amount a little over 25 percent is in the Great Lakes (40). While desalinization of ocean water remains an attractive possibility, it has thus far not proved to be economically feasible.

Recent changes in farming technology have produced staggering pollution effects. This is caused in part by the livestock wastes which now drain into the waterways. One head of cattle produces waste equivalent to 16.9 humans. Whereas a few decades ago an acre of land supported one or two head of grazing cattle, a herd of 500 are now concentrated on an acre and managed by controlled feedings. This is equivalent to a human population of 8500 per acre without sewage treatment in terms of the organic waste (41). For the grazing herd, this organic residue was recycled into the soil; the overwhelming majority now is added to the organic pool in the waterways. The consequence of this high level of organic residue is a sharp increase in the biochemical oxygen demand (BOD). Because bacterial decomposition of organic materials in water consumes oxygen, the dissolved oxygen level drops to very low levels in water which has a high organic content. As fish life is completely dependent on dissolved oxygen, this rising BOD sharply alters all life patterns. The trout, for example, requires greater than 5 parts per million dissolved oxygen and is one of the most vulnerable fish species to rising BOD. Once the dissolved oxygen level becomes sufficiently low, anaerobic decomposition begins: instead of the carbon dioxide-water by-products of aerobic decomposition, the by-products are methane gas, hydrogen sulfide, and the mercaptans, all of which cause offensive odors and additional destruction of aquatic life.

This increasing organic content also contributes to a third major concern—eutrophication. Eutrophication is more directly related to the high concentrations of inorganic chemical fertilizers which result from modern farming techniques. The result is super-fertile water in which algae and other plant forms increase explosively. As these plants pass through their life cycle, there is a sharp rise in organic residue adding another demand for oxygen and triggering a similar chain of events to that which follows increased extra-aquatic organic debris.

Occasionally a critical combination of super-fertile water, algae overgrowth, temperature, sunlight, and other unknown factors occurs, and a bloom takes place. Typical of such a bloom is the development of a red tide. The catabolic processes of these organisms produce a potent toxin which affects not only fish life in the vicinity but is absorbed and concentrated by clams and oysters. When these shellfish are eaten, serious respiratory problems develop in humans.

A fourth health concern is the accumulation of heavy metals as trace elements and radioactive debris. Although these may be toxic when concentrated in humans, they are being discarded into the earth's water in increasing quantities. At least eight such elements are known to be carcinogenic in animals. Berg and Brubank (42) have made a careful statistical analysis of the occurrence of these metals in water supplies and the cancer mortality rates for a wide variety of specific neoplastic lesions. The strong relationship between cadmium concentrations and esophageal and large bowel cancers was particularly striking in their study.

Some stimulating, if unclear, negative correlations have also been noted between hard water and hypertension (43), degenerative vascular diseases (44), and coronary artery disease (45). The effects of trace elements on human health warrants increased investigation.

CONCLUSIONS

Reordering our priorities to deal effectively with the changes which have taken place within medicine and society as a whole presents a serious dilemma. Our preoccupation with disease, a medical profession trained primarily to deal with disease, and a health care system designed to respond to the consequences of disease, have left us with few models to effectively study health or bring to bear the multidisciplinary skills and concerns necessary for an appropriate analysis of the major effects of environmental influences. Contributing to the dilemma is a surprising lack of real information with which we can analyze these problems. The situational determinants of health and the specific ways in which various environmental influences interact to cause disease have been studied in only a most preliminary and general way.

Such studies as have been done present suggestive evidence of a wide variety of hazards to human health in the environment. But these data only aggravate the dilemma; they do not solve it. If it requires long-range chronic exposure to potentially harmful environmental factors to give rise to disease, tolerable exposure limits may not be determinable. It will take many years to accumulate the evidence which will permit setting of rational standards and exposure limits. In the meantime, man must act; he must set standards based on the available inadequate evidence, and some major efforts are possible in the light of present information. We have the technological capability of developing transportation systems which are at once safe, efficient, and of low pollution hazard. That we continue to resist doing so while accidents become an increasing cause of direct mortality and morbidity in our culture is hard to justify. The long-range effects of effluents from internal combustion engines can be significantly reduced without waiting to ascertain the full nature of their consequences for health.

But uncertainty remains; this uncertainty engenders emotional, subjective arguments from all sides. Those who believe there is high risk from low exposures to environmental pollutants lobby with vigor for restrictive standards, standards which may be far beyond those necessary to protect human health. The industrial sector which contributes to much of the atmospheric and water pollution can similarly argue that no clear evidence has been developed which conclusively incriminates the current level of pollution. In the absence of any solid information, the arguments remain emotional, heated, and irresolvable. Aesthetic issues also confuse the problem, for there are those who insist that whether or not pollution affects human health, if it's ugly or unpleasant, it needs to be controlled or eliminated.

For the present, man must act without all of the evidence. Society must develop a mechanism by which interim decisions can be made for the regulation of our environment in the interests of human health while the scientific community works to build the data base from which more rational long-range decisions can be made. In the extremely complex setting in which general community pollution interacts with human health, the techniques for building that data base are sadly lacking. The most successful directions for the next phase of scientific progress call for the development of tools of inquiry for studying these problems in the general population while we intensively investigate those selected industrial populations where specific pollutants occur in sufficiently high concentrations to allow clarification of the hazards they present.

REFERENCES

1. Dublin L. I., Lolka, A. J., and Spiegelman, M. *Length of life.* New York: Ronald Press, 1949, Chapter 3.
2. Adamson, J. A., and Folland, H. *Shepherd of the ocean.* London: Botley Head, 1969, p. 221.
3. Donne, J. Elegy: The Autumnal.
4. *Vital Statistics of U. S.*, U. S. DHEW, PHS, US6PO, 1968, Vol. II, Table 1-25, pp. 1-101.
5. Psalm 90:10.
6. Dubos, R. *Mirage of health: Utopias, progress, and biological change.* New York: Harper & Brothers Publishers, 1959.
7. Fuller, R. B. *Operating manual for spaceship earth.* Carbondale: Southern Illinois University Press, 1968.
8. Purdom, P. W., ed., *Environmental health.* New York and London: Academic Press, 1971.
9. Goldsmith, J. R. Effects of air pollution on human health. In *Air pollution and its effects*, A. C. Stern, ed., New York and London: Academic Press, 1968, Chapter 14, pp. 547-615.
10. Man's impact on the global environment. Report of the study of environmental problems, MIT. Cambridge, Massachusetts: The Massachusetts Institute of Technology Press, 1970.
11. National Air Pollution Control Administration. *Danger in the air.* Washington, D.C.: Government Printing Office, DHEW, Publication #1, May 1970.
12. Man's impact on the global environment. Report of the study of critical environmental problems, MIT. Cambridge, Massachusetts: The Massachusetts Institute of Technology Press, 1970, p. 68.
13. Environmental quality: First annual report of the Council on Environmental Quality. Washington, D. C.: U.S. Government Printing Office, August 1970, p. 99.
14. Steiner, P. E. *Cancer: Race and geography.* Baltimore, Maryland: Williams and Wilkins, 1964.
15. Haenszel, W., and Taeuber, K. E. Lung cancer mortality as related to residence and smoking history. II. White women. *J. National Cancer Institute*, 1964, *32*, 803-823.
16. Bueckley, R., and Dunn, J. Excess lung cancer-mortality rates among Mexican women in California. *Cancer,* 1957, *10*, 66.
17. Winkelstein, W., Jr., and Gay, M. L. Suspended particulate air pollution. Relationship to mortality from cirrhosis of liver. *Arch. Environ. Health*, 1971, *22*, 174-177.
18. Winkelstein, W., Jr., and Kantor, S. Stomach cancer: Positive association with suspended particulate air pollution. *Arch. Environ. Health*, 1969, *18*, 545-547.
19. Winkelstein, W., Jr., and Kantor, S. Prostatic cancer: Relationship to suspended particulate air pollution. *Amer. J. Public Health*, 1969, *59*, 1134-1138.

20. Firket, J. *Bull. Acad. Roy. Med.* Belg., 1931, *11,* 683, quoted by J. R. Goldsmith, Effects of air pollution on human health. In *Air pollution and its effects.* A. C. Stern, ed., New York and London: Academic Press, 1968.
21. Wehrle, P. F., et al. Pediatric aspects of air pollution. *Pediatrics,* 1970, *46,* 637-639.
22. Douglas, J. W. B., and Waller, R. E. Air pollution and respiratory infection in children. *Brit. J. Prev. Soc. Med.,* 1966, *20,* 1.
23. Air Pollution Control Office. Air quality criteria for nitrogen oxides. Washington, D. C.: Environmental Protection Agency, Publication No. AP-84, 1971.
24. Colley, J. R. T., and Reid, D. C. Urban and social origins of childhood bronchitis in England and Wales. *Brit. Med. J.,* 1970, *2,* 213.
25. Bates, D. V. Air pollutants and the human lung. *Am. Rev. of Resp. Dis.,* 1972, *105,* 3-15.
26. Lave, L. B., and Seskin, E. P. Air pollution and human health. *Science,* 1970, *169,* 723-733.
27. Lave, L. B., and Seskin, E. P. Air pollution, climate, and home heating: Their effects on U. S. mortality rates. *Am. J. Pub. Health,* 1972, *62,* 909-916.
28. Goldsmith, J. R. Effects of air pollution on human health. In *Air pollution and its effects,* A. C. Stern, ed., New York and London: Academic Press, 1968, p. 583.
29. Weill, H., Ziskind, M. M., et al. Recent developments in New Orleans asthma. *Arch. Environ. Health,* 1965, *10,* 148.
30. Hammond, E. C., and Horn, D. Smoking and death rates. Report on 44 months of follow-up of 187,783 men. *J. Amer. Med. Assn.,* 1958, *166,* 1294-1308.
31. Goldsmith, J. R., and Landau, S. A. Carbon monoxide and human health. *Science,* 1968, *162,* 1352-1359.
32. Schulte, J. H. Effects of mild carbon monoxide intoxication. *Arch. Environ. Health,* 1963, *7,* 524-530.
33. Goldsmith, J. R., and Rogers, L. H. Health hazards of automobile exhaust. *Public Health Reports* (U.S.), 1959, *74,* 551-558.
34. Bird, D. *New York Times,* February 26, 1973, p. 23.
35. Environmental quality: First annual report of the Council on Environmental Quality. Washington, D. C.: U.S. Government Printing Office, August 1970, p. 67.
36. Zemactis, W. L. Water and waste water. In *Environmental Health,* P. W. Purdom, ed., New York and London: Academic Press, 1971, Chapter 4, p. 149f.
37. Andersson, et al. Outbreak of giardiasis: Effect of a new anti-flagellate drug, Tinidazole. *Brit. Med. J.,* 1972, *5,* p. 449.
38. Moore, G. T., et al. Epidemic giardiasis at a ski resort. *New England J. Med.,* 1969, *281,* 402.
39. National Commission on Community Health Services. *Changing environmental hazards: Challenges to community health.* Report of Task Force on Environmental Health, 1966, 27-28.

40. Wasserman, L. P. Sweetwater pollution. *Science and Technology*, 1969, 20-27.
41. Patrick, R. Use without abuse of our water resources. In *Environment, man, survival*, L. H. Wullstein, ed., Salt Lake City: University of Utah, 1971, 87-95.
42. Berg, J. W., and Burbank, F. Correlations between carcinogenic trace metals in water supplies and cancer mortality. *Ann. N. Y. Acad. Sciences*, 1972, *199*, 249-264.
43. Perry, H. M., Jr. Hypertension and the geochemical environment. *Ann. N. Y. Acad. Sciences*, 1972, *199*, 202-216.
44. Lynd, F. T. Other degenerative diseases of blood vessels. *Ann. N. Y. Acad. Sciences*, 1972, *199*, 229-235.
45. Correa, P., and Strong, J. P. Atherosclerosis and the geochemical environment: A critical review. *Ann. N. Y. Acad. Sciences*, 1972, *199*, 217-228.

12

Occupational Health: Working Yourself Sick

John M. Peters

Many possible modifications of the environment could prevent disease and promote health; however, certain areas appear more responsive to interference than others. For a number of reasons, occupational health looms as one focus of concern which may yield great returns for efforts expended. It represents an area of great need, but one in which there exists a very real possibility of altering conditions to prevent needless mortality and morbidity. One can separate the potential victim from his source of danger; one can keep high-risk individuals from exposing themselves to potentially harmful work experiences.

On another level, occupational medicine may be the most appropriate testing ground for exploring the health threat of numerous suspected environmental toxins. It stands to reason that if manifestations of disease are not found in persons exposed to levels of a pollutant manyfold greater than that found in the ambient atmosphere, one would not expect to see much illness resulting from lower concentrations among the general public. Thus the study of occupational diseases may serve as a first line of investigation of environmental effects among the public at large. In addition to more intense exposures in the working environment, exposures can be more easily studied because they usually occur one at a time.

For example, concern over the many potential toxic effects of sulfur oxides might first be explored through a study of workers in an industry with heavy exposure to miscellaneous compounds. If these men are found to suffer from certain maladies at rates in excess of the general population (of similar age, sex, and other characteristics), and if other known factors (e.g., smoking habits) cannot account for these differences, then it would be appropriate to launch the sophisticated (and expensive) epidemiologic studies to test the relationship between pollution by SO_2 and ill health. On the other hand, if no increased disease is found among those exposed to high pollutant levels, much time and effort can be saved.

It should not be surprising to learn that in a society in which productivity is as highly valued as it is in the United States, occupational health is a problem of no small magnitude. At least 24,000 Americans are killed each year because of their jobs. Some 14,000 die traumatically while another 10,000 deaths are directly traceable to occupational disease. This latter figure represents a conservative estimate based on known effects of known occupational exposures, mostly physical or chemical in nature; there is a very strong possibility that it would be substantially higher if we knew more about the subtle effects of various other exposures. Morbidity figures are more difficult to obtain but are nonetheless impressive; for example, seven million American workers are regularly exposed to hazardous noise levels. While we are beginning to generate some estimates of the morbidity and mortality wrought by some physical and chemical agents, other surfaces have not even been scratched. We are just beginning to focus attention on less obtrusive factors like psychological effects of working; few investigators have examined the dangers of stress or boredom. Needless to say, even less has been done to explore the potential synergistic relationships between these psychological factors and various physical or chemical stresses.

One might rationalize that these 24,000 known deaths and uncountable others pale in significance when compared to the morbidity and mortality produced by cigarette smoking or automobile accidents. However, the situations from the standpoint of prevention are very different. The prevention of occupational disease depends largely on other than personal factors. It is almost always possible to engineer a work environment that is safe and healthy without relying on the behavior of the worker. On the other hand, reducing the devastation from automobile accidents or from cigarette smoking requires major changes in personal habits. Inducing people to change their behavioral patterns is not easy and, so far, attempts to do so have defied systematic approaches. In contrast, once problems are found in the area of occupational health, the institution of preventive measures is conceivable and practicable. Because most of the diseases produced by the working environment are chronic and untreatable, it is especially important and logical to prevent them.

Occupational health is one area of community medicine in which new knowledge has immediate application and in which prevention can and will work.

In addition to the many chemical insults possible in the working environment, occupational stresses can also be physical as well as psychological. Even the relatively simple problems of assessing the effects of specific chemical or physical agents on the human body are in many cases inadequately understood, especially with regard to chronic diseases and chronic exposures. The rather remarkable mobility of the work force complicates this further. If a specific exposure does not produce a chronic disease until 20 to 30 years have elapsed, the discovery of such a relationship is delayed by the rapid turnover of labor. This turnover phenomenon may retard the understanding of the connection between chronic exposure and chronic disease, but it may also be an inadvertently useful device to protect the worker. On the other hand, multiple exposures could be theoretically worse than a sustained dose if they produce additive or synergistic effects. The number of potential variables which might be considered in various combinations becomes rapidly overwhelming. Small wonder then that solution of an occupational health problem requires a multidisciplinary approach wherein the disciplines involved are dictated by the nature of the problem.

Confronted with a problem or potential problem, the investigator usually follows three basic steps: 1) identifying and quantifying the stress (be it chemical, physical, or psychological); 2) determining the effect of the stress on health; and 3) establishing proper control or preventive measures. This process can be readily illustrated with examples drawn from traditional occupational health problems.

The first step is concerned with establishing the parameters for exposure or stress. Let us assume, for example, that a group of workers is exposed to some dust. As this constitutes an airborne exposure with the lung as the route of entry, it would be important to know how much dust the workers breathed and where in the respiratory system the dust would be deposited. The general approach would be to quantify the dust concentration in the air in the worker's breathing zone and to determine the size distribution of the particles so that the deposition in the lung could be estimated. The industrial hygienist is responsible for this step. He is usually an engineer or a chemist with additional training in biology and toxicology. On the other hand, if the occupational health problem involves radiation, a physicist would provide pertinent exposure information.

The second step usually involves the physician and the identification of the effects of the exposure or stress on health. It may be necessary to employ toxicology, physiology, psychology, or other disciplines, depending on the nature of the problem. The example of dust exposure could involve physiology (pulmonary function tests) if the dust has a primary effect on the lung, or it could involve toxicology if it had a primary effect elsewhere. Once it has been ascertained that the situation has produced unhealthful effects, it must be determined at what levels of exposure these effects are produced. With these two pieces of information the next step can be undertaken.

The third step involves control of the problem. In the case of a dust exposure, the industrial hygienist is called upon again to "engineer" the control. Obviously, controls vary depending on the nature of the problem. For example, ventilation is the most likely mode of control for dust exposure.

CURRENT SURVEILLANCE SYSTEM IN THE UNITED STATES

Would an employer knowingly allow the existence of a working environment that could produce a chronic occupational disease in a worker? Would a worker knowingly take a job that could affect his health adversely? Would the federal government permit these things to happen? Are the universities failing to provide the training and research information necessary to make meaningful decisions about working environments? The answer to all these questions is an unfortunate yes. And in this answer lie most of the reasons why occupational disease still occurs with appalling regularity in the United States.

If this seems dramatic, it ought to. Until very recently there were more federal game wardens in the United States than federal industrial safety and health inspectors; the abuse of birds and game has received more attention than the working conditions of humans. Should an industry that provides jobs be allowed to persist if its workers suffer disease because of their jobs? Who will make that decision?

While significant strides have been made in removing health hazards to workers, and while some large industries have acted admirably in this respect, an inexcusable amount of abuse of the worker's health and safety is still being perpetuated by private industry. This happens for many complex reasons. Some of the simpler ones include:

1. *Size and number problems.* In the United States there are 3.5 million employers of 80 million workers. Of these, 3.1 million employers have fewer than 20 workers. Only 26,000 employers have more than 250 workers. There is an inverse relationship between the size of the industry and the rate of occupational disease among its employees; the larger an industry, the better it can afford to secure the expert service it needs to provide safe and healthful working conditions.

2. *Competition.* Because safe working conditions require financial investment, the industry that de-emphasizes safety and health could theoretically undersell the more conscientious industry. This translates into money and profits—the hallmark of American industry.

Moreover, there are major economic dis-incentives against a corporation even acknowledging that an illness may be work related for fear of incurring severe penalties through workmen's compensation. The mine owners of West Virginia have refused to recognize the relationship between pneumoconiosis, or black lung, and working in the coal mines. The companies operating uranium mines have refuted all efforts to link higher rates of lung cancer to such radioactive exposures.

Once the causal link is established between occupational exposure and illness, the company becomes liable for the costs of maintaining the employee affected as well as the costs of his care. The threat of such potentially vast liability should serve as an impetus to seek more effective preventive measures. Too often it stimulates more intense defensive litigation instead.

3. *Diffusion of responsibility.* The stockholder owns the company, but the management runs the company and is expected to produce a profit. Few companies are willing to go into the red to pay for environmental controls to protect their workers. However, it is difficult to identify the person at fault when a worker is made chronically ill by his work. The responsibility is diffused among the several echelons of management and ownership, to say nothing of the role of the unions.

Traditionally, workers and members of trade unions have not been very interested in protecting their own health. The general reaction of the worker when confronted with a hazardous job has been to request and receive hazard pay. This is changing, perhaps in response to the general environmental awakening. The worker, like all other human beings, is beginning to question the effects of his job on his life and his future. Even prior to the Occupational Safety and Health (OSH) Act of 1970, the International Union of

Rubber Workers (IURW) negotiated for and won the establishment of an occupational health research fund to be given to an outside institution to conduct research relating to occupational hazards in the rubber industry. The first such three-way agreement was signed in 1971 by IURW, the B. F. Goodrich Company, and the Harvard University School of Public Health. This occupational medicine landmark represents the cooperation, interest, concern, and teamwork that are necessary to do the job that so far has not been done. The achievement of occupational health in America rests more with the worker than with any other sector of industry. If the worker stays concerned and interested, he will get the working conditions he deserves.

4. *Manpower.* Even if an industry wanted to supply the best and safest working conditions for its employees, it is sometimes difficult to find the necessary experts to institute them. Occupational medicine is not a popular specialty; in 1972 there were fewer than 300 physicians with specific training in this field. This deficiency may be caused in part by the expectations of industry in regard to industrial physicians. Too often they are placed in a position in which their loyalties to their patients and their employers are divided. Too often this field seems to attract the less competent physicians. Unfortunately, many of the same deterrents appear to apply to the field of industrial hygiene as well.

Universities have also been negligent in that most medical schools teach little or no occupational medicine and have almost no specialists in occupational medicine on their faculties. While many medical schools are developing programs in community medicine, not many of them include occupational health problems in their purview. Schools of public health have done only slightly better, but the number of full-time academic persons interested primarily in occupational medicine is small indeed. This may be due in part to lack of federal support for research in this area, lack of access to industrial problems, and a general lack of interest on the part of academicians. Again, the OSH Act of 1970 should produce changes in this area.

5. *Insufficient governmental surveillance.* Until the passage of the OSH Act of 1970, the federal government was minimally involved in occupational disease surveillance.

The most remarkable thing about state surveillance has been its complete lack of uniformity. Some industrialized northern and eastern states have had good state programs; most southern states have not. This variance has resulted in some rather appalling adventures to the detriment of the worker. One example will illustrate this: A large eastern state outlawed the production of beta naphthylamine because it produced bladder cancer in many workers. The factory closed only to reopen in a southern state where no such ban existed, much less an occupational health surveillance system. As a result, southern workers have been developing bladder cancer at an unconscionable rate. Lack of uniformity in workmen's compensation laws has also been a paramount feature of our patchwork state pattern. The OSH Act of 1970 promises wholesale change in both areas because it supplies the machinery to eradicate the problems described above. However, accomplishing its successful enforcement will require many years, much money, and much manpower.

The OSH Act, with its far-reaching health and social implications, ostensibly was promulgated because ". . . personal injuries and illnesses arising out of work situations impose a substantial burden upon, and are a hindrance to, interstate commerce in terms of lost production, wage loss, medical expenses, and disability compensation payments."

The Act provides for the preservation of human resources by:

> . . . authorizing the Secretary of Labor to set mandatory occupational safety and health standards applicable to businesses affecting interstate commerce, and by creating an Occupational Safety and Health Review Commission for carrying out adjudicatory functions under the Act;
> . . . providing for research in the field of occupational safety and health, including the psychological factors involved, and by developing innovative methods, techniques, and approaches for dealing with occupational safety and health problems;
> . . . providing medical criteria which will assure insofar as practicable that no employee will suffer diminished health, functional capacity, or life expectancy as a result of his work experience;
> . . . providing for training programs to increase the number and competence of personnel engaged in the field of occupational safety and health;
> . . . providing for the development and promulgation of occupational safety and health standards;
> . . . providing an effective enforcement program which shall include a prohibition against giving advance notice of any inspection and sanctions for any individual violating this prohibition;

> . . . encouraging the States to assume the fullest responsibility for the administration and enforcement of their occupational safety and health laws by providing grants to the States to assist in identifying their needs and responsibilities in the area of occupational safety and health, to develop plans in accordance with the provisions of this Act, to improve the administration and enforcement of State occupational safety and health laws, and to conduct experimental and demonstration projects in connection therewith; and
> . . . providing for appropriate reporting procedures with respect to occupational safety and health which procedures will help achieve the objectives of this Act and accurately describe the nature of the occupational safety and health problem.

The Act provides for inspections, citations, and penalties. It also established the National Institute of Occupational Safety and Health (NIOSH) within the Department of Health, Education and Welfare (HEW). The Secretary of HEW has the following responsibilities which are in turn delegated to NIOSH:

1. The development of . . . research, experiments, and demonstrations relating to occupational safety and health, including studies of psychological factors involved, and relating to innovative methods, techniques, and approaches for dealing with occupational safety and health problems.
2. The development of . . . criteria dealing with toxic materials and harmful physical agents and substances which will describe exposure levels that are safe for various periods of employment, including but not limited to the exposure levels at which no employee will suffer impaired health or functional capacities or diminished life expectancy as a result of his work experience.
3. The exploration of . . . problems . . . created by new technology . . . including research into the motivational and behavioral factors relating to the field of occupational safety and health.
4. The prescription of . . . regulations requiring employers to measure, record, and make reports on the exposure of employees to substances or physical agents which . . . may endanger the health and safety of employees.
5. The establishment of . . . programs of medical examinations and tests as may be necessary for determining the incidence of occupational illnesses and the susceptibility of employees to such illnesses.

6. The publication of . . . [an annual] list of all known toxic substances by generic family or other useful grouping, and the concentrations at which such toxicity is known to occur.
7. The conduction and publication of . . . [annual] industry-wide studies of the effect of chronic or low-level exposure to industrial materials, processes, and stresses on the potential for illness, disease, or loss of functional capacity in aging adults.

If adequately carried out, the OSH Act of 1970 would circumvent most of the problems attributed to private industry, governmental agencies, universities, and workers. This important and significant piece of health legislation will require much effort to implement. It represents the beginnings of what might someday be adequate surveillance.

Safe Exposure Limits

Today, approximately 5000 chemical substances are in common use in American industry. Each year our technology introduces about 500 new ones. From a toxicologic standpoint we know very little about many of these compounds. The American Conference of Governmental Industrial Hygienists (ACGIH) has seen fit to promulgate threshold limit values (TLVs) for about 500 substances.

TLVs refer to time-weighted, airborne concentrations which are set to protect "nearly all workers" who may be exposed eight hours a day, 40 hours a week, and presumably for a working lifetime. The ACGIH describes TLVs as "guides in the control of health hazards." Interestingly, these values were adopted by the Occupational Safety and Health Act of 1970 as interim legal limits for exposure until the National Institute of Occupational Safety and Health (NIOSH) could develop its own criteria and standards.

A consideration of the basis for the TLVs will illustrate the depth (or lack) of knowledge concerning the effects of chronic exposure to many materials, even to substances that have been around for many years. Approximately 38 percent of the TLVs are based on human experience and give consideration to the chronic effects of exposure. If one examines the data from which these numbers are derived he will find that many lack the support of sound epidemiologic studies. Certainly, to set valid TLVs one would need adequate exposure information together with ample data on the health effects of exposure. Sometimes the two are available, but not commonly from the same study.

Eleven percent of the TLVs are based on experiments involving human volunteers. These studies necessarily relate to acute toxicity because an investigator cannot expose a "volunteer" for 40 years; therefore, they essentially exclude the possibility of studying chronic effects. For example, the effects of SO_2 on human beings have been studied in the laboratory under acute exposures. The TLVs are in part derived from these experiments. To this day no adequate study has been conducted to determine the chronic occupational effects of SO_2. On the other hand, SO_2 is a common atmospheric pollutant, thought by some to produce chronic effects in the general population.

What is even more appalling is that 51 percent of the TLVs are based only on animal experiments (27 percent) or set by chemical analogy (24 percent). Even assuming that animal data apply to man, which is a large assumption, most animal experiments on toxicity are either acute or subacute in nature and do not examine adequately the question of chronic effects. This is not to blame the ACGIH or anyone else but to point out the severe limitations of our knowledge regarding hazards which confront the worker who might be exposed. The worker is essentially a guinea pig.

In addition to the TLVs being as questionable as they are, there are several other toxicologic possibilities that may not even be considered when they are set. For example, it is clear that if we do not know very well what one substance will do, we have little chance of predicting what the interactions of two or more might be. By the same token, we have little ability to monitor the doubling, tripling, or even tenfold increase of an uncommon tumor in a relatively small group of workers. For example, the discovery of excess bladder cancer in the leather industry required the most sophisticated epidemiologic techniques, even when the risk of the leather worker is an unsubtle 20 times that of another working group. How many less overt risks are we likely to overlook even when seeking them specifically? It is even more difficult to discover the mutagenic and teratogenic effects that can be anticipated from chemical exposures.

Clearly, we are relying more on the inherent toughness and resiliency of man than on knowledge of occupational exposures and their effects.

PREVENTION AND THE STRATEGY OF CONTROL

Despite the gaps in our current knowledge about the totality of risks posed by the occupational environment, there is a logical sequence of steps to control occupational hazards. As is often the case, the most instinctive reaction is not always the best. The use of a protective respirator to solve a problem of airborne pollution should remain a last resort rather than a primary response. Whenever possible, the following priorities should be observed:

Substitution. If a worker is exposed to a toxic chemical, first consideration should be given to substituting a substance that is less toxic within the range of the industrial process under consideration. A good example of how simple substitution can solve a serious problem is the replacement of benzene (benzol), which produces aplastic anemia and leukemia, with toluene or xylene, which does not. Similarly, fiberglas has recently been substituted for asbestos, a potent fibrogenic and carcinogenic agent.

Enclosure or isolation. If substitution is not possible, and it frequently is not, the next priority in control consists of constructing a barrier between the exposure and the worker. This principle is illustrated by the enclosure of a noisy machine or by the use of closed systems in chemical processing. In steel processing, for example, heat is an important problem and very difficult to control. Special air-conditioned booths or cubicles (mini-environments) can be constructed for the worker in such a setting.

Ventilation. If substitution, enclosure, or isolation is not possible, ventilation is the next consideration for dust, gas, vapor mist or smoke problems. Control by ventilation includes both local exhaust and general ventilation. If one has a workroom with a single source of occupational exposure, for example, a tank full of solvent, the obvious way to handle this would be by local exhaust ventilation of the tank rather than general ventilation of the room. Situations in which general ventilation would be superior are easy to imagine. An important, but often ignored, principle of ventilation is the need to take the offending material away from the breathing zone of the worker. All too frequently one finds an exhaust system in which the worker must spend time with his nose between the pollution source and the exhaust hood. This obviously can be worse for the worker than no ventilation at all.

Personal protection. Only when it is not possible to control an occupational hazard by the mechanisms described above should personal protective devices be considered. Certain working conditions preclude control by other than personal protection—fire fighting, for example. The fire fighter rarely knows what environmental conditions he will encounter. Each burning building he enters offers a multitude of possible exposures including various combinations of low oxygen, high carbon monoxide, heavy smoke particulates, irritant gases, and heat. The best protection for the fire fighter is for him to carry his own environment with him (protective hat, coat, boots, and air supply).

As a means of respiratory protection, masks are hot and uncomfortable, require special fitting to avoid leakage, and increase breathing resistance. This latter point can be a very significant factor, depending on either the man's health or the physical demands of the job. For example, an asbestos worker with early asbestosis and some shortness of breath is going to have difficulty tolerating a respiratory device that increases his work of breathing. By the same token, the worker with normal lungs who must perform significant work will also find the mask an impediment. For these and other reasons, the worker may be unlikely to wear his respiratory device and, hence, this means of protection may not be generally successful.

Medical surveillance. Ideally, the working environment should be so controlled that medical surveillance is not necessary. For example, if a noise source is controlled to the extent that no worker is exposed to more than 80 decibels, then it is not necessary to survey the workers with audiograms. Such control is not always possible. In most situations, control is not easily accomplished, and a medical surveillance procedure is required to measure the impact of the environmental factors. However, medical monitoring is only a secondary adjunct and should not be considered part of the basic control process. It should be viewed only as a means of verifying the success rate of any control procedure.

CLASSIFICATION OF OCCUPATIONAL DISEASE

In the search for the etiology of a patient's problem, it may well behoove today's practitioner to suspect the occupational environment as an important possible cause. The contemporary physician, however, is at an extreme disadvantage on several counts. First, he usually knows little about industry or its possible exposures; second, the fact that he sees patients one at a time means that he would detect only gross epidemics; and third, he is usually taught little or nothing about occupational diseases or how to take an occupational history. The remainder of this chapter will attempt to provide information which, at least in part, will help correct these deficiencies.

Agents Producing Occupational Disease

It is clearly beyond the scope of this chapter to list and describe all the known occupational diseases. The interested reader is referred to Donald Hunter's *Diseases of Occupations,* or the International Labor Office's two-volume encyclopedia, *Occupational Health and Safety.* However, an outline of some of the well-defined occupational health problems, along with some of the features of each, is presented here to give some idea of the scope and breadth of today's problem. Table 1 classifies some of the well-described occupational diseases by etiologic agent.

OCCUPATIONAL HISTORY

A frequently neglected part of the clinical work-up is obtaining the occupational history. This information is important for at least three reasons: 1) to establish the correct diagnosis; 2) to advise the patient about the risk of returning to work after treatment; and 3) to correct the working conditions so that other cases are prevented. The last action is all too seldom carried out. In most states, occupational illness is a reportable disease. Because many occupational diseases (the occupational lung diseases especially) are chronic diseases for which there is no satisfactory treatment, it is obviously very important to prevent them. Unless the physician is willing to initiate corrective action, the likelihood of more cases is high. In many states all that may be required is a telephone call to the responsible state agency.

An adequate occupational history requires the history-taker to have: 1) a strategy for unearthing all appropriate information, and 2) a working knowledge of clinical conditions which can be caused by occupational exposure.

Taking an Occupational History

The procedure for acquiring a complete occupational history is to ascertain, beginning with the time the subject first left school, all of his full-time jobs, the locations and names of the companies, the title of the jobs and the exposures involved, and the duration of employment in each job. Unfortunately, workers are not always

TABLE 1

CLASSIFICATION OF OCCUPATIONAL DISEASE BY ETIOLOGIC AGENT

I. CHEMICAL AGENTS

A. Metals

Agent	*System(s) Affected*	*Principal Manifestation(s)*	*Diagnostic Laboratory Tests*
Lead	Gastrointestinal Neuromuscular Hematopoietic Central nervous	Abdominal pain (colic) Palsy (wrist drop) Anemia Encephalopathy	↑Urine and blood Pb ↑ΔALA—urine ↑Coproporphyrin III
Mercury	Central nervous Oral mucous membranes Renal	Stomatitis and gingivitis Tremor Erethism	↑Urine and blood Hg Depressed renal function
Cadmium	Pulmonary Renal	Pulmonary edema (acute) Emphysema (chronic) Nephritis	Characteristic urinary protein
Chromium	Respiratory Cutaneous	Dermatitis Skin ulcers Nasal septal perforation Lung cancer	
Beryllium	Pulmonary Other	Pulmonary granulomatosis and fibrosis	Beryllium in urine (acute) Beryllium in tissue (chronic)
B. Solvents			
Benzene (benzol)	Hematopoietic Central nervous	Aplastic anemia Leukemia Narcosis	↑Phenol in urine ↓Blood count
Carbon tetra-chloride	Hepatic Renal	Toxic hepatitis Oliguria or anuria	Function tests, renal and hepatic
Carbon disulfide	Central nervous Renal	Mania Acceleration of atherogenesis Chronic renal disease Parkinsonian syndrome	↑Cholesterol and lipids Renal function tests
Methyl alcohol	Ocular	Blindness	Acidosis

Agent	*System(s) Affected*	*Principal Manifestation(s)*	*Diagnostic Laboratory Tests*
Irritants	Respiratory*	Upper respiratory irritation Bronchospasm Pulmonary edema Chemical pneumonitis	X-ray Pulmonary function tests
Examples: Ammonia Hydrochloric acid Hydrofluoric acid	Upper	Irritation	
Sulfur dioxide Chlorine Fluorine	Middle	Bronchospasm (Pulmonary edema or chemical pneumonitis in high dose)	
Ozone Nitrogen dioxide Phosgene	Lower	Delayed pulmonary edema (as a rule 6-8 hours following exposure)	
Asphyxiants			
Simple asphyxiants**	Central nervous	Anoxia	$\downarrow O_2$ in environment
Chemical asphyxiants: carbon monoxide	Blood-oxygen transport	Headache Dizziness	Carboxyhemoglobin
hydrogen sulfide	Respiratory center paralysis	Hypoventilation Irritation of respiratory tract	$\downarrow pO_2$
cyanide	Cellular enzymes (cytochrome oxidase)	Anoxia	

*Site of action in respiratory system depends on H_2O solubility—the less soluble the gas the deeper the irritant effect and the more delayed the effect.

**Have no specific toxic effect; act by displacing O_2. Examples: N_2, H_2, CH_4.

(Continued)

CLASSIFICATION OF OCCUPATIONAL DISEASE BY ETIOLOGIC AGENT, Continued

D. Dusts

Agent	*System(s) or Organs Affected*	*Principal Manifestation(s)*	*Diagnostic Laboratory Tests*
Inorganic			
Silica	Pulmonary	Nodular fibrosis (silicosis) Chronic obstructive lung disease	X-ray Pulmonary function tests
Asbestos	Pulmonary Peritoneum	Diffuse fibrosis (asbestosis) Lung cancer Mesothelioma	X-ray Pulmonary function tests Asbestos bodies
Talc	Pulmonary	Fibrosis Pleural thickening	X-ray Pulmonary function tests
Coal	Pulmonary	Chronic obstructive lung disease Coal workers' pneumoconiosis	Pulmonary function tests X-ray
Others: Kaolin Mica Diatomaceous earth Aluminum	Pulmonary	Fibrosis	Pulmonary function tests X-ray
Organic			
Cotton	Pulmonary	Chronic obstructive lung disease (byssinosis)	Pulmonary function tests (no specific X-ray change)
Detergent enzymes	Pulmonary	Bronchitis Pneumonitis Asthma	Pulmonary function tests X-ray
Hay	Pulmonary	Granulomatous reaction (farmer's lung)	X-ray Pulmonary function tests
Sugar cane	Pulmonary	Granulomatous reaction (bagassosis)	X-ray Pulmonary function tests

E. Some Carcinogenic Chemicals

Agent	*Organ Affected*	*Type of Cancer*
Benzene	Bone marrow	Leukemia
Nickel	Lung	Lung cancer

Asbestos	Lung Peritoneum	Lung cancer Mesothelioma	
Arsenicals	Skin	Skin cancer	
Coal tar	Skin Lung	Skin cancer Lung cancer	
Analine dyes* Beta naphthylamine Alpha naphthylamine Benzidine Auramine Magenta	Bladder	Bladder cancer	

II. SOME PHYSICAL AGENTS PRODUCING OCCUPATIONAL DISEASE

A. Noise

Agent	*Organ(s) or Systems Affected*	*Principal Manifestation(s)*	*Diagnostic Laboratory Tests*
Noise	Ear Central nervous system	Deafness Stress	Audiometer
B. Radiation			
Ionizing (alpha, beta, gamma, X-ray and neutrons)	Bone marrow	Leukemia	Bone marrow or blood studies
	Eye Bone	Other cancer (Lung cancer in uranium miners or bone cancer in radium dial painters, for example) Cataracts	Slit lamp exam Chest X-ray
Non-ionizing			
Ultraviolet Infrared Microwaves	Eye Skin	Corneal irritation Cataracts Cancer of skin	Slit lamp

*Excluding analine itself, which is not carcinogenic.

(Continued)

CLASSIFICATION OF OCCUPATIONAL DISEASE BY ETIOLOGIC AGENT, Continued

C. Temperature

Agent	*Organ(s) or Systems Affected*	*Principal Manifestation(s)*	*Diagnostic Laboratory Tests*
Heat and cold	Temperature regulation	Hypo- or hyperthermia "Cold injury" or "heat stress"	

D. Pressure

High and low pressure	Hollow cavities Bone	"Squeeze" Air embolism Bone necrosis (caisson disease)	X-ray of bones

III. BIOLOGICAL AGENTS

A. Bacteria

Agent	*Disease*	*Groups Commonly Affected*
B. anthracis	Anthrax	Wool workers Cattle breeders
M. tuberculosis	Tuberculosis	Nurses, doctors, other hospital workers
Brucella melitensis	Brucellosis	Veterinarians Farmers Meat packers Laboratory workers

B. Rickettsia

Coxiella burneti	Q fever	Abbatoir workers Meat packers Stock handlers

C. Viral

Viral	Hepatitis	Doctors, nurses, and other hospital personnel

aware of their exposures. This lack can be overcome in part by the physician acquiring more knowledge of industrial processes and potential exposures, especially of those in the geographic area of his practice.

It is important to also record hobbies and moonlighting jobs. The worker will often give a vague name for a product that he has worked with or he might mention an occupational title that is foreign. If one suspects that there is a relationship between the occupation and the disease, or wants to rule out that possibility, the state agency responsible for industrial hygiene may be helpful or the company for which the man works might provide useful information. It is often necessary to trace the product in question to the original producer. At times the producer will not voluntarily reveal the chemical nature of his material, but under the OSH Act of 1970 he can be required to divulge this information.

COMMON CLINICAL CONDITIONS WITH POSSIBLE OCCUPATIONAL CAUSE

Lung Cancer. Everyone thinks of cigarette smoking in association with pulmonary cancer, but there are several occupational exposures that produce lung cancer as well, often in conjunction with cigarette smoking. In terms of numbers, asbestos probably produces more lung cancers than any other occupational exposure. It is interesting that workers (for example, pipe coverers or insulation workers) who smoke increase their risk of lung cancer very dramatically—their risk of developing a tumor is 90 times greater than that of a nonsmoking nonasbestos-exposed worker. The lung cancer incidence in uranium miners is also very high and, again, cigarette smoking has an additive or synergistic effect. The bronchogenic carcinoma of uranium miners is produced by alpha radiation of the radon daughters. The co-carcinogenic effect of smoking probably relates directly to the alpha radiation of polonium 210, a natural constituent of cigarette smoke. Chrome, nickel, and arsenic are known occupational causes of lung cancer as well.

Pulmonary edema. Noncardiac causes of pulmonary edema must be considered in the differential diagnosis. Pulmonary irritants should receive particular attention. Because of the delay between exposure and onset (usually 6–8 hours, sometimes as long as 24 hours), it is difficult to connect the exposure with the disease unless the physician is aware of the possibility and inquires into it. Some of the pulmonary irritants which should be considered are nitrogen dioxide, phosgene, ozone, and the halogen gases (Cl_2, Br_2, F_2). However, some more unusual substances may cause pulmonary irritation; for example, fermenting silage yields nitrogen dioxide which may cause a form of pulmonary edema called silo-filler's disease. Exposure can also occur in more common situations such as welding or fire fighting.

Hepatitis. Halogenated hydrocarbons, especially carbon tetrachloride but also DDT, should be considered as possible causatives. Serum or infectious hepatitis can also be job related in hospital occupations, for example.

Abdominal pain. One should always consider the possibility of lead poisoning in the differential diagnosis of abdominal pain. The principal occupations known to involve lead exposure which should be familiar to surgeons include babbitt working, battery making, enamel making or using, lead mining, milling and smelting, painting, plumbing, pottery working, ship dismantling, soldering, and welding.

Aplastic anemia and leukemia. Either diagnosis should prompt the physician to inquire into the possibility of the patient having been exposed to benzene. Recently, small shops where furniture is refinished have been found to have high benzene exposures from the solvent in the stripping material used. Usually the user does not know to what solvent he is exposed. Benzene is also often a contaminant of less harmful solvents such as toluene (toluol) and xylene (xylol). Radiation exposure must also be considered.

Acute psychoses. Psychiatrists especially should be familiar with toxic psychoses, some of which can have a work-related cause. Such substances as lead (especially organic lead), mercury (especially methyl mercury), carbon disulfide (used in viscose rayon production), and several other solvents can induce acute psychic disturbances.

Sarcoidosis. Salem sarcoidosis was first diagnosed in Massachusetts in the 1940s and clustered in persons engaged in fluorescent lamp manufacture; beryllium was later incriminated as the cause. Today beryllium is widely used, especially in many metal alloys. Machinists, particularly, are at risk even when working with metals containing as little as 1 percent beryllium. Beryllium must always be considered in the differential diagnosis of diffuse fibrotic or granulomatous pulmonary diseases.

Chronic obstructive pulmonary disease. Easily the most important factor contributing to this syndrome is cigarette smoking. However, certain occupational exposures must also be considered. The end stage of chronic cotton dust exposure (grade III byssinosis) is indistinguishable from cigarette-induced chronic bronchitis and/or emphysema. Polyurethane manufacture involves exposure to toluene diisocyanate which appears to produce, after prolonged exposure, chronic obstructive lung disease in some cases. Cadmium has also produced emphysema on chronic exposure, and chronic low-level exposure to pulmonary irritants, including SO_2, Cl_2, and welding fumes, are suspected but not yet proven causes.

Bladder cancer. About 20 to 40 percent of bladder cancer can be attributed to occupational exposure. The leather and rubber industries in particular are associated with bladder cancer. The dyestuffs industry has also produced many cases, especially from exposure to beta naphthylamine, benzidine, auramine, and magenta, but not analine.

Pulmonary fibrosis. There are several important occupational causes of pulmonary fibrosis. The classic condition of nodular fibrosis is, of course, silicosis, resulting from exposure to silica. In the United States there are still 3000 new cases of silicosis each year, since hard rock miners, foundry workers, granite workers, construction workers, and even coal miners frequently develop this chronic, serious, untreatable disease. While nodular fibrosis is the usual pattern in silicosis, linear fibrosis occurs in asbestos workers. As noted earlier, chronic disease caused by beryllium exposure can also take the form of chronic fibrosis. Other less commonly encountered occupational exposures which can also induce a fibrotic reaction include, for example, those caused by talc, mica, diatomaceous earth, and aluminum dust.

Peripheral neuropathy. The differential diagnosis of peripheral neuropathy must include investigating exposure to certain heavy metals (lead and mercury) as well as carbon disulfide.

Cataracts. Exposure to sources of both ionizing and nonionizing radiation should be considered. Neutron exposure especially, but also gamma or x-rays, will produce cataracts. Infrared and microwave exposures will also induce cataractogenic effects.

A CASE ILLUSTRATION

Occupational disease is a large problem in the United States. Perhaps the scope of occupational health can best be illustrated by the following story. I was asked to visit an industrial plant in rural Massachusetts which manufactured crushed velvet. The plant manager was concerned about several episodes of illness among the workers. He himself had developed symptoms including chest pain and cough, with an abnormal electrocardiogram and elevated enzymes. His diagnosis was acute myocardial infarction and, after spending several days in the hospital, he remained at home six weeks before returning to work. Another worker had been hospitalized twice with a diagnosis of acute viral illness. Still another worker had consulted his private practitioner with complaints of cough, dry throat, pain in the chest, weakness, fever, and chills; he was referred to a neurologist and later to a psychiatrist, but no definitive diagnosis was made by any of these physicians.

The first step in evaluating this problem was to gain an understanding of the industrial process involved. I considered the toxicity of each of the basic materials used to make the crushed velvet and then followed the process from beginning to end, noting where exposures might take place and where the affected employees had been working. No processes or materials appeared particularly toxic or hazardous; none seemed potentially responsible for the symptoms that the three workers had described. However, the workers with symptoms handled the material after it had been dipped in a substance which was used to act as a water and stain repellent. This particular chemical was a fluoropolymer hydrocarbon containing fluorine. In no place was this material heated above 340° F. (It is usually considered that this material must be heated to about 500° F. to produce any toxic products which could possibly be responsible for the conditions described.)

With only this one unsatisfactory lead, I interviewed all workers in this particular part of the plant and identified a constant and characteristic factor. Typically the worker would feel perfectly well on arrival at work, only to note, after two or three hours, the onset of dryness in the throat, dry hacking cough, pain in the chest, shaking chills, weakness of the legs, and sometimes nausea and headache. Of the 14 workers interviewed, 7 described such experiences. After the symptoms and other data gathered on these workers were displayed in tabular form, it could be seen that the 7 affected workers were smokers, while the 7 unaffected workers were nonsmokers. The picture was consistent with polymer fume fever secondary to the fluoropolymer used in the process. Further questioning revealed that the onset of symptoms frequently occurred shortly after smoking a cigarette. As a cigarette burns at approximately 800° F, a cigarette contaminated with fluoropolymer could readily produce the polymer fume to cause the disease; it is estimated that as little as 1 mg on a cigarette will produce the necessary toxic material. In this case, I made one recommendation—that the workers wash their hands before smoking. This recommendation was carried out with the subsequent disappearance of polymer fume fever in this factory.

The foregoing story has relevance to occupational medicine because it illustrates several important points. A disease indistinguishable from a short, flu-like illness was caused by an occupational exposure. It is clear that in the three cases initially described, the physicians failed to identify the occupational cause of the illness This is certainly understandable. In the first case, the plant manager unnecessarily lost eight weeks of work and had suffered an untold amount of anxiety concerning a possible heart attack. (It was later ascertained that his ECG abnormality had been present on his induction into the Navy 20 years earlier.) The second worker who had been hospitalized twice with allegedly acute viral illness ran up a considerable medical bill and again suffered undue anxiety and apprehension as a result of this illness. The third worker saw three physicians and paid three medical bills with no satisfactory solution to his problem. The ease with which the problem was solved once it was understood stands in striking contrast.

Many new materials are being introduced into the environment at an accelerating rate. At this point, it is reasonable to assume that the use of water and stain repellent materials in the home could similarly produce problems among unsuspecting persons through the same process of contaminated cigarettes. The polymer fume fever would again be indistinguishable from a short, severe, flu-like illness. Polymer fume fever is an acute disease from which recovery is thought to be complete and, as such, is certainly a less important occupational disease than most, which are chronic and untreatable. Nonetheless, this story illustrates some of the complexities facing not only the worker, but also the physician and, potentially, each of us as consumers in a technological society. Occupational disease does exist and is frequently unrecognized when it presents in the doctor's office. An interest and awareness of this possibility on the part of practitioners would do much toward reducing occupational disease today.

RECOMMENDED READING

Books of General Interest

1. *Asbestos and Enzymes.* Paul Brodeur, Ballantine Books, New York, 1972. Paperback, $1.25. An interesting, well-written account of the asbestos and detergent enzyme problems including health, social, political, and economic ramifications. Originally appeared in *New Yorker* magazine.
2. *Occupational Epidemic. The Ralph Nader Task Force Report on Job Health and Safety.* Joseph A. Page, Mary-Win O'Brien Center for Study of Responsible Law, Washington, D. C., 1972. A thorough account of conditions as they exist today in the working environment. Includes a commentary on the Occupational Safety and Health Act of 1970.
3. *The President's Report on Occupational Safety and Health.* U.S. Government Printing Office, Washington, D. C. 20402, 1972, $1.75.
4. *Exploring the Dangerous Trades.* Alice Hamilton, Augustus M. Kelley, Clifton, New Jersey, 1972. A fascinating autobiography of the American leader for reform in occupational health practices. First female faculty member at Harvard, Dr. Hamilton recounts her adventures with industrial leaders of 50 years ago to improve working conditions.
5. *De Morbis Artificum (Diseases of Workers) 1713.* Barnardino Ramazzini, New York Academy of Medicine, Harper Publishing Co., New York, 1914. Translated from the Latin text of 1713, this book describes many of the occupational diseases of today with amazing accuracy. This means that either Ramazzini was very perceptive, or we haven't made much progress, or both. Diseases associated with over 50 occupations ranging from wet nursing to blacksmithing are described.
6. *Work Is Dangerous to Your Health.* J. Stellman and J. Daum, Pantheon, 1973. Written for workers, this book describes human physiology and exposures that affect it.

Books with Specific Information about Occupational Diseases

1. *The Diseases of Occupations.* Donald Hunter, Little, Brown & Co., Boston, 1969. The most complete textbook describing occupational diseases to date. Written with considerable historical perspective. Some parts are a little out of date but in general it is extremely useful.
2. *Toxicity of Industrial Metals.* E. Browning, Appleton-Century-Crofts, New York, 1969. An excellent book on the practical toxicology of metals found in industry. Includes review of the literature and clinical aspects of each metal's toxic effects.
3. *Toxicity and Metabolism of Industrial Solvents.* E. Browning, Elsevier Publishing Co., Amsterdam-London-New York, 1965. As above except that the focus is on solvents.

4. *Occupational Diseases: A Guide to Their Recognition.* U.S. Department of Health, Education and Welfare, U. S. Government Printing Office, Washington, D. C., 1964. $2.25. This book summarizes a tremendous amount of material, but does not include much detail. Describes the major disease processes associated with various exposures and outlines the occupations in which these exposures may be encountered.
5. *Encyclopedia of Occupational Health and Safety.* International Labor Office, Geneva, 1971, McGraw-Hill. One of the best places to begin to find out about an occupational health problem. It is well organized and includes information on treatment for various occupational diseases.

13

Psychosocial Factors in the Genesis of Disease

John Cassel

The dramatic changes that have occurred in the nature of the diseases afflicting Western society over the last hundred years have been well documented, but the extraordinary regularity with which these changes have occurred in countries which have undergone industrialization has been less well recognized. In all countries for which we have data it would appear that the earliest health consequences of industrialization and the concurrent urbanization have been an intensification of diseases which have historically been the plagues of mankind, namely the infectious diseases. Thus in Great Britain and the United States, industrialization was initially accompanied by an increase in tuberculosis rates. This disease reached its peak over a period of some 50 to 75 years and then began to decline. It is worth noting that this decline took place before the discovery of the tubercle bacillus and several decades before any organized antituberculosis program was initiated. Furthermore, the decline in incidence has continued at about the same rate over the last 75 to 80 years notwithstanding the discovery of new and important drugs for the treatment of this disease (1). As tuberculosis began to decline it was replaced as a central health problem in both Britain and the United States by major malnutrition syndromes. In Britain rickets was the scourge, in the United States, pellagra. For reasons that also are only partially understood, these disorders, in turn, reached a peak, declined and were themselves replaced by some of the diseases of early childhood. These, too, waxed and then waned largely, but not entirely, under the influence of improvements in the sanitary environment and through the introduction of immunization programs, to be replaced between the two world wars by an extraordinary increase in the rate of duodenal ulcer, particularly in young men. This phenomenon, while more marked in Britain, occurred in the United States as well and was accompanied by a marked shift in the male-female ratio of the disease (2). Gradually, for totally unknown reasons, these rates have declined and have been replaced by our current epidemics of coronary heart disease, hypertension, cancer, arthritis, diabetes, mental disorders, and the like. There is some evidence that some of these disorders have reached a peak and are now declining. Death rates from hypertensive heart disease, for example, apparently have been declining in the United States since about 1940–1950 (3).

A NEW INTERPRETATION

Despite intensive research, the explanations for the genesis of these changes in disease patterns have so far proved to be relatively unsatisfactory. Attention has been focused on the introduction of new pollutants and toxicants into the air and water and on the reduction of old ones, on the increasing amount of ionizing radiation in the environment, and on the hazards associated with pesticides and food additives. Changes in plant and animal life and the changing nature of the microorganisms with which man comes into contact have also received considerable attention. The influence of certain aspects of behavior—exercise, diet, cigarette smoking, and alcohol consumption have been studied in some detail. None of these changes, however, has afforded a very satisfactory explanation for the occurrence of the new diseases or for the decline of the old ones. One of the consequences of dissatisfaction with the more orthodox explanations has been an awakening of interest in the possible role of social and cultural stress factors as determinants of disease. This interest has been reinforced by the realization that changes in the social structure and in the values, attitudes, and beliefs which accompanied the industrial revolution have occurred equally as rapidly as have the changes in technology and in the physical and biological environment, and that they may have equal importance in determining the forms of health problems manifest in any society. Thus, while there is still general agreement with the notion that man's health is to a large extent influenced by the nature of his environment, the ideas about the causative factors in this environment have been broadened from the physicochemical and biological to include the presence of other members of the human species.

Evidence to support this point of view comes from animal behavior studies, small group experiments, and epidemiologic investigations. (Clinical case studies are also reported in the literature, but these have not been included in this discussion.) Perhaps the most convincing evidence comes from the animal studies. To a large extent, these have been concerned with variations in the size of the group in which the animals interact and in situations which lead to confusion over territorial control. For example, a number of investigators have shown that as the number of animals housed together increases, but all other factors such as genetic stock, diet, temperature, and sanitation are kept constant, maternal and infant mortality rates rise, the incidence of arteriosclerosis increases, resistance to a wide variety of insults, including drugs, microorganisms, and x-rays decreases, and there is an increased susceptibility to various types of neoplasia (4–12). Lack of territorial control has been shown to lead to the development of marked and persistent hypertension in mice, to increased maternal and infant mortality rates, and also to reduced resistance to bacterial infections and decreased longevity (13).

In addition to demonstrating the health effects of variations in the social milieu, further animal studies have provided clues as to the processes through which they may be produced. Changes in group membership and the quality of group relationships have been shown to be accompanied by neuroendocrine changes, particularly—but not exclusively—by changes in the pituitary and adrenal-cortical systems (14,15). The changes in some of these hormones, such as the 17-hydroxycorticosteroids and the catecholamines, especially if prolonged, can in turn markedly alter the homeostatic mechanisms of the body and its resistance to a wide variety of stimuli.

The evidence then from a series of such studies would seem to be sound methodologically and reasonable from a biological point of view; but convincing as this evidence would appear to be, the relevance of these findings to human health is as yet unproved, and considerable doubt exists as to the appropriate analogues in the human social system. For example, attempts to demonstrate that increased population density and crowding are related to poorer health status in humans have been unconvincing and have led to confusing and often conflicting results (16). A careful review of some of these studies taken in conjunction with the animal work would suggest that for future research in this area to be profitable, we should abandon a search for the direct human counterpart to animal crowding or territorial confusion and concentrate instead on some more general principles, or hypotheses, that can be derived from these data. In my view, four such principles seem worth considering.

The Consequences of Crowding

The first of these can perhaps best be stated as a hypothesis. This would hold that the social process linking high population density to enhanced susceptibility to disease is not the crowding per se but the disordered inter-individual relationships that, in animals, are inevitable consequences of such crowding. While being manifest by a wide variety of bizarre and unusual behavior, these relationships often have in common a failure to elicit anticipated responses to what were previously appropriate cues and an increasing disregard of traditional obligations and rights. Thus habitual acts of aggression (including ritualized aggression), subordination, or cooperation on the part of one animal fail to elicit appropriate reciprocal responses on the part of another. Characteristic obligations and responsibilities become blurred (e.g., female rats cease caring for their young and male-female relationships become disturbed to a point where the equivalent of gang rapes have been reported in rats under conditions of high population density). The failure of behavior patterns to accomplish their intended results (i.e., to lead to predictable responses on the part of others) leads to one of three types of responses on the part of the animals involved, the most common of which is a repetition of the behavioral acts. Such acts are of course always accompanied by profound neuroendocrine changes, and presumably their chronic repetition leads eventually to the permanent alterations in the level of the hormones and autonomic nervous system arousal described under conditions of animal crowding. The fact that these behavioral acts are in a sense inappropriate in that they do not modify the situation can be expected to enhance such changes. Under these conditions it is not difficult to envisage the reasons for the increased susceptibility to environmental insults displayed by such animals.

An alternative response on the part of some animals is to withdraw from the field—to remain motionless and isolated for long hours on end. It is apparently not uncommon, for example, to observe mice under crowded conditions crouched in most unusual places—on top of the razor thin edge of a partition or in the bright light in the center of the enclosure—completely immobile and not interacting with other animals. Such animals apparently do not exhibit the increased pathology demonstrated by the interacting members (4).

The third alternative is for some animals to form their own deviant groups, groups that apparently ignore the mores and codes of behavior of the larger group. Thus, gangs of young male rats have been observed invading nests, attacking females, involved in homosexual practices, and so on. I am not aware of any data on the health status of these gang members but, according to this hypothesis, they also should not exhibit any increase in pathology.

This hypothesis then would suggest that in human populations the circumstances in which increased susceptibility to disease would occur would be those in which, for a variety of reasons, individuals are not receiving any evidence (feedback) that their actions are leading to desirable and anticipated consequences. In particular this would be true when these actions are designed to modify the individual's relationships to the important social groups with whom he interacts. Such circumstances might occur in a variety of situations. First, it is highly probable that when individuals are unfamiliar with the cues and the expectations of the society in which they live (as in the case of migrants to a new situation, or in those individuals involved in rapid change of the social scene, such as the elderly in an ethnic enclave caught up in the process of urban renewal), their actions would be unlikely to lead to the consequences they anticipate and thus cause the chain of events suggested above; they should be more susceptible to disease than are those for whom the situation is familiar. Some circumstantial evidence supporting this point of view exists. Thus Scotch (17,18) found that blood pressure levels among the Zulu who had recently migrated to a large urban center were higher than for those who had remained in their rural tribal surroundings and for those who had lived for over ten years in the urban setting. In two independent studies Syme (19,20,21) has demonstrated that occupationally and residentially mobile people have a higher prevalence of coronary heart disease than those in stable populations and that individuals who display greater discontinuity between childhood and adult situations, as measured by occupation and place of residence, have higher rates than those in which less discontinuity could be determined. Tyroler and Cassel designed a study in which death rates from coronary heart disease, and from all heart disease, could be measured in groups which were themselves stable but around which the social situation was changing in varying degree. For this purpose they selected 45-54-year-old white male rural residents in various counties of North Carolina and classified those counties by the degree of urbanization occurring in that locality. Death rates for coronary heart disease and all heart disease showed a stepwise increasing gradient with each increase in the index of urbanization of the county (22). In a further study, Cassel and Tyroler (23) studied two groups of rural mountaineers, one of which was composed of individuals who were the first of their family to engage in industrial work, while the second comprised workers in the same factory drawn from the same mountain coves and doing the same work for the same pay as the first group, but who were the children of previous workers in this factory. The underlying hypothesis was that the second group, by virtue of their previous experience, would be better prepared for the expectations and demands of industrial living than the first and would thus exhibit fewer signs of ill health. Health status was measured by responses to the Cornell Medical Index and by various indices of sick absenteeism. As predicted, the first group had higher Cornell Medical Index scores (more symptoms) and higher rates of sick absenteeism after the initial few years of service at each age than had the second.

A second set of circumstances in which it would be unlikely that the individual was receiving any feedback that his actions were effectively modifying the situation might occur where there is some evidence of social disorganization. This, while still being far from a precise term that can be accurately measured, has proved to be a useful concept in a number of studies. For example, in the hands of several investigators, various indicators of social or familial disorganization have been related to increased rates of tuberculosis (24), mental disorders (25), deaths from stroke (26), and prevalence of hypertension (27). Clearly, more work needs to be done in clarifying and quantifying this concept, but until there is recognition of what needs to be clarified or quantified, little progress can be anticipated.

Susceptibility to the Effects of Social Processes

The second general principle which emerges from the animal work is that not all members of a population are equally susceptible to the effects of these social processes. Systematic and regular differences have been observed with the more dominant animals showing the least effects and the subordinate ones having the most extreme responses (28). These differences are manifest in the magnitude of the endocrine changes as well as in increased morbidity and mortality rates. Conceivably, these findings may, in part, explain the high levels of blood pressure found in American Negroes who not only usually occupy a subordinate position in society but whose lives are frequently characterized by considerable evidence of social and familial disorganization.

Protective Factors

The third principle is concerned with the available protective factors, those devices which buffer or cushion the individual from the physiological or psychological consequences of social disorganization. These factors would seem to be of two general categories, biological and social. Under biological would be included the adaptive capacities of all living organisms, the capacity, given time, to adjust physiologically and psychologically to a wide variety of environmental circumstances. In animals this is illustrated by the higher responses of laboratory-naive animals to given stimuli than of veteran animals (29), and to the much lower rate of pathology in animals born and reared in crowded conditions than in animals transferred to these conditions some time after birth (30). In humans, the finding that death rates from lung cancer in the United States, when controlled for cigarette smoking, are considerably higher in the farm born who migrated to cities than in lifetime urban dwellers (despite the longer exposure of the latter to atmospheric pollution) (31) would seem to be evidence of the same phenomenon.

In addition to these biological adaptive processes, various social processes have also been shown to be protective. Chief amongst these are the nature and strength of the group supports provided to the individual. In rats, for example, the efficacy with which an unanticipated series of electric shocks (given to animals previously conditioned to avoid them) can produce peptic ulcers is determined to a large extent by whether the animals are shocked in isolation (high ulcer rates) or in the presence of litter mates (low ulcer rates) (32). The territorial conflict which led to the elevated blood pressures quoted above (13) was produced by placing mice in intercommunicating boxes. Hypertension only occurred, however, when the mice were strangers. Populating the system with litter mates produced none of these effects. In humans, small group studies have shown that the degree of autonomic arousal that can be produced by requiring solutions to what in reality are insoluble tasks is more extreme if the group is made up of strangers than when it is made up of friends (33). Modern studies on the epidemiology of tuberculosis in the United States and Britain have shown that the disease occurs more frequently in marginal people, that is, in people who, for a variety of reasons, are deprived of meaningful social contacts (24,34).

If these three principles, or hypotheses, are correct, the implication would be that health changes which are dependent upon the presence of other members of the same species will not be universal, affecting all people in the same manner. A more adequate formulation would hold that such consequences will be dependent on:

1. The importance or salience of the interpersonal relationships that become disordered;
2. The position of the individuals experiencing such disordered relationships in the status hierarchy;
3. The degree to which the population under study has been unprepared by previous experience for this particular situation (i.e, has had insufficient time to adapt); and
4. The nature and strength of the available group supports.

Effect of Group Relations on Susceptibility

The final general principle that can be derived from the animal experiments relates to the manifestations of ill health that might be anticipated under conditions of social change and disorganization. The model of disease causation provided by the germ theory has accustomed us to think in mono-etiologic specific terms. Accordingly, much of the work concerned with social or psychological antecedents to disease has attempted to identify a particular situational set (usually labeled "stress" or "a stressor") which would have a specific causal relationship to some clinical entity, analogous to the relationship between the typhoid bacillus and typhoid fever. Such a formulation would appear to be clearly at variance with the animal data, a striking feature of which is the wide variety of pathologic conditions that emerge following changes in the social milieu. A conclusion more in accordance with the known evidence would be that such variations in group relationships, rather than having a specific etiological role, would enhance susceptibility to disease in general. The specific manifestations of disease would be a function of the genetic predisposition of the individuals and the nature of the physicochemical or microbiologic insults they encounter. This concept of generalized susceptibility would be consistent with the situation in the United States where it has recently been demonstrated that regions of the country that have the highest death rates from cardiovascular disease (age, race, sex specific) also have higher than expected death rates from all causes, including cancer and infectious diseases (35). This illustration, of course, does not necessarily document that social processes are responsible for such an increased susceptibility, but does lend credence to the view that variations in generalized susceptibility may be a useful concept. Somewhat more direct evidence is provided in an industrial study in the United States which has shown that managers in a company who, by virtue of their family background and educational experience, were least well prepared for the demands and expectations of executive industrial life had the highest rates of all diseases—major as well as minor, physical illness as well as mental, long-term as well as short-term (36).

Presumably, then, the causes of disease may vary under different conditions. In preindustrialized societies where people live in small, tightly organized communities, the exposure to highly potent disease agents may account for the major part of disease causation. Under these circumstances, variations in susceptibility caused by social processes may be of relatively little importance. With increasing urbanization, populations become increasingly protected from such disease agents but simultaneously exposed to the social processes discussed above. Variations in susceptibility now assume greater importance in the etiological picture and the concomitant changes in such factors as diet, physical activity, and cigarette smoking will facilitate the emergence of new manifestations of such susceptibility.

SUMMARY

In summary then, it is postulated that one of the more important features of our environment that affects susceptibility and resistance to disease is the presence of other members of the same species. Specifically, it is suggested that man, in common with all social animals, engages in many forms of behavior designed to establish his position in relationship to important others in his environment. When these behaviors do not lead to the anticipated responses (or when the responses are unclear or conflicting), chronic alterations in the neuroendocrine homeostatic mechanisms occur. Stated in other words, it is suggested that when the behavior of individuals is inappropriate in kind or amount to affect the situation eliciting such behavior, the biological consequences will include marked alterations in these homeostatic mechanisms.

It is further suggested that such inappropriate behavior will not lead to the emergence of any specific clinical disease entity. Rather, such circumstances will enhance susceptibility to a wide variety of physicochemical and biological insults (disease agents). The particular manifestations of this increased susceptibility will vary, being dependent on the genetic composition of the individuals involved, the nature and type of the disease agents to which they are exposed, and their particular state of physiological and psychological balance resulting from their prior experience. Thus, research attempts to link psychosocial stresses, particularly those generated by inappropriate behavior and lack of feedback, to specific clinical disease entities are unlikely to be satisfactory. Furthermore, the consequences of such disordered relations (as far as susceptibility to disease is concerned) are likely to be modified by the strength of the group supports and the position of the individual in the status hierarchy.

Such a formulation, it is believed, may explain the cyclical variations of susceptibility to diseases that accompany periods of rapid social and cultural change. Those members of society who are the first to become involved in such change will be the first to manifest such increased susceptibility. With the passage of time such members will have learned how to order their relationships with important others in the new situation and, consequently (until new changes occur), their susceptibility should decrease. As other segments of society become increasingly involved in such changes they too will begin to show various manifestations of increased susceptibility. Such a formulation could explain the otherwise puzzling finding that two to three decades ago coronary heart disease mortality rates were higher among the more urbanized affluent members of society. In more recent times, rates in urban populations seem to be stabilizing or falling, while rates among rural and less affluent groups are rising (37).

Finally, it is suggested that to test such a formulation, new research strategies will have to be developed. It will no longer be adequate to search for the psychosocial antecedents of any single clinical entity in representative samples of the population. If representative samples are to be used, a wide variety of diseases will have to be included as possible consequences of these psychosocial factors. If a single disease entity is to be the outcome variable, the populations will have to be selected on the basis of characteristics which would indicate clearly that they are at risk of manifesting an increased susceptibility to that disease entity.

REFERENCES

1. Grigg, E. R. N. The arcana of tuberculosis. *Am. Rev. TB.*, 1958, *78*, 151-172, 426-453, 583-703.
2. Suser, M., and Stein, Z. Civilization and peptic ulcer. *Lancet*, 1962, *1*, 115-119.
3. Paffenberger, R. A., Jr., Milling, R. N., Poe, N. D., et al. Trends in death rates from hypertensive disease in Memphis, Tennessee, 1920-1960. *J. Chron. Dis.*, 1966, *19*, 847-856.
4. Calhoun, J. B. Population density and social pathology. *Sci. Amer.*, 1962, *206*, 139.
5. Ratcliffe, H. L., and Cronin, M. T. I. Changing frequency of arteriosclerosis in mammals and birds at the Philadelphia Zoological Garden. *Circulation*, 1958, *18*, 41-52.
6. Swinyard, E. A., Clark, L. D., Miyahara, J. T., and Wolf, H. H. Studies on the mechanism of amphetamine toxicity in aggregated mice. *J. Pharmacol. and Exptl. Therap.*, 1961, *132*, 97-102.
7. Davis, D. E., and Read, C. P. Effect of behavior on development of resistance in trichinosis. *Proc. Soc. Exp. Biol. Med.*, 1958, *99*, 269-272.
8. Ader, R., and Hahn, E. W. Effects of social environment on mortality to whole body—x-irradiation in the rat. *Psychol. Rep.*, 1963, *13(1)*, 211-215.
9. Ader, T., Kreutner, A., and Jacobs, H. L. Social environment, emotionality and alloxan diabetes in the rat. *Psychosom. Med.*, 1963, *25*, 60-68.
10. King, J. T., Lee, Y. C. P., and Visscher, M. B. Single versus multiple cage occupancy and convulsion frequency in CH mice. *Proc. Soc. Exp Biol. Med.*, 1955, *88*, 661-663.
11. Andervont, H. B. Influence of environment on mammary cancer in mice. *J. Nat. Cancer Inst.*, 1944, *4*, 579-581.
12. Christian, J. J., and Williamson, H. O. Effect of crowding on experimental granuloma formation in mice. *Proc. Soc. Exp. Biol. Med.*, 1958, *99*, 385-387.
13. Henry J. P., Meehan, J. P., and Stephens, P. M. The use of psychosocial stimuli to induce prolonged hypertension in mice. *Psychosom. Med.*, 1967, *29*, 408-432.
14. Mason, J. W. Psychological influences on the pituitary-adrenal-cortical system. In *Recent Progress in Hormone Research*, G. Pincus, ed., 1959, *15*, 345-389.
15. Mason, J. W., and Brady, J. V. The sensitivity of the psychoendocrine systems to social and physical environment. In *Psychobiological approaches to social behavior*, D. Shapiro, ed. Palo Alto: Stanford University Press, 1964.
16. Cassel, J. Health consequences of population density and crowding. Chapter 12 in *Rapid Population Growth*, prepared by the National Academy of Sciences. Baltimore: Johns Hopkins Press, 1971, pp. 462-478.

17. Scotch, N. A. Sociocultural factors in the epidemiology of Zulu hypertension. *Am. J. Pub. Health,* 1963, *52,* 1205-1213.
18. Bibile, S. W., et al. Variation with age and sex of blood pressure and pulse rate for Ceylonese subjects. *Ceylon J. Med. Sci.,* 1949, *6,* 80.
19. Syme, S. L., Hyman, M. M., and Enterline, P. E. Some social and cultural factors associated with the occurrence of coronary heart disease. *J. Chron. Dis.,* 1964, *17,* 277-289.
20. Syme, S. L., Hyman, M. M., and Enterline, P. E. Cultural mobility and the occurrence of coronary heart disease. *Health and Human Behavior,* 1965, *6,* 178-189.
21. Syme, S. L., Borhani, M. O., and Buechley, R. W. Cultural mobility and coronary heart disease in an urban area. *Am. J. Epid.,* 1965, *82,* 334-346.
22. Tyroler, H. A., and Cassel, J. Health consequences of culture change: The effect of urbanization on coronary heart mortality in rural residents of North Carolina. *J. Chron. Dis.,* 1964, *17,* 167-177.
23. Cassel, J., and Tyroler, H. A. Epidemiological studies of culture change, I: Health status and recency of industrialization. *Arch. Envir. Health,* 1961, *3,* 25.
24. Holmes, T. H. Multidiscipline studies of tuberculosis. In *Personality stress and tuberculosis,* P. J. Sparer, ed. New York: International Universities Press, 1956.
25. Leighton, D. C., Harding, J. S., Macklin, D. B., MacMillan, A. M., and Leighton, A. H. *The character of danger.* New York: Basic Books, Inc., 1963.
26. Neser, W. B., Tyroler, H. A., and Cassel, J. Stroke mortality in the black population of North Carolina in relation to social factors. Presented at the American Heart Association Meeting on Cardiovascular Epidemiology, New Orleans, March 1970.
27. Harburg, E., et al. Stress and heredity in Negro-White blood pressure differences. Progress report to National Heart Institute, 1969.
28. Christian, J. J. The potential role of the adrenal cortex as affected by social rank and population density on experimental epidemics. *Am. J. Epid.,* 1968, *87,* 255-264.
29. Mason, J. W., Brady, J. V., Polish, E., et al. Concurrent measurement of 17-hydroxycorticosteroids and pepsinogen levels during prolonged emotional stress in the monkey. *Psychosom. Med.,* 1959, *21,* 432.
30. Kessler, A. Interplay between social ecology and physiology, genetics, and population dynamics of mice. Doctoral dissertation, Rockefeller University, 1966.
31. Haenzel, W., Loveland, D. B., and Sirken, M. G. Lung cancer mortality as related to residence and smoking histories. *J. Nat. Cancer Inst.,* 1962, *28,* 947-1001.
32. Conger, J. J., et al. The role of social experience in the production of gastric ulcers in hooded rats placed in a conflict situation. *J. Abnorm. and Soc. Psych.,* 1958, *57,* 216.
33. Bogdanoff, M. D., Back, K., Klein, R., Estes, E. H., and Nichols, C. The

physiologic response to conformity pressure in man. *Ann. Int. Med.*, 1962, *57*, 389-397.

34. Brett, G. Z., and Benjamin, B. Housing and tuberculosis in a mass radiography survey. *Brit. J. Prev. and Soc. Med.*, 1957, *11*, 7-9.
35. Syme, S. L. Personal communication.
36. Christenson, W. N., and Hinkle, L. E., Jr. Differences in illness and prognostic signs in two groups of young men. *J. A. M. A.*, 1961, *177*, 247-253.
37. Cassel, J., et al. Incidence of coronary heart disease by ethnic group, social class, and sex. *Arch. Int. Med.*, 1971, *128*, 901-906.

14

Behavioral Sciences: A Focus on People and Organizations

Rodney M. Coe

We are in the midst of a rapidly growing movement—if not revolution—for change in medical education. In medical schools all over the United States changes are taking place in policies and practices of recruitment of faculty and students, in the length of programs, in content and emphasis of the curriculum, and in recognition of the institution's commitment to the broader community as well as to the students it trains. A major concomitant of this movement is the rising demand for the services of behavioral scientists as full-time members of the faculty and staff of medical schools and health care institutions. This chapter suggests some contributions of behavioral scientists to the education of medical students and to the delivery of health services.

A recent project of the Medical Sociology Section of the American Sociological Society (1) indicated that social or behavioral scientists are becoming increasingly important both in teaching medical students and in conducting research in medical centers. Responses from the deans of 74 medical schools to an initial questionnaire showed that all but three institutions provided some instruction in the behavioral sciences. There was, to be sure, considerable variation in amount, scope, and duration of the subject matter presented. Furthermore, there were differences as to which department division, section, or office had responsibility for preparation and presentation of behavioral science material. Some presentations involved only a few lectures by social scientists during the year. Other schools reported year-long, intensive courses for introducing behavioral science concepts and methods to medical students. Most schools fell somewhere between those extremes. Behavioral science content was most often the responsibility of departments of psychiatry, community medicine or community health, or preventive medicine.

In view of the persistent confusion over nomenclature, it may be useful to state briefly what behavioral or social sciences cover. Most writers tend to use the terms behavioral and social interchangeably. There seems to be general agreement, however, that whichever label is used, the science includes psychology, sociology, anthropology (at least cultural or social anthropology), economics, and political science. In addition, some writers include history, geography, law, and the behavioral aspects of biology. It is noteworthy that the term behavioral sciences is frequently found, but behavioral science almost never. The latter term would seem to imply a single, all-encompassing set of interrelated theoretical concepts and methods resulting in a unified scientific discipline. Since this is not yet a reality, the plural of the term is more accurate. At the same time, one does talk about a behavioral scientist, a designation which usually refers to a specialist in one of the disciplines noted above but who also has some working knowledge of and interest in one or more of the other disciplines.

Another kind of distinction can be made between basic and applied research efforts on the part of behavioral scientists who work in or with medical schools. Some investigators work toward developing concepts and testing theories within their own discipline (or at least within the behavioral sciences) while others emphasize putting the results of their studies to work to alleviate distress, solve technical problems, or promote solutions to broad social problems. Both approaches are important and, in fact, interrelated. Seldom is research in the behavioral sciences completely pure or completely applied. To paraphrase Straus (2), a distinction can be made between behavioral sciences in medicine and behavioral sciences of medicine. The former term refers to work in which the main purpose is to solve practical problems related to some issue in medical care service or delivery. The latter term could refer to the same kind of project, but one in which the emphasis is in the development or testing of concepts in a medical context.

The balance of this chapter will include an overview of the historical antecedents of the present movement to incorporate behavioral sciences into the medical school curriculum, a description of some specific contributions of the behavioral sciences, and a discussion of issues in the integration of social science concepts into medical curricula and medical practice.

SOME HISTORICAL ANTECEDENTS OF PRESENT CONVERGENCE[1]

A number of observers have commented on the importance of the behavioral sciences to medical education and to medical practice (3); in fact, one of the earliest statements was published more than 75 years ago (4). Nonetheless, it has only been since the mid-twentieth century that collaboration among the disciplines has become remarkable. Throughout the history of medicine there has always been some recognition of social, psychological, economic, and political factors in the etiology, diagnosis, and treatment of diseases. However, toward the end of the nineteenth century with its great scientific achievements in the biological and physical sciences, the distinction between the science of medicine and the art of medicine became more apparent and, from the perspective of medical educators, the greater importance lay with developments in the science. During the first half of the twentieth century, laboratory sciences became the great tradition in medicine and in medical education.

Meanwhile, many new developments were also taking place in the behavioral sciences. Psychology and economics were already recognized academic fields by the end of the nineteenth century—about the time that sociology and social anthropology were getting underway. Although there were differences in points of time at initiation and in rates of development, the behavioral sciences had in common an impetus towards becoming scientific disciplines and, in this regard at least, were developing their concepts and methods on the same model of science that guided the growth of the biological and physical sciences before them. Except for psychology, which has always had close ties with medicine, the behavioral sciences tended to look elsewhere for substantive areas in which to apply their concepts and methods. Sociology was nurtured on issues resulting from urbanization, social class differences, family organization and functioning, and deviant behavior. Early anthropologists concentrated on primitive societies as an area in which to develop and test concepts of human interaction. Similarly, political science and economics focused attention on fields other than medicine. As a consequence, during the last quarter of the nineteenth century and the first half of the twentieth, there was a

[1]A fuller discussion of these factors may be found in Coe, R. M. *Sociology of Medicine*, especially in chapter 1. New York: McGraw-Hill, 1970.

parallel, but almost independent growth of the behavioral sciences and of medicine. In all the fields involved, there has been a tremendous expansion of a body of verified knowledge, further development of theoretical paradigms, and a sharpening of research designs and methodological tools and procedures.

The Scientific Base of Behavioral Science

This growth and development has been in large part responsible for the present push for collaboration between the medical and behavioral sciences. The first requisite for collaboration for mutual benefit would seem to depend upon an ability to conduct scientifically sound studies which could lead to verification of theoretical concepts on the one hand and to resolving practical problems on the other. For some fields within medicine, these criteria were met shortly after the turn of the nineteenth century. Achievement of status as a scientific discipline has come later to most of the behavioral sciences, but recognition of this level of accomplishment is now generally acknowledged.

Changing Patterns of Disease

A second reason for convergence has been the change in the patterns of morbidity (and mortality) resulting at least in part from the scientific achievements in medicine. Perhaps the most spectacular changes have occurred in efforts to prevent or at least control communicable diseases. Thus, tuberculosis, influenza, and pneumonia which were major killers in 1900 have been replaced by heart disease, cancer, and stroke. In the process, the crude death rate for the United States has been reduced from about 17 deaths per 1000 population in 1900 to about 9 deaths per 1000 in 1970 (5). In most modern industrialized nations in which scientifically developed public health practices have been employed along with modern medical practices, epidemic diseases such as smallpox, cholera, typhoid fever, poliomyelitis, tuberculosis, and even rubella have all but disappeared.[2] There has been a subsequent rise in average length of life and consequently an increase in the proportion of elderly people in the population. Along with increasing age come increased incidence and prevalence of chronic, debilitating dis-

[2]Some important exceptions, however, especially the venereal diseases, continue to increase despite availability of effective medication and preventive procedures.

eases which have not yet responded dramatically to scientific developments in medicine. More to the point, efforts to understand the implications of chronicity for the individual patient, his family, and the provider agencies in the community would seem to be more in the sphere of the behavioral than the biological sciences. Even where there is biologically based knowledge about prevention of diseases, there is need for a behavioral science evaluation of human motivations to use (or not to use) the knowledge available. In summary, the outcomes of early achievements in medical research have resulted in the rise of different kinds of health problems the solutions to which cannot evolve solely from the application of physical and biological sciences. On the contrary, an increasingly stronger role will fall to the behavioral sciences in the resolution of these problems.

Both medical and behavioral science have applied the principles of epidemiology to problems of chronic diseases. The procedures for identifying causes of epidemic diseases have been broadened to include long-term, noncommunicable diseases and physical handicaps. In fact, investigators of problems of social deviance such as alcoholism, drug abuse, mental illness, and so on also have made use of these procedures. Because of the broadened scope of his field, the epidemiologist finds his theoretical and methodological interests merging with those of social psychologists, demographers, and sociologists.

More often than not communicable diseases could be traced to a single organism which, when identified, could be prevented from attacking the potential human host. Chronic diseases and disabilities, however, are more often the result of multiple causes, at least some of which are social in nature. That is, major contributors to health problems in old age, for example, are habits associated with different life styles. They may be class-linked, related to one's occupation, or to such personal habits as smoking, drinking, or dietary practices. In this regard, note should be taken of the role of psychiatry in promoting the convergence of psychology and neurology in the study of psychosomatic diseases and the important contribution of psychoanalytic and other psychiatric theories in pointing out that mental illnesses can have a distinctly social etiology (6). In any event, the overlap in interests of the medical practitioner and the medical researcher with those of behavioral scientists is apparent.

Behavioral science may also concern itself with the assessment of medical organization. It bears repeating that all human groups, regardless of cultural heritage or economic resources, develop institutions and institutionalized ways of meeting their needs including—and perhaps even especially—those related to medical care. In modern societies this refers to the organization of medical resources, including practitioners and their assistants, and to hospitals and other supporting services. In an area which might be labeled administrative medicine, the behavioral sciences would seem uniquely qualified to make a contribution to medicine. Thus issues of medical economics—fee-for-service versus other forms of payment; the cost of care in general; comprehensive health insurance versus other forms—are subjects of study for economists. Effectiveness and efficiency of organization of service modalities in clinics and hospital settings are evaluated by industrial engineers as well as behavioral scientists. The distribution of manpower, the effects of continued specialization, the development and organization of different levels of care—acute, extended, and custodial—are also areas in which expert advice to medical directors can be and is provided by behavioral scientists.

Medical Care Services Delivery

Finally, but not exhaustively, a third reason for convergence between medicine and the social sciences—besides internal developments and changes in the pattern of morbidity—is the rising criticism of medical care services in the United States. The criticisms are coming not from segments of the medical profession, but from behavioral scientists and, most importantly, from consumers. Furthermore, consumers look to practitioners of behavioral sciences not only to criticize the present delivery system, but to propose ways of correcting the problems. Again, many members of the medical profession are turning more and more to behavioral scientists for these suggestions.

In summary, the fact of convergence of behavioral sciences and medical administration, practice, and research can be traced to the prior development of theoretical concepts and methodological tools, to the changing picture of morbidity, and to the increasing inadequacies and inequities in the delivery of medical care services. Further, it can be noted that specific areas of convergence include: 1) an identification and understanding of social factors in etiology and distribution of diseases in human populations; 2) knowledge of the influence of such factors as attitudes and values on the behavior of individuals in response to illness or disease and, from the provider's perspective, the influence of attitudes, values, and training on the behavior of the professional towards the patient; and 3) an evaluation of the effectiveness and efficiency of the organization of health services in the community (7).

SOME CONTRIBUTIONS OF BEHAVIORAL SCIENCES

We have suggested that one important factor in the rising importance of the behavioral sciences in medicine has been the maturation of the various disciplines in terms of scientifically verifiable hypotheses, research design and methodology, and the expansion of a body of knowledge. In the paragraphs that follow, each of these areas will be briefly examined and illustrated by means of a current research project in community medicine.

We can describe the behavioral sciences as the study of man with regard to human systems of social relationships. This permits an examination of the theoretical frameworks of each of the disciplines and their points of overlap in terms of the individual, of human groupings, and of institutions. Generally speaking, psychology is the science most concerned with the individual and thus with the "internal environment." That is to say, knowledge of processes of cognition, perception, learning, and motivation are all special contributions of psychology. Disturbance in these processes, and their relationship with physiological processes such as psychopathology, are important issues in the field of medicine. Sociology and anthropology can be differentiated from psychology because of their focus on interaction between individuals, particularly in different kinds of human groups from the dyad to communities and nations. Forms of interaction, i.e., behavior, and their antecedents in terms of attitudes and values and how they are transmitted from one generation to another, how change occurs and how groups control behavior are key concepts. Conceptualization at the institutional level is the principal focus of economics, political science, and history. It bears repeating, however, that dividing lines between the disciplines are not sharp and, in fact, one of the threads of contemporary educational processes is to blur further the distinctions through interdisciplinary training and teamwork in practice.

Along with development of concepts has come increased sophistication in research methods and analytic procedures. In this regard, there is close correspondence between behavioral sciences and medical sciences as both are derived from the same rules of scientific investigation and employ the same techniques. For example, the case study approach—whether by observation or inquiry or both—is a familiar feature of clinical teaching and research, as well as an approach of psychological studies. The case study is also a method in other behavioral sciences where the case may be a particular human group or an organization or even a whole community. The study of human groups in interaction may take place in contrived settings such as small group laboratories modeled after the laboratories in the physical and biological sciences, in natural settings such as homes, schools, factories, hospitals, or in communities such as primitive villages. A procedure that is becoming more popular is the survey which employs sophisticated sampling methods, highly developed interviewing skills (or substitute forms), and data collection devices. In addition, secondary sources of information are used in historical investigations and for background information about particular subjects, for example, data from the census of the United States in community studies. The important point here is not that there are research methods which are unique to the behavioral sciences, but that the methods commonly associated with them are not only shared by other fields, but are derived from the same scientific ethos.

The most apparent contributions of the behavioral sciences, quite naturally, lie in expansion of the body of verified knowledge about human behavior in the context of health and disease. Although there have always been a few scholars interested in applying their disciplinary skills to the field of medicine, it has only been during the last 20 to 25 years that there has been a widespread effort to expand this area of knowledge. The success of this effort is attested to by the enormous volume of information that has been published, and while we cannot begin to mention even the major works (8), we can identify the principal areas of contribution. Briefly, these are: 1) identifying social factors in etiology and distribution of diseases in the human population, including individual factors such as habits or group factors such as social class, place of residence, or occupation; 2) tracing the influence of attitudes and values on perception and response to disease and illness, especially factors related to seeking help from lay and professional resources in the community; 3) evaluating effectiveness and economics of the various forms of organizational and institutional settings in which health care services are delivered, ranging from the individual practitioner working alone to organized clinics and hospitals and their support agencies; and 4) describing the various alternative ways of organizing the different parts of the health care system in terms of delivery of services in an efficient and economical, but effective fashion.

EXAMPLES OF BEHAVIORAL SCIENCES APPLIED TO MEDICAL CARE ISSUES

A project which attempted to assess the impact of the Medicare program may illustrate some of the above principles. This project, which was begun in 1966 before the federal program was initiated, employed a before-after design in terms of establishing a baseline of attitudes, values, and behaviors of individuals in different settings along with an assessment of organizational relationships among community agencies providing some health-related services to older people. In 1968, after the program had been in operation for two years, a second wave of data collection took place (9). The purpose of the project was to evaluate the impact of this large-scale federal program on the provision of health care services by community resources and the utilization of those services by residents in the selected research sites.

The study focused on Medicare as an innovation in paying for medical services to beneficiaries of the program (10). In part, the study evaluated the economic assumption which predicted rapid overutilization of community resources by older people because the care would be free. However, from a behavioral science perspective, it was hypothesized that utilization (i.e., behavior) would not change until some antecedent conditions were satisfied. Thus, employing some principles which have been demonstrated empirically many times over, it was expected that behavior of older people would change only after there had been a change in the perception of symptoms as indicative of illness and in the norms defining those symptoms as warranting the attention of medical professionals. It was thought also that some provisions of the program, such as extended care and home health services, might lead to a revised definition of the sick role compatible with the characteristics of chronic diseases.

It was also hypothesized that in anticipation of increases in utilization, community resources—both individual and organizational—would first react by shifting present resources of personnel, equipment, and space to meet those needs. Eventually however (we thought within two years), there should have occurred a reorganization of community resources—physicians and other personnel, hospitals, extended care facilities, nursing homes and home health services, not to mention supporting services—for better coordination and distribution of services required by older people in the community especially, but generally for everyone.

To test these general themes the investigation pursued parallel lines of inquiry. One was a survey of more than 2000 older residents (including a control group) in each of five communities representing metropolitan areas, large cities, and rural medical care trade centers. This survey involved detailed interviews with randomly selected respondents with regard to their attitudes, perceptions and behaviors related to medical care and, of course, their social and demographic background information. The other line of investigation, community resources, involved interviews with physicians practicing in these five communities and with managers of hospitals, extended care facilities, and nursing homes, and with directors of home health agencies. In addition, secondary sources of data such as census materials, other research reports, and special studies of the communities involved were also employed.

The findings of this first evaluation of Medicare are somewhat anticlimactic. By now, it is common knowledge that older people did not dramatically change their customary patterns of utilization in terms of hospital admissions (although for some segments, utilization rates increased because of the extensiveness of medical care needs), but the idea of the Medicare program itself received overwhelming acceptance by beneficiaries. Also during that first two-year period, there was almost no coordination of services in any of the facilities and little, if any, change in the ways in which doctors practiced medicine, or organizations conducted their business.

Through the case approach method (i.e., types of communities, and surveys in households and organizational settings, plus observations and reference to secondary sources), data were collected, processed, and analyzed to test hypotheses derived from general social science practices. In the process, some information was collected on the prevalence and distribution of diseases in this particular age group in the population and on the influence of attitudes, values, and perceptions of older residents on their illness behavior. Moreover, separate community agencies were evaluated in terms of the quality of service rendered, the achievement of organizational objectives, and the agency's relationship to other service or supporting organizations in the community. That information, and the present follow-up, are being assessed to determine where resistance to change is located in the system and what means can be used to bring about a creative realignment of personnel, equipment, and space to meet more fully the continuing health care needs of the population in these communities and elsewhere in the country.

Another example of contributions of behavioral scientists—this time illustrating the influence of attitudes and values on professional behaviors—may be drawn from a study of physicians' office practices (11). In this case, a nationwide random sample of nearly sixteen hundred general practitioners and internists was interviewed about their attitudes and practices with respect to preventive medicine, the aging processes, adult patients, and preventive health care services. Other information collected included the nature, type, and operation of the respondents' office practices and related professional activities.

Among the several related objectives of this investigation were: 1) assessment of degree to which practitioners provided preventive health care services to adult patients in comparison with standards of good practice as devised by a panel of experts in preventive medicine; 2) evaluation of the influence of attitudes, values, and beliefs of the physician on his "behavior," i.e., provision of services; and 3) development of a model of good preventive health care in terms of the relationship between attitudes, behaviors, and characteristics of these physicians.

As indicated, data were collected by means of personal interviews with the respondents. In addition to a standard occupational interview, some specially designed questions were used to assess the variables of central interest. For example, the level of preventive health services was measured in terms of laboratory tests and examination procedures employed by the respondent in routine physical examinations along with counselling activities and cooperation with other providers in the community. There also was a special test of the doctors' knowledge about normal and disease-related conditions of aging and a battery of items on attitudes toward older people drawn from previously developed instruments. Supplemental questions were employed to assess the rationale for use of tests and procedures, perspective on the aging process, and so on.

The findings of the study are of some importance not only because they describe an area of activity which has not been studied enough, but also because some basic social science theories provided the explanation of the observed variations in professional behaviors. Thus, the major finding was that this sample of physicians routinely employed about 50 percent of the tests and procedures recommended by the panel of experts, but there was considerable variation in the number of procedures used and in the rationale for using them. Most of the variation could be explained in terms of the practitioner's definition of and attitude toward preventive medicine and his knowledge of the normal and disease-related conditions of aging. As predicted, the more positive the doctor's attitude toward preventive medicine and the more likely he was to define it in terms of a cooperative venture between himself and his patient, then the more closely he would come to the standards set by the experts (i.e., the higher his score on provision of services).

Similarly, the more accurate was the doctor's knowledge of conditions of aging, the better was his performance on the provision of services. However, the practitioner's attitude toward older patients had no effect on his practices with those patients. In other words, attitudes and values (which one, after all, developed in the medical education process) that have professional relevance—such as attitude towards preventive medicine—do influence one's behavior, while professionally irrelevant attitudes—such as stereotypes of older people—even when negative do not affect professional practices. Finally, it may be noted that these findings taken together did provide a description of models of physician practices in which two of the key variables were age of the practitioner and degree of specialization. Generally speaking, younger specialists performed better on preventive care practices than older nonspecialists.

It is possible to describe some general features of behavioral scientists' roles in medical school settings. In the first place, behavioral scientists, like their faculty colleagues, can and do participate in the traditional activities of teaching, research, and service. The first two of these activities are more or less obvious although the form and content may vary from one place to another. Instruction may focus on basic principles of a social science (and therefore be similar to other basic science courses) or an application of social science principles to specific health problems (as in the clinical sciences). Likewise, research may be focused on a behavioral science problem or on a broader issue where the intent is a practical solution to a problem. In both functions, behavioral scientists may work alone, with other behavioral scientists, or with a multidisciplinary team which includes health professionals. The service function of behavioral scientists is somewhat different in that direct medical care—the laying on of hands—is not performed. However, behavioral scientists do give consultations in relation to providing information about, and sometimes techniques for, solving health-related problems. These may involve matters of family relations, housing and local government, community organization, the environment, education, and so on. This service function goes beyond the traditionally defined services of a medical school and could be considered a service in response to the community, or at least some segments of it, and their demands for help with health as well as medical problems.

The role of behavioral scientists can be more specifically noted in terms of their contributions to the perspectives of medical students (and practicing physicians as well) (12). Behavioral sciences, for example, continually emphasize the human dimension of patient care, i.e., that the patient is a person and not just a disease-bearing organism. All too often this perspective becomes lost in the emphasis on biological and physical sciences and in the employment of medical gadgetry. Second, the repersonalization of the patient includes the knowledge that attitudes and values which guide behavior are derived from group interaction and that knowledge about the nature and influence of the group is important to the practitioner in terms of diagnostic and therapeutic procedures. It is often not apparent to practitioners that their attitudes and values are also derived from group interaction and also influence their behavior, both professional and personal. Third, it is clear that the practice of medicine (and the training process for it) requires the cooperation and collaboration of many individuals and organizations. Thus another contribution of behavioral scientists is a knowledge and understanding of the structure and function of many types of practice settings for the delivery of direct medical services and the types of agencies which support those services.

REFERENCES

1. American Sociological Society. Study for teaching behavioral sciences in schools of medicine. Contract HSM 110-69-211, C. R. Fletcher, Ph.D., Project Director.
2. Straus, R. The nature and status of medical sociology. *American Sociological Review*, 1957, *22*, 200-204.
3. See Leavell, H. R. Contributions of the social sciences to the solution of health problems. *New England Journal of Medicine*, 1952, *247*, 885-897; Straus, R. A role for behavioral sciences in a university medical center. *Annals of the American Academy of Political and Social Sciences*, 1963, *346*, 99-108; and, more recently Kendall, P. L., and Reader, J. G. Contributions of sociology to medicine. In *Handbook of medical sociology*, 2nd ed. H. E. Freeman, S. Levine, and L. G. Reeder, eds. Englewood Cliffs, New Jersey: Prentice-Hall, 1972, 1-29.
4. McIntire, C. The importance of the study of medical sociology. *Bulletin of the American Academy of Medicine*, 1894, *1*, 425-434.
5. U.S. Department of Commerce. *Statistical Abstract of the United States, 1970*. Washington, D. C.: Government Printing Office, 1971.
6. See Leighton, A., Clausen, J., and Wilson, R. N. *Explorations in social psychiatry*. New York: Basic Books, 1957.
7. Mechanic, D. Sociology and public health: Perspectives for application. *American Journal of Public Health*, 1972, *62*, 146-151. See also McKinlay, J. B. The concept "patient career" as a heuristic device for making medical sociology relevant to medical students. *Social Science and Medicine*, 1971, *5*, 441-460, and Polgar, S. Health and human behavior areas of interest common to the social and medical sciences. *Current Anthropology*, 1962, *3*, 159-205.
8. General texts include Coe, R. M. *Sociology of medicine*. New York: McGraw-Hill, 1970; Freeman, H. E., Levine, S., and Reeder, L. G., eds. *Handbook of medical sociology*, 2nd ed., Englewood Cliffs, New Jersey: Prentice-Hall, 1972; Mechanic, D. *Medical sociology, A selective view*. New York: Free Press, 1968; Jaco, E. G. *Patients, physicians and illness*, 2nd ed., New York: Free Press, 1972. In addition, the following periodicals also report results of research in behavioral sciences in health: *American Journal of Public Health, Public Health Reports, Health Services Research, Inquiry, International Journal of Health Services, Journal of Health and Social Behavior, Medical Care, Medical Care Review, Social Security Bulletin*, and *Social Science and Medicine* to name only ten.
9. Coe, R. M., and associates. *Medicare report: Evaluation of the provision and utilization of community health resources*. Kansas City: Institute for Community Studies, Inc., 1970, reports the results of these two data collection periods. In addition, a third wave was conducted in 1971, the data for which are presently (1972) undergoing evaluation.

10. For details of the insurance program and an economic analysis, see Myers, R. J. *Medicare.* Bryn Mawr, Pennsylvania: McCahan Foundation, 1970.
11. Coe, R. M., and Brehm, H. P. *Preventive health care for adults: A study of medical practice.* New Haven: College and University Press Services, Inc., 1972.
12. American Sociological Society. Study for teaching behavioral sciences in schools of medicine. Contract HSM 110-69-211, C. R. Fletcher, Ph.D., Project Director, pp. 73-75.

15
Population, Politics, and Public Health

Jonathan B. Weisbuch

Childbearing and the provision of adequate food, housing, and resources for survival are the oldest forces in nature. To assure survival, man must now curb his reproductive drive and reverse his headlong destruction of the environment or he will find himself on a planet depleted of resources necessary to sustain life. The increased rate of resource utilization parallels the increase in population. The sharply rising curve of world population shown in Figure 1 can virtually be superimposed on the curves describing fossil fuel production, food consumption, water usage, or other indices which define man's exploitation of his physical environment.

Careful analysis is necessary to unveil the factors and forces which influence human fertility and to determine the means by which these forces may be controlled.

From a demographic point of view, excess fertility is very different in the developed industrial countries as compared to the developing areas of the world. In industrial nations, the impact of excess fertility is not felt directly by society as a whole, but rather by the individual groups and families whose personal resources are constrained by the demands to feed, clothe, and educate their children. In general, the burden of excess fertility in the Western nations is carried by the poor who are unable to prevent excess births. The social and personal costs associated with high levels of fertility among the poor are expressed in high infant and maternal death rates (1), high levels of malnutrition (2), and high levels of pregnancy out-of-wedlock (3). The only visible impact excess fertility makes on most members of a developed society is the increasing

Figure 1

GROWTH OF HUMAN NUMBERS

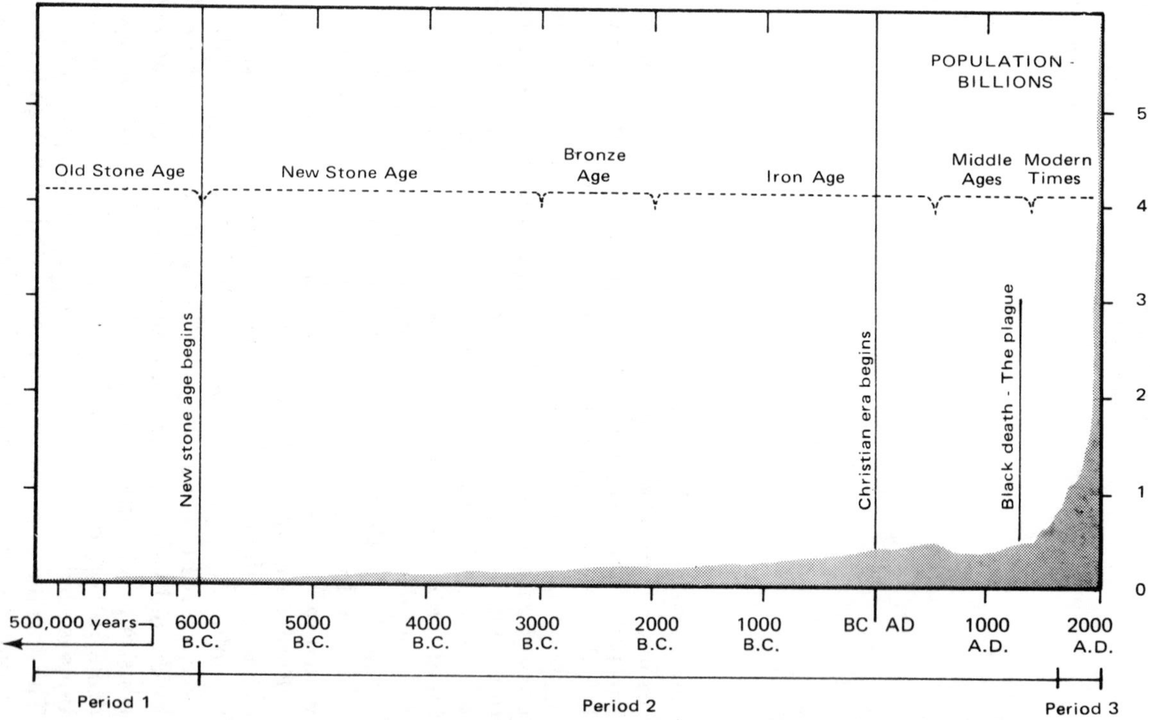

POPULATION - BILLIONS

Old Stone Age
New Stone Age
Bronze Age
Iron Age
Middle Ages
Modern Times

New stone age begins
Christian era begins
Black death - The plague

5
4
3
2
1
0

500,000 years
6000 B.C.
5000 B.C.
4000 B.C.
3000 B.C.
2000 B.C.
1000 B.C.
BC AD
1000 A.D.
2000 A.D.

Period 1
Period 2
Period 3

cost of welfare and other social services; the poor housing, malnutrition, and poor health are almost invisible to society at large.

But wherever the family lives, the impact of too many children in a family is the same. Family structure is placed in jeopardy: the father cannot provide for his children, the mother cannot care for them adequately. The very old and the young who cannot provide for themselves become burdens. Malnutrition, disease, despair, and death accompany the family whether it lives in Calcutta or New York. For humanistic as well as social and economic reasons, the prevention of excess fertility in every corner of the globe has become a requirement for survival.

The prevention of any human ill requires an understanding of the epidemiology of that problem. A problem needs clear definition and accurate measurement. Its distribution as to time, place, and persons needs delineation. The factors which determine its occurrence must be clarified. The epidemiology of population growth and excess fertility is presented below.

DEFINITIONS AND INDICES OF MEASUREMENT

Most nations perform total censuses at regular intervals in order to determine a precise baseline population figure. Then by keeping a record of births, deaths, immigration, and migration for any interval, usually on an annual basis, the aggregate population can be approximated at any time between census dates. The change in population size, or the growth of the population, is the sum of the difference between births and deaths plus the net change through migration. As migratory movements into and out of most nations are small, we may neglect them and define another term, the natural increase, as the change in population brought about by the difference in the number of births and deaths.

The *natural increase* value is the figure usually quoted to measure the rate of change in the population with time. Migratory movements are usually of minor significance and allow the rate of natural increase and the growth rate to be used synonymously. But both natural increase and growth rate are only crude estimates of population change; other measures are needed to qualify the situation.

The *general fertility rate* (GFR) is an estimate of probability of a woman giving birth in a given year:

$$\text{GFR} = \frac{\text{total births per specified time period}}{\text{total number of females in the childbearing age group (usually 15 to 44 years old)}} \times 1000$$

The age-specific prevalence histogram (commonly called a *population pyramid)* shown in Figure 2 gives a picture of age and sex distribution of a population.

Excess fertility is the delivery of more children by a woman than she, her husband, or her family desires (4). This definition does not define the term from a national perspective; to extrapolate, national excess fertility is the birth of more children than the nation can feed, house, clothe, and educate in ways consistent with accepted cultural values. In either case, national or individual, the excess level of fertility is that number of births greater than the presumed ideal number of births. The nation that wishes to hold its crude birth rate at 25 births per 1000 people experiences excess fertility when the birth rate rises above that value; the individual family whose ideal size is three children, experiences excess fertility when the fourth pregnancy is gestating.

Another set of measures often used in demographic analysis are those relating to *knowledge* of contraceptive methods, *attitudes* toward their use, and *practice* with regard to usage, of available devices. The KAP studies, as they are often called, determine through personal interviews with a representative sample of child-bearing women the frequency of accurate knowledge, the current attitudinal profile, and the behavior of people in the area under consideration. While fraught with the many problems attending population survey methods, reports of KAP studies do give valuable information. The attitudinal section often will present data on concepts of ideal family size, by age, race, religion, husband's occupation, social class, and other social parameters. These data are essential for planning any delivery system to provide contraceptive services (5) or for monitoring changes on the national scene.

THE EPIDEMIOLOGY OF POPULATION, POPULATION GROWTH, FERTILITY, AND EXCESS FERTILITY

The population of the world in 1972 was over 3.7 billion human beings (6). The average crude death rate in the world is 14 per 1000; the crude birth rate is 34 per 1000, resulting in births exceed-

Figure 2
Population Pyramids

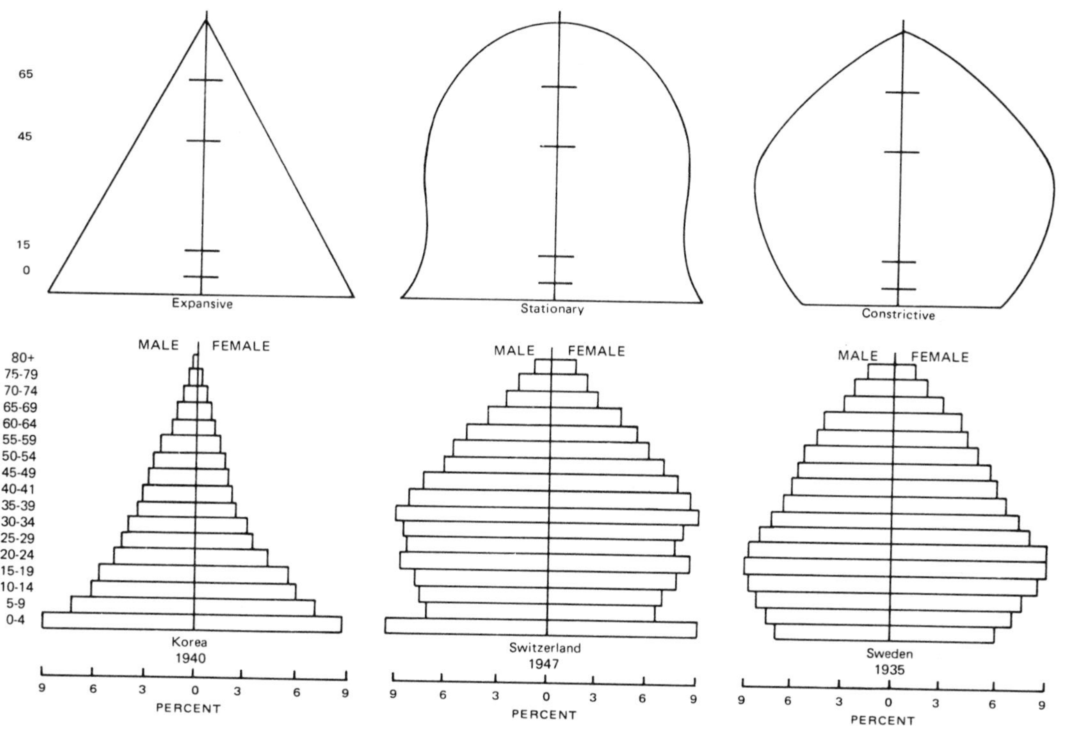

Source: Petersen, W. *Population*. New York: The MacMillan Company, 1961, p. 628.

ing deaths by 20 per 1000 per year, a world population increase of 2 percent per annum (7). The death rate continues to fall as new technology is introduced into the underdeveloped world. In the face of a death rate decline, the natural increase can be diminished in only one way: by reducing births. A rapid perusal of birth rates and per capita income in various nations indicates that the poorest nations (on a per capita income scale) are those with the highest births rates. Similar correlations between poverty and birth rate exist in the United States and other nations in which the relationship has been studied (8).

Deeper analysis of the data complicates the simple hypothesis that the problem of excess fertility is simply a problem of poverty. Urban living and income levels are also factors that affect fertility. Demographic analysis in the United States demonstrates marked variations in fertility between religious groups which are independent of differences in social class (9). The wide fluctuations in the U.S. birth rate and marriage rate shown in Figure 3 indicate how complex the relationship is between the economic cycle, other social changes (postwar), marriage rates, and fertility. Developed nations as well as undeveloped nations demonstrate fertility variations as a function of social change.

Industrialization and urbanization are prime movers in altering the social pattern from a traditional culture to a modern one. The shifts from traditional values and beliefs to a contemporary set of social attitudes is another factor in changing fertility patterns. The traditional society, based on rural agriculture, is characterized by many variables which encourage high fertility: 1) the extended family, necessary for optimizing limited economic resources, reduces the cost of children and allows for the relatively inexpensive support of the elders; 2) the demand for inexpensive manpower to till, sow, and reap encourages large families, as does the demand for semiskilled manpower to produce cottage industry output; 3) religious and cultural values toward early and universal marriage, mores against contraception, and values which favor female fecundity are common in traditional societies; 4) the absence of adequate environmental hygiene, the paucity of medical care, and the prevalence of infectious illness results in high levels of mortality, especially infant mortality, and encourages high rates of pregnancy; and 5) the traditional role of women as homemakers and mothers plays an important role in keeping fertility high. These factors change as individuals leave the land, migrate to the cities, adopt an independent life style, work in industry for a daily wage, and move

Figure 3
Vital Statistics for the United States, 1920–1970

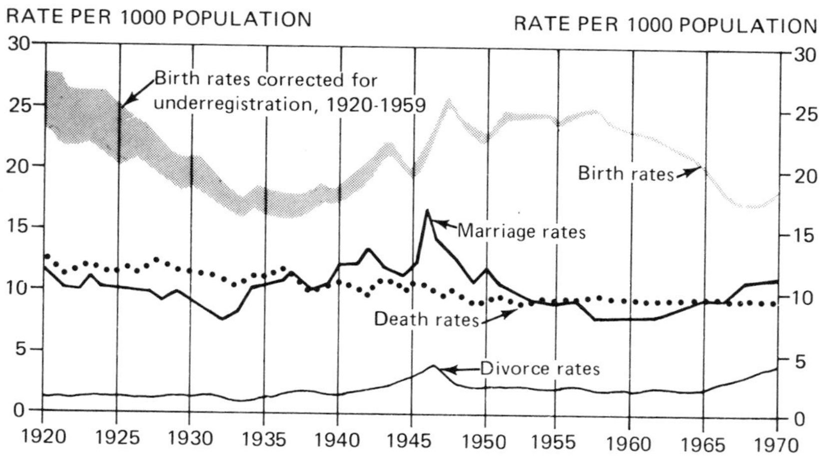

Source: Chart prepared by Department of Commerce, Bureau of the Census. Data from Department of Health, Education, and Welfare, Public Health Services.

away from the close family ties of the past. Men and women in this situation may marry later and have fewer children than before these changes occurred.

A general reduction in fertility did occur in the Western developed nations as they became urbanized and industrialized (10,11). Limited evidence seems to indicate that a similar phenomenon may be occurring in the developing world. In the short run, urbanization, industrialization, and economic development tend to exacerbate the problem of population increase, even while helping to reduce individual fertility. This seeming paradox occurs because two initially independent forces are at play. Net population increase is a simple function of births less deaths; but the factors which affect fertility are very complex and not immediately dependent on those forces which help lower the death rate. A major result of economic and technologic development is the ability of a society to lower the death rate, an option rarely rejected. The new technology has supplied numerous tools to combat disease, to increase social services, and to improve education, the environment and agriculture, all of which have an immediate impact on lowering the crude death rate, specifically by reducing that fraction of deaths caused by infectious diseases, diseases of children, and deaths associated with parturition and malnutrition.

The rapid drop in death rates, particularly infant death rates, causes the sharp divergence between births and deaths. The impact on the birth rate is not as immediate. The birth rate remains high during the initial phases of the technologic revolution, resulting in a rapid increase in the population growth rate.

A number of hypotheses have been proposed to explain how human fertility is modulated by the environmental, social, and biologic factors described above. A few of these theories are presented in the next section.

PREVAILING HYPOTHESES RELATING TO POPULATION CHANGES

The various theories of population growth fall into three categories: 1) Population growth is directly related to the means of subsistence. 2) Population growth is principally affected by changes in birth rates and death rates. 3) Numerous factors in the complex web of human society affect both the means of subsistence and the levels of births and deaths which then, secondarily, result in changes in the natural increase of the population.

Malthus is probably the most famous theorist arguing that a change in the levels of subsistence is the prime factor in population growth; his entire thesis was that to remove the constraints of want and deprivation from the laboring poor was to unbridle their reproductive instincts which lead to overpopulation (12). There is ecological data to indicate that all biologic species do achieve equilibrium with their environment in time, so that the population of each species in the ecosystem remains relatively stable (13). Whether such a state exists for the human organism is not clear.

The economic arguments relating goods and resources with population changes are primarily variants of the hypothesis that the level of subsistence is the primary factor determining population dynamics. But economics is not the only factor dictating changes in human behavior, especially behavior related to fertility. The subsistence hypotheses do not explain all available data.

The hypotheses which relate human population growth to changes in birth rates and death rates are exemplified by the theory of the demographic transition (14). The theory explained much of the data available in the postwar period for Western nations whose birth rates and death rates had been fairly well documented for at least 150 to 200 years. The essential facts are pointed out in

Figure 4
The Demographic Transition in Western Europe and the United States

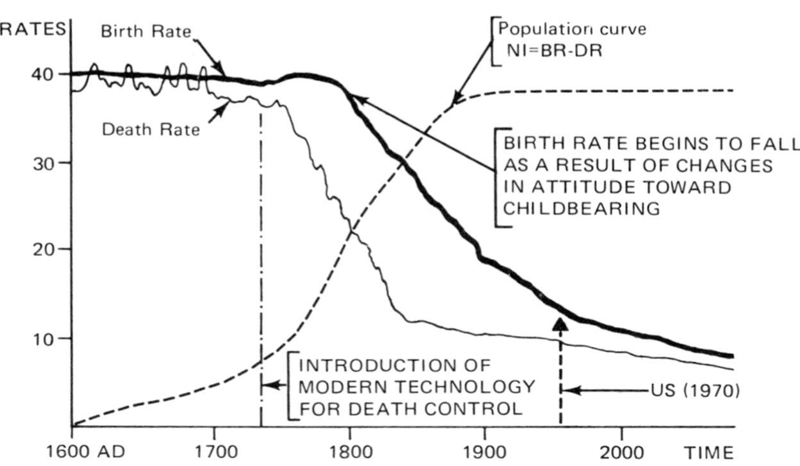

Figure 4, which shows the change in recorded birth and death rates in Western Europe and the United States for the past 300 years.

An important aspect of the demographic transition model is that during the process important demographic changes take place in society: 1) birth rates and death rates fall to low levels; 2) the population increases manyfold; and 3) the structure of the population pyramid changes. Prior to the transition, the broad-based population pyramid is common (see Figure 2): many children and young people, relatively low average life expectancy, and very few elders. At the end of the process, with low fertility, the shape of the pyramid is much squarer: few children, many middle-aged and older adults, and a relatively large number of elders.

The demographic transition model is a reflection of the changes that have taken place and are taking place in various nations during the past few centuries. The model seems to apply to a few developing nations, but whether it will apply to all emerging nations is not clear. What is clear is that death rates and birth rates in the underdeveloped world were very high 25 to 30 years ago; today with the application of modern death control methods death rates have dropped. Birth rates still remain high, and in some cases higher than before. No one can be sure that fertility will fall in accordance to theory.

The weakness in the transition theory is that specific aspects of the economic development process have not been delineated as having a greater or lesser impact on fertility. As originally stated, a developing nation undergoing industrialization and technologic change would experience a drop in fertility. But this theory is not very helpful for the nation desiring to lower its birth rate, because no specific aspect of the theory indicates what to emphasize to gain the most impact on fertility. A nation invests in many areas to promote economic development. For a demographic theory to be valuable, it should at least delineate particular areas into which resources should be channeled which would accomplish both the goal of economic growth and a rapid decline in fertility.

Toward this end, a number of unified theories on population change have been advanced. Factors which affect fertility may include health care delivery, agriculture, transportation, and the other aspects of national development (15). To these may be added macro-social changes, internal family psychology, and the changes in individual self-image and life style (16). They operate on individuals and on the family so that married couples make specific decisions which in the aggregate affect the overall population of the nation. Social changes which affect the roles of women are important levers in lowering fertility.

Again, further research is needed to tighten the numerous hypotheses which have been formulated to describe population change.

EPIDEMIOLOGIC SURVEYS TO TEST POPULATION HYPOTHESES

Studies suggest that the availability of birth control methods is helpful in reducing the birth rate only if women of the area are motivated to use the materials (17,18). As the concept of ideal family size regresses toward one or two children, the utilization of contraceptive methods by younger and younger women will occur.

Cultural factors also promote high fertility, for example, the desire for a male heir. The proof of virility—the *machismo* phenomenon—is another profound drive for children (19). Given this set of cultural variables, plus a perception that 50 percent of the children may die before their fifth birthday, family desire for relatively large families and high fertility will take precedence over other social forces mitigating for a reduced level of childbearing. Cultural and social norms are very difficult to change quickly. Because these factors have a strong impact on fertility levels, changes in birth rates do not occur quickly.

Environmental changes which have an impact on infant and child mortality are more readily implemented and result in a rapid decline in death rates. Relatively simple public health—improved water supply, sanitation engineering, better housing, immunization and feeding programs, the elimination of infectious diseases such as malaria, yaws, endemic syphilis—all have a marked effect on infant death. As the death rate falls, the perception of a high death rate also falls but only after a measurable time lag. Women who realize they no longer need to have eight pregnancies to produce four surviving children will begin to seek means for limiting their reproductive capacity. But the drop in the infant death rate will increase the number of excess births. The number of excess children will affect the behavior pattern of women who will then take action to reduce the excess. Without a sense of excess, the demand for fertility reduction will be minimal. But the process takes time.

The precise relationship between mortality levels and fertility has not been defined. Descriptive studies have shown a positive relationship between the two variables (20). Two significant observations emerge: 1) the rate of natural increase of a population is maximal at moderate levels of mortality; and 2) the number of births per woman does not drop markedly until low levels of mortality are achieved. Figure 5 is an attempt to demonstrate the changing effects that various systems in society have at different phases in the transitional process on the reduction of natural increase. The changing role of agriculture, health systems, urbanization, and education bear witness to the complexity of the factors in the network of human reproduction. These imply a need for the combined efforts by agro-industrial economists; cultural anthropologists; demographers and social scientists; and health care specialists with expertise in public health, preventive medicine, and contraceptive services. The overlap of intellectual skills in these spheres of endeavor is essential to bring about optimal reduction in fertility. Overemphasis in any one sphere may exacerbate the problem of population growth rather than mollify its impact.

The role of community medicine is as much to solve problems as to determine truth; it may not be necessary to know everything about human fertility before we can initiate programs to diminish excess fertility and bring absolute fertility down to reasonable levels in every nation. No one approach will apply for all areas: each program must be skillfully designed to meet the sociocultural, environmental, and biological needs of the people in the area. Multidimensional problems require multidimensional solutions which are designed to distribute resources in a balanced manner.

Figure 5

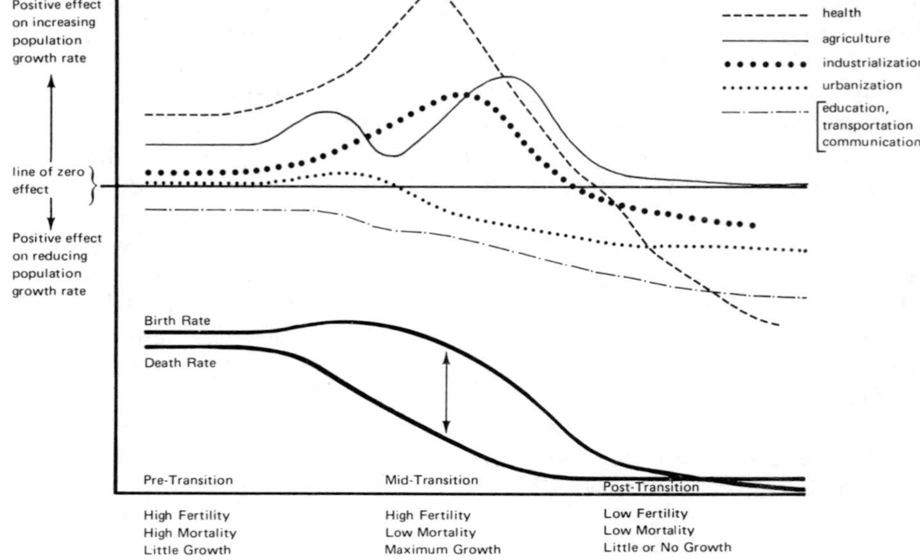

PRESENT PROGRAMS: METHODS FOR CURBING EXCESS FERTILITY

Programs to help women limit excess fertility span the globe. In many cases programs are designed to encourage families to have a specifically defined number of children. A few nations still persist in a public policy of proscription of birth control information; but even in these countries the solution to the problem of excess population is sought.

In each nation the problem can be distilled to two primary goals: 1) excess fertility must fall to zero; and 2) the gross reproduction rate should fall to between 2 to 3 offspring. The first objective relieves the family of too many mouths to feed; the second will presumably answer the national problem of rampant population growth. If excess fertility could be brought to zero and the age-specific fertility rates brought to a level of bare replacement immediately, the population would increase by at least 50 percent before stability occurred. If the time dimension required for the fall in birth rates were 15 years, the population would increase 2 1/2 times before zero growth stabilization would occur (21). Demographic transition takes time to stabilize regardless of the methods exploited to achieve the goals.

In order for every woman to be able to limit excess fertility, she must have full control over her normal biological mechanisms. She must have effective contraceptive methods available to her; and she must use these methods. Abstinence, contraception, sterilization, abortion, infanticide all have been exploited from earliest time to reduce excess birth. All that is new in modern medicine is the degree of sophistication employed in interrupting the normal reproductive processes.

All available forms of biologic interruption require cooperation of the participants; for this reason contraceptive devices are effective in reducing only excess or unwanted births. Legal controls are not strong enough to require women and men to use the pill, the condom, the IUD, or to accept sterilizing surgery. Massive programs to provide family planning materials to an entire population have been relatively unsuccessful in the developing areas of the world whose levels of mortality are still moderately high; these areas remain nonindustrialized, nonurban with low levels of literacy, and with mothers who still desire between four and five offspring.

By contrast, in developed industrial societies where the individual desire to limit family size is profound, governmental antinatal programs are not needed. The availability of effective contraceptive methods, including abortion, in the developed world has been followed by marked reductions in birth rate with a decline in the population growth rate to less than one percent per annum.

In contrast to the Western nations with low growth rates and no national birth policies, the underdeveloped world, with high growth rates, have frantically sought national policies which will stem the tide. In the face of extraordinary efforts, biologic approaches dictated through legislation to control fertility have not achieved the objective of reducing the ideal family size below three children. On the other hand, without an adequate system to deliver biologically effective contraceptive methods, the reduction of individual excess fertility proceeds very slowly even when desired by the people.

After the war, the Japanese passed a law legalizing the practice of abortion on demand. The birth rate in Japan has fallen in the 25 years since the passage of the law from 32.3 to 19 (22). Other governmental policies in Japan also promoted a drop in birth rates. Massive economic development with governmental support brought the urbanization and industrialization to a feverish level. The cultural changes which have taken place in Japan since 1948 have been profound: shifts from rural to urban dominance, from agriculture to industry, from the extended to the nuclear family; the development of an economically consuming population; a growth of social legislation with nearly complete state support of health services and care for the elderly; and a generally higher educational attainment—all these work toward decreasing fertility. The availability of abortion on demand and other highly effective methods of fertility control have enhanced the decline of the birth rate. Abortion and effective contraception became the vehicle for change, but probably not the cause.

Other nations have taken national positions on fertility control and population growth. Today, India, with a population of over 500,000,000 people (14 percent of the world total), has one of the largest state-run family planning programs in the world. National policy in India identifies family planning to be at the very center of planned development (23). A major input of this campaign is mass communication praising the value of small families. The investment in the program is approximately $30 million per year during the current fourth 5-year plan (24). The program includes the provision of all forms of contraception, sterilization, education, and the use of incentives to lower fertility. Official reports indicate a reduction in birth rates from an estimated annual rate of 41 in the decade 1951 to 1960 to below 30 births per 1000 per year in some of the urban centers in 1965-1970 (23), but unofficial sources indicate the reported reduction may be false.

If governmental planning, policy, and legislation can affect the fertility of the people, the programs in India will be successful. The success of a nation in achieving economic independence is tied to success in limiting population expansion. The results are not yet tabulated; a decade or more will be needed to determine the effect of the various programs. Past history gives no basis for an optimistic prediction, for governmental efforts to modify human behavior have almost always failed; however, the modern world is a complex environment which has invariably demonstrated the errors of demographic predictions (25).

LONG-RANGE PLANS: CONCLUSIONS

The world will be troubled by a rapidly rising population (at or near the annual increase of 2 percent) for many decades to come. The momentum of population growth cannot be avoided (21). The picture is neither as bleak as some alarmists maintain, nor as sanguine as other pundits would hope. Parts of the globe, the developed nations, will see their population achieve stasis and will then be confronted with the problem of maintaining economic growth without the support of population growth. Other parts of the world will have to commit vast efforts to stabilize their populations. This latter group of nations will exist for a long time.

The problem of population growth must be viewed in light of the personal attitudes which define excess fertility. If fertility is not viewed by the people as resulting in unwanted children, programs to limit national growth are doomed to failure. Excess fertility becomes a problem to parents as mortality levels begin to fall. When faced with a set of alternatives, people make decisions based on the relative values of the expected outcomes; the "costs" of action are part of the decision process. The choice to avoid excess fertility is possible even in the most primitive societies: abstinence from sexual contact, induced abortion, and even infanticide are available alternatives, although the relative costs of such action may be quite high.

The capability of a population to limit excess fertility to zero is still no assurance that population growth will fall if desired family size remains high. India, for example, would continue to grow at a little less than 2 percent per year even if women could limit their completed family size to four children. For a nation to reduce its growth rate, it is not sufficient to limit excess fertility, for in most developing areas the desired family size is still extremely large. The preference for a smaller family size must occur if a nation is to reduce its growth rate to one percent or less. Massive family planning programs do not necessarily accomplish this objective, even though they may help in reducing the crude birth rate. Total social, cultural, and economic change must take place for families to modify their sense of the ideal family.

During the process of change, family planning services must be available in order to give the people the capacity to biologically control their fertility. A health system that provides comprehensive services, including all the modern methods for effective contraception, is an essential element in the overall control of population; but it is clearly not the only element needed. If the program is backstopped with a system that allows therapeutic abortion on demand, families will have complete biologic control over their reproductive cycle. When total biologic control is available, the social, economic, environmental, and cultural forces which change individual preferences will be most effective. A very rapid fall in growth rate is not an unreasonable expectation, if all these factors are operative. In the absence of major elements, little if any change can be expected.

Complete reproductivity control may not be necessary if the average desire for children is between one and three per couple. The changes in the environment that promote better housing, better communications, better education, better water systems and sanitation services can be strong motivators to reduce the desired number of children. The drive toward industrialization, equal status for women, urbanization, increases in leisure time with growing per capita income also help to lower fertility through modification of the attitudes toward family size and structure.

This chapter has attempted to demonstrate which human social systems relate to the problem of population and which can be influenced to change present human behavior. We began the discussion by alluding to the fact that the balance on which man's existence rests is threatened by his own headlong rush to procreate. Initially, both the procreative force and the desire to dominate the environment helped to assure the continuation of man as a species. Today, both primal forces pull in opposite directions, toward overpopulation and environmental destruction. Self-preservation over the next 100 years will require careful planning and deliberate action. Man must learn to work within his environment, helping to regenerate it on the one hand, but at the same time, allowing it to supply the necessary resources for a much larger population than now exists. For the population to stabilize, the social structure of man's community must influence people to reduce the consequences of the procreative impulses to very low levels. The ticket to survival is not an easy one. But it never has been.

REFERENCES

1. Lerner, M. Social differences in physical health, Chapter 3 in *Poverty and health: A sociologic analysis*, J. Kosa, A. Antonovsky, and K. Zola, eds. Cambridge, Mass.: Harvard University Press, 1969, pp. 69-112.
2. *Hunger U. S. A.* Report by the Citizens Board of Inquiry into Hunger and Malnutrition in the United States. Boston: Beacon Press, 1969, p. 37: "Magnitude: available evidence indicates that the percentage of poor affected by hunger and malnutrition range between one-third and one-half of the poor."
3. Moynihan, P. *On understanding poverty.* New York: Basic Books, 1968, p. 234.
4. Whelpton, P. K., Campbell, A. A., and Patterson, J. E. *Fertility and family planning in the United States.* Princeton, New Jersey: Princeton University Press, 1966, pp. 235-236.
5. Beasley, J. D. View from Louisiana. In *Family Planning Perspectives,* 1969, *1*, 2-15.
6. *World Population Prospects 1965-85.* United Nations Population Division Working Paper No. 30, December 1969.
7. *1972 World Population Data Sheet.* Washington, D. C.: Population Reference Bureau, Inc., 1972.
8. Freedman, R., Coombs, L. C., and Friedman, J. Social correlates of fetal mortality. *Milbank Memorial Fund Quarterly*, 1966, *44*, 327-344.
9. Westoff, C. F., and Ryder, N. B. Methods of fertility control in the United States: 1955, 1960, and 1965. In *Family and fertility*, William T. Lin, ed. Notre Dame, Indiana: Notre Dame University Press, 1967.
10. Heer, D. M. Economic development and fertility. *Demography*, 1966, *3*, 423-444.
11. Whelpton, P. K. Industrial development and population growth. *Social Forces,* 1928, *1*, 458-467, 629-638.
12. Malthus, T. *A summary view of the principle of population*, initially published in 1830, reprinted 1960 in *On population; three essays by Thomas Malthus, Julian Huxley, and Frederick Osborn.* New York: New American Library.
13. Dice, L. R. *Man's nature and nature's man: The ecology of human communities.* Ann Arbor: University of Michigan Press, 1955.
14. Davis, K. *Human society.* New York: Macmillan, 1949, pp. 603-608.
15. Taylor, C. E., and Hall, M. F. Health, population and economic development. *Science,* 1967, *157*, 651-657.
16. Rosen, B. C., and Simmons, A. B. Industrialization, family fertility: A structural-psychological analysis of the Brazilian case. *Demography,* 1971, *8*, 49-69.
17. Wyon, J. B., and Gordon, J. E. *The Khanna study, population problems in rural Punjab.* Cambridge, Mass.: Harvard University Press, 1971.
18. Beasley, J. D., Frankowski, R. F., and Hawkins, C. M. Orleans Parish

family planning demonstration program: A description of the first year. *Milbank Memorial Fund Quarterly*, 1969, *46*, 225-253.
19. Lewis, O. *La vida*. New York: Random House, 1966.
20. Hill, J. R., Stycos, J. M., and Back, K. W. *The family and population control*. Chapel Hill: University of North Carolina Press, 1959.
21. Keyfitz, N. On the momentum of population growth. *Demography*, 1971, *8*, 71-80.
22. Taeuber, I. B. Fertility and research on fertility in Japan. *Milbank Memorial Fund Quarterly*, 1956, *34*, 129-149.
23. Raina, B. L. India. In *Family planning and population programs*, B. Berelson, R. K. Anderson, O. Harkavy, J. Maier, W. P. Mauldin, and S. J. Segal, eds. Chicago: University of Chicago Press, 1966. Pp. 111-121.
24. Chandrasekhar, S. *India's population: Facts, problems and policy*. New Delhi: Meenakshi Prakashan, 1967.
25. Heer, D. *Society and population*. Englewood Cliffs, New Jersey: Prentice-Hall, 1968, pp. 10-11.

APPENDIX

An Approach to the Teaching of Epidemiology

Hugh S. Fulmer

Because epidemiology lies within the larger framework of community medicine, which, in turn, should be viewed in the still larger context of medical education, the teaching of epidemiology should be placed in proper perspective. First, it would be well to define some terms and concepts.

Community medicine has had many meanings for many people ever since the first department bearing that title was created in an American medical school in 1960 (1). A useful working definition states that community medicine, when defined as an academic discipline, deals with the identification and solution of community health problems. This implies that it is not just the clinical practice of medicine in the community or in the community hospital, although it includes a study of each; nor is it simply the management of the ills of the community, although it includes that, too. For just as in clinical medicine, diagnosis must precede therapy, so in community medicine, identification or community diagnosis must be emphasized and come before management or therapy of community health problems.

When one analyzes the definition further, the whole concept may be derived. A community is a population of individuals and, although they each have their particular hereditary background, they share several common subcultures. These individuals are continually interacting with their total environment, which includes physical, biological, and social components; they have a specific disease status, a dynamic and ever-changing expression of this genetic-environmental interaction. Health professionals and their associates (working as individuals, groups, agencies, and institutions, using certain facilities, applying their biomedical technology, delivering their services to the people) determine the health services system. Thus, the four components of community medicine may be viewed as a population of people, in an environment which includes everything "outside of the skins" of that population, interacting to produce a pattern of disease, or health status, which is modified by the health service system of the community. In turn, the system tends to be modified as the health status changes, so that community medicine may be viewed as a dynamic, changing interaction among these four major variables:

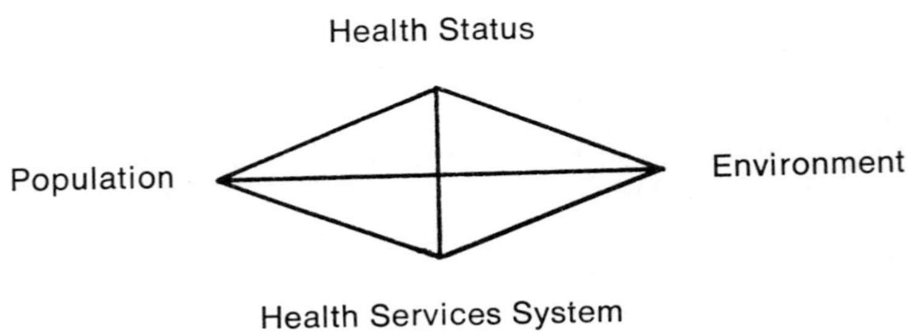

In sketching the place of community medicine as an academic discipline in medical education, one must always bear in mind how community medicine is defined and conceptualized, so that its relevance to the daily practice of medicine and health care is under continual scrutiny and review.

A physician practicing in a given community is concerned with the entire spectrum of disease: he should be promoting and maintaining health, preventing disease, and rehabilitating patients at the same time that he is treating sick individuals. Moreover, there are differences between caring for individual patients and dealing with the health status of communities from which those patients come. The latter implies the exercise of health leadership based on a sense of responsibility for the entire community; it requires knowledge of how a community and its health services system are organized, how they function, and how they may be changed by voluntary methods as well as by working through the legislative process. And in addition, it is based upon a knowledge of available health resources so that a physician may call upon them for his patients and his community. It implies a knowledge of clinical epidemiology and how all factors that bear on the health of the individual and the family can be assessed and, if need be, modified. Thus a prime objective in the education of medical students should be the development of a perspective on the responsibility of the future physician for his community, as well as the traditional responsibility for his individual patients, with all of the knowledge, skills, and attitudes that such a goal implies.

COMMUNITY MEDICINE IN MEDICAL SCHOOLS

Too frequently in medical schools the educational area encompassing the foregoing dimension, traditionally called public health or preventive medicine, has been inadequately taught. There are many reasons for this, from uninspired teaching and understaffing, to minimal support by the administration, lack of interest by the medical students, and unimaginative conceptualization of what the subject is and how it should be taught. One result has been that most medical students in the past have placed public health or anything akin to it low on their preference lists for career choice. But, more importantly, they have not seen its relevance for the practice of medicine.

The first department of community medicine initiated an educational program which appears to have general applicability.* Its premise was that medical students should study communities with the same degree of curiosity, intensity, and rational thought that they learned to employ in studying individual patients in hospital beds. The community assignment was the key; it was through a student-centered, faculty-guided experience in a community that students finally grasped the epidemiologic concepts and principles presented earlier in the classroom.

Each student in the senior year of medical school was assigned to a particular community and told: "This community is your patient; we want you to diagnose it and propose management for it as if it were an individual patient." Students were assigned to communities of all types, from urban to rural, affluent to disadvantaged, throughout the state and they worked in them for extended periods of time.

Several tasks were set for the students to accomplish under the

*This community medicine program is described in detail in Tapp, J. W., Jr., and Deuschle, K. W. The community medicine clerkship—a guide for teachers and students of community medicine. *Milbank Memorial Fund Quarterly*, 1969, *47*, 411-447.

sort of faculty tutelage that they would have expected had they been making rounds on hospital wards. They had to diagnose the pattern of disease in the community in an attempt to ascertain its health status. They had to describe what management was being given through the health services system to deal with this disease pattern. They were asked to propose how the elements of the concept of community medicine might be modified to improve the health status. In order to understand the usefulness of epidemiology, they also had to study a single health problem in depth, such as heart disease, accidents, or how a physician's practice works. In this way they took the scientific approach to disease problems in a population and to their solutions.

To become familiar with the way families function in their home settings, the students were also asked to study a spectrum of families, from rich to poor, in which different types of health problems existed, in order to understand how their way of life influenced their diseases, how their health needs were cared for—based on their social and economic circumstances—and what their attitudes were toward health care. This was an exercise in applied clinical epidemiology. Finally, they were required to examine individual patients in order to get a quantitative sense of the pattern of disease as it expressed itself in the community clinical setting, in contrast to what they might have seen in the university hospital. This multifaceted approach enabled them to grasp the essentials of community medicine, including the basic sciences of epidemiology and medical care.

Because epidemiology, like the other medical sciences, is of practical significance to the student of medicine largely in relation to what he will do later, as a physician, the way in which it is taught may be fruitfully examined.

EPIDEMIOLOGY AND THE DENOMINATOR CONCEPT

Whether in textbooks such as MacMahon's *Epidemiology* (2), Paul's *Clinical Epidemiology* (3), a monograph such as Pickles' *Epidemiology in Country Practice* (4), or an article such as Stewart's "Epidemiological approach to assessment of health" (5), the importance of the concept of the denominator in epidemiological thinking is repeatedly expressed. Most medical students have learned only about the numerator; i.e., they have learned only about sick patients. And they have not been aware that they have learned about only a numerator, for the sick patients are not ordinarily referred to as a numerator. Physicians have not been trained to think quantitatively about the populations from which their patients come. Those who have entered the field of community medicine have generally come in through the back door. One might say that opening the back door consists of recognizing the existence and meaning of the denominator. As Stewart has stated, the first concept in epidemiology is simple: the denominator (5). But this statement is deceptively simple. Epidemiology is the science of denominators and as such it is the counterbalance of clinical training, which is preoccupied with numerators. It is as important as the invention of the wheel, and as revolutionary. However, it is in the teaching of this simple, yet revolutionary, concept that much of the difficulty that exists in the teaching of epidemiology arises.

Students don't really learn about denominators until they actually face them, work with them, and think about them. That is why epidemiology is rarely taught until the student has had to confront the healthy population in the community, as well as those who are diseased. Most of the medical student's experience occurs either in the wards of a university hospital or a community hospital, where he examines patients who are critically ill, be they medical, pediatric, surgical, or psychiatric, or in the outpatient clinic. In the community, however, the student may be disciplined to observe the healthy population, the worried well, the early sick, and the chronically ill, in addition to the acutely ill, and may be led to consider the denominator as well as the numerator. The denominator of the total population at risk of ill health, in conjunction with the numerator of those sick, whether they are in bed or walking around, may best be comprehended by apprenticeship in the community.

One of the educational benefits of viewing the community at large in terms of its health status as compared to looking at a patient in a hospital bed is the denominator concept as illustrated by the realities of community needs and demands. White outlined what might be found quantitatively in studying illness generated in a population of adults over a month's period of time in a normal community (6). He found that in a month, 750 out of 1000 people would have an illness of some sort. Of course, an overwhelming majority of these illnesses would be minor. Most of them would be upper respiratory infections, gastrointestinal upsets, minor injuries, and so on. But, surprisingly, 250 people, or one out of four, will have seen a physician during that month. Of these 250, five would be referred to another physician, a specialist; another nine would be admitted to the community hospital. Only one would have an illness requiring admission to a university hospital. The medical student who is used to learning about the world of medicine in the university hospital will, if he thinks critically, be able to compare and contrast what he has now seen in the community with what he has come to know in the university hospital. And, of course, this contrast will be striking. What he has seen in the university hospital would be seriously ill patients with rather complicated or unusual diseases requiring specialized care. In the community, however, he is disciplined to think about the 1000 healthy people and the amount of illness that can ensue in a month, out of which only one would have been a patient on the university hospital ward. And he may be challenged to ask: How do the health professionals and society handle the denominator of 1000? What is the health services system, how does it work, and how should it work?

Thus, if the average medical student does not get out into the community, he tends to develop a distorted picture of the reality of disease as it afflicts communities, because he is likely to perceive the community as reflecting the sum of university hospital patients, and the practice of medicine as concerned mostly with the care of those he has seen there.

On the university hospital ward, the student emulates his clinical teacher. He gains a sense of responsibility in the care of the patient. He learns the meticulous application of scientific principles in the diagnosis and care of the individual. This is all to the good and is not to be decried. But he is focusing on the individual and he has not had time to think about the community because the community is not there in front of him. But when he is in the community, as a student under the guidance of community medicine faculty, he must think about it. Finally, the meaning of the denominator hits home. The great health issues of the day, concerned with the numbers and distribution of sick people, the organization and delivery of medical care, are seen from a holistic and scientific vantage point, given the necessary careful faculty guidance.

COMMUNITY MEDICINE CURRICULUM AND EPIDEMIOLOGY

To reach the objective of the development of a perspective on the responsibility of a future physician for his community, consider the curriculum in community medicine at a new medical school (the University of Massachussetts) and contrast it to that formerly in effect at the school which pioneered in the field program (the University of Kentucky). The field experience mentioned above occurred in the senior year. It had been deliberately placed there on the assumption that the student would by then be well grounded in the fundamentals of the clinical approach to the patient. He might therefore more closely identify as a near-member of the medical profession. He could represent a doctor as a visiting student in the community. The climate of the times at present, however, is such that the student can hardly wait until his senior year for his community medicine experience. He needs an earlier introduction.

Certainly times have changed. Students are much more socially oriented than they were five years ago. Often they demand that faculty come to grips with the health issues of the day. Many have even had academic or service experiences in the community during their premedical years. Most first-year students are ready to view the health problems in the community. They won't do it with the degree of medical sophistication that they might in their senior year, but it is important for medical faculties to seize upon the activist attitude of today's students and initiate the process of producing informed students of community medicine right at the outset. This should not consist of merely classroom exercise, although that may be a valuable additional exposure, but an arrangement whereby each student spends a block period of time in the community, under guidance, is the key. Such a first-year program has been set up and is functioning effectively at the University of Massachusetts medical school.

Along with the pioneering fourth-year field program, a second-year course in epidemiology at Kentucky was a model that could be profitably reviewed in planning programs for other schools. It consisted of 15 to 25 weekly sessions of three hours each in which, serially, the students covered the approach, strategy, methods, content, and uses of epidemiology, ranging from infectious and noninfectious diseases to accidents, to population problems, mental health, and so on. This course was so oriented that community medicine was seen to have a scientific underpinning and content. It utilized educational techniques that put learning at a premium as opposed to teaching. At each three-hour session, faculty presented lectures which were followed by at least two hours of seminar in which the students would not only review the best (and sometimes the worst) in scientific literature related to epidemiologic problems, but could also discuss, as the group saw fit, points that were raised in a particular session.

However, this second-year course did not include a detailed

consideration of the management of community ills—a topic that might be entitled "medical care and its connotations." Therefore, at Massachusetts the second-year course includes diagnosis and management of community-health problems in a classroom course. This gives students ample opportunity to learn the scientific approach to diagnosing and managing disease problems in the community after being exposed to these problems during the first-year field program. The second-year course is given in the second half of that year. It is introduced at a time when the students are well along in their pathology course and will have completed a course in microbiology. Such timing is important.

When the methods and principles of epidemiology are taught before medical students have actually had any courses concerned with disease, the overall outcome tends to be weaker than if placed later in the curriculum. Before epidemiology can be made to come alive, students ought to know something about disease. When we have tried to teach the course without their having such knowledge, we discovered we were spending an inordinate amount of time in defining and discussing disease and disease processes —giving them a particular clinical picture—before we could talk about the epidemiology of the disease. Also, students were more desirous of learning the clinical features of a particular disease problem, not its epidemiology. As the subject concerned numerators in relation to denominators, and as they knew very little about the characteristics of the numerator, it was difficult to talk about denominators, rates, and associations. Epidemiology should be taught when the time is ripe, and the time may not be ripe until the latter part of the second year (as many medical curricula are now structured).

During the second-year course the basic concepts and principles of epidemiology may be presented. If students know something about the numerator, the concept of the denominator can be brought home again and again by numerous examples. The place of epidemiology in the investigation of disease; the epidemiologic concept of cause; the strategy of epidemiology (that is, how one may conceptually begin by describing a disease in a population according to time, place, and person parameters, progress to testing for hypothesized factors in causation through analytic approaches, and then attempt to confirm hypotheses through experimental epidemiology) may be outlined. Measurement of disease frequency; sources of mortality and morbidity data; characteristics of people by age, sex, or ethnic group; and consideration of diseases in different places and over different time periods are repeatedly covered as the student sequentially progresses from the easier-to-understand problems of infectious disease to those of chronic disease causation via case-control and cohort studies or experimental studies. If the course is given at the same time that students are being introduced to clinical medicine, and after they have had considerable experience in laboratory medicine, they may be able to see the relationship between the laboratory, the clinic, the bedside, and the community.

Discussions about the relationship of human attitudes and behavior as major determinants of disease can be brought out in regard to any particular disease problem. The fact that this is an applied science, and that it is through the practical application of existing knowledge that disease is controlled in a community, is something that should be repeatedly emphasized. Whenever the concept of causation is introduced, multifactorial causation should receive full discussion. The other principle to be stressed in such a course is that facts should determine action. Although in the epidemiologic approach the hypothesis is central, before knowledge can be applied to control disease in a population, knowledge must be available.

One benefit of a major course in epidemiology is that it affords opportunity to examine priorities in medicine. The answers that epidemiology gives to questions about priorities in medical care, in terms of incidence, prevalence, high-risk groups, cost-efficiency, diagnosis, treatment, and so on, are scientific answers which command respect. As Stewart notes, for primary prevention of diseases that are the result of cultural deprivation and alienation, and when "affluence and prejudice jostle unemployment and nihilism as the setting for social diseases," we cannot rely as much on basic or clinical science as we can on social and educational enlightenment (5). In addition, secondary and tertiary prevention depend upon early diagnosis, counseling, and prompt effective treatment. If this conception of comprehensive medicine is to come from the practicing primary physician, he has to be better prepared than his predecessors have been. In order to prepare him, a significant proportion of his medical education has to be concerned with the area of community medicine, particularly its basic sciences of epidemiology and medical care, for priorities rest on quantitative reasoning as well as on a particular value system.

The third year may be the best time to emphasize clinical epidemiology. As the student works with patients in the hospital and in the clinic, he should begin to imitate the approach of the clinical epidemiologist. This could more readily be done if members of the clinical departments also viewed their patients in an epidemiologic sense. Until most clinical teachers embrace epidemiology in their thinking and teaching, it will remain the role of a department of community medicine to supplement clinical teaching with clinical epidemiology. As students study individual patients, they should review the principles of viewing the family as the basic biosocial unit of society, replete with factors that bear on disease problems in the individual patient, and which in turn reverberate on the family. This may be done in many ways, such as having the student carry out a family study with every third, fourth, or fifth patient that he works up. It might be done throughout clinical clerkships on medicine, pediatrics, psychiatry, obstetrics, gynecology, and surgery. In case presentations, the student should be ready to review the home and community situation in its relationship to the patient. The fundamental need is for conjoint teaching between the department of community medicine and the other clinical departments. Similarly, second-year epidemiology could be taught in an integrated manner with the introduction of medicine. It could be interdigitated to the degree that students learn epidemiologic content in relation to the same specific diseases they are learning from the clinical perspective.

The fourth-year field program at Massachusetts is similar to the senior year program described above. That is, students study total communities and their health problems and learn to understand how these problems are being met and what might be done to improve the situation. In addition, they study particular disease problems in detail via the epidemiologic approach. They apply clinical epidemiology in the home situation as it bears on the individual and family disease problem seen by community physicians or other health workers, and they perform a descriptive epidemiologic study of the pattern of disease in the community. This is done in conjunction with other student health workers. For example, nursing students, social work students, and students from the allied health fields may all work together, observing community health problems from their various vantage points; they may work in communities as teams in order to learn to appreciate their respective roles and how teamwork might function in the future.

CRITICAL QUESTIONS IN DESIGNING THE EPIDEMIOLOGY COMPONENT OF A MEDICAL SCHOOL CURRICULUM

The foregoing discussion outlines the way community medicine and its basic sciences of epidemiology and medical care are taught in some medical schools—a small and biased sample. In conclusion, there are certain considerations that ought to be made when proposing a program in epidemiology for any medical school (7).

In the development of an epidemiology course, the first question that should be asked is: What are the proposed goals of the course? Specifically, what types of changes are sought in medical students with regard to knowledge, skills, and attitudes? In the case of knowledge, what information should they have in epidemiology? Should they have a minimal amount or should they have enough to give them a critical understanding of the entire field? In regard to skills, should they become acquainted only with the fact that an epidemiologist goes through a certain strategic approach as he unravels a problem? That is, should the aim be for them to develop a personal capacity to utilize epidemiologic techniques for specific purposes? Or that they merely be well acquainted with this approach? With regard to attitudes, when they finish the course should they have developed a particular philosophy which might be viewed as the epidemiologic approach to thinking about disease in the individual as well as the community? Should they have developed a particular value system which affects their personal priorities both in the private practice of medicine and as they relate to the health problems of the larger community?

Having decided the types of changes that are desirable in these three areas and the degree of change that should be expected in students, would such changes be sought in the average student, all students, or just a handful of them? Would the aim be for them to pursue a career in family medicine or community medicine or to make them better practicing physicians in whatever clinical area they may go into?

Secondly, what components would be assembled for the development of this course? One of the components, of course, would be the set of proposed goals outlined above. But would the knowledge to be gained be covered by a set of major topics, within which subtopics are chosen, or would the waterfront be briefly surveyed, or would a couple of topics be covered in great and elaborate detail in an attempt to influence attitudes and develop skills? Would this be accomplished through the exploration of a few specific situations or a wide variety? What materials would be used? Would textbook assignments be made? Would the entire range of audiovisual aids, including motion pictures, slides, programmed learning, case materials, and operating models be employed? Would methods independent of the material be used, for example, role playing or interviewing?

Thirdly, what constraints would there be in setting up the course? At the beginning, how much education will the students already have had? Will they be required to have had biostatistics before entering medical school? If not, will a course in biostatistics be presented before epidemiology? Or with it? What have they had in the social sciences? Will these be taught in conjunction with epidemiology or community medicine? Will they be a part of the course in epidemiology? Not only what education have the students had before medical school, but what experience have they had? Have they, like some of our students now, worked in communities as premedical students? How mature are they? How do they compare with the students of five years ago? Basically of course, there would be concern with their intellectual capacity, their achievement ability, their motivation, and how they relate to other students.

Should the consumer of medical education, that is, the medical student, be involved from the beginning in planning and in evaluating course work? If we are to help the student initiate a process of lifelong self-education, then the principles of self-scrutiny, criticism, and evaluation should be imbued from the beginning. Along this line, what kind of an evaluation mechanism should be established? Whether there is a division of medical education for the school or not, there is need for an evaluation process whereby content, teaching methods, demands on faculty and students, administrative organization and arrangement for teaching programs, and the place of the teaching program in the curriculum as a whole undergo a continual process of evaluation and review.

What limitations would there be in choice of methods and materials available? That is, will there be any administrative decision that would limit use of video tapes or programmed instruction? Will there be times in which equipment is not available? How much money will the students and faculty be able to spend on something that would require expenses such as the field program? And what is the limitation in budget for the course in terms of the faculty, the staff, and available facilities and equipment? One other constraint that cannot be forgotten is the possible opposition from administration or other chairmen or faculty or even students as to what is being done and therefore why this amount of time should be made available.

Fourthly, the actual selection of components requires a careful review of goals. Will those who are chosen to teach be interested and inspiring teachers? Will lecturers or discussion leaders be sufficiently stimulating? Will assigned readings be of high quality? Will there be any training in the skill of asking questions when interviewing, in designing questions, or in logic? Will the student be shown examples of skills used in dealing with complex social problems such as those that arise out of complicated case histories in medical sociology or administration? Will a combination of teaching methods such as lectures, textbook assignments, and the use of problem materials and programmed instruments be employed? And will the idea that the course focuses on a learning experience, rather than simply content transmission, be emphasized? Will such procedures as handing out written copies of lectures be considered? Will the class be divided into small groups for some of their learning and experience? What will be the sequence of courses in the curriculum? Will there be consideration that it might be more desirable for the student to have biostatistics, pathology, and microbiology before classroom epidemiology? Where would the field experiences best be placed if they were being considered?

Revisions of course objectives may well be necessary in light of the answers to these questions. A likely outcome is that more will have been planned than the allotted time allows and that paring will be necessary. The expectations for achievement of knowledge, skills, and attitudes by the students may have to be curtailed. Rather than watering down a particular aspect of the course, should that section be dropped? Sometimes a little is not worth doing. If the presentation would be superficial, that part of the course may better be omitted.

After all these years, there are still few people devoted to the review and research of educational methods—an ironic fact when one considers the stature of our educational institutions. But it would be especially tragic if, in light of the need for continual review and updating of teaching methods that is necessitated by the rapidly changing health issues and problems that confront us, those who teach epidemiology should fail to apply their science to the study of how it should be taught. And as an applied science, how effectively can epidemiology be taught if divorced from the classroom of application, the community?

REFERENCES

1. Deuschle, K., Fulmer, H., McNamara, M., and Tapp, J. The Kentucky experiment in community medicine. *Milbank Memorial Fund Quarterly,* 1966, *44,* 9-22.
2. MacMahon, B., and Pugh, T. F. *Epidemiology—Principles and methods.* Boston: Little, Brown and Company, 1970.
3. Paul, J. *Clinical epidemiology.* Chicago: The University of Chicago Press, 1966.
4. Pickles, W. N. *Epidemiology in country practice.* Baltimore: Williams and Wilkins Company, 1939.
5. Stewart, G. T. Epidemiologic approach to assessment of health. *Lancet,* 1970, ii, 115-119.
6. White, K. L., Williams, T. F., and Greenberg, B. G. The ecology of medical care. *New England Journal of Medicine,* 1961, *265,* 885.
7. Penchansky, R., ed. *Health services administration—Policy cases and the case method.* Cambridge, Massachusetts: Harvard University Press, 1968.

ADDITIONAL READINGS

Epidemiology

1. Anderson, J. A. D. *A new look at social medicine.* London: Pitman Medical Publishing Company, Ltd., 1965. Chapter 6, pp. 55-64, Social medicine as an instrument of research; Chapter 7, pp. 65-75, Teaching social medicine.
2. Bothwell, P. W. *A new look at preventive medicine.* London: Pitman Medical Publishing Company, Ltd., 1965.
3. Clark, D. W., and MacMahon, B., eds. *Preventive medicine.* Boston: Little, Brown and Company, 1967. Part I, Methods in preventive medicine, Chapters 2-7, pp. 11-104.
4. Fox, J. P., Hall, C. E., and Elveback, L. R. *Epidemiology: Man and disease.* London: The Macmillan Company, 1970.
5. Kilbourne, E. D., and Smillie, W. G., eds. *Human ecology and public health.* London: The Macmillan Company, Collier-Macmillan Ltd., 1969. Chapter 1, pp. 7-28, Demography, culture, and economics and the evolutionary stages of medicine; Chapter 6, pp. 125-150, Epidemiology.
6. King, M., ed. *Medical care in developing countries.* London: Oxford University Press, 1966. Chapter 5, An approach to public health.
7. Morris, J. N. *Uses of epidemiology,* 2nd ed. Baltimore: William and Wilkins Company, 1967.
8. Sartwell, P. E., ed. *Preventive medicine and public health.* New York: Appleton-Century-Crofts, 1966. Chapter 1, pp. 1-9, Epidemiology;

Chapter 2, pp. 20-44, Statistical reasoning; Chapter 3, pp. 45-75, The health of a population; Chapter 4, pp. 76-106, General epidemiology of infections.

9. Susser, M. *Causal thinking in the health sciences*. New York: Oxford University Press, 1973.

Biostatistics

1. Arkin, H., and Colton, R. R. *Tables for statisticians*, 2nd ed. New York: Barnes and Noble, 1969.
2. Bancroft, H. *Introduction to biostatistics*. New York: Paul B. Hoeber, Inc., 1957.
3. Hill, B. *Principles of medical statistics*, 8th ed. New York: Oxford University Press, 1967.
4. Huff, D. *How to lie with statistics*. New York: W. W. Norton and Company, Inc., 1954.
5. Maroney, M. J. *Facts from figures*, 3rd ed. Great Britain: Penguin Books, 1951.
6. Oldham, P. D. *Measurement in medicine*. Philadelphia: J. B. Lippincott Company, 1968.
7. Wallis, W. A., and Roberts, H. V. *The nature of statistics*. New York: The Free Press, 1968.
8. Witts, L. J. *Medical surveys and clinical trials*, 2nd ed. London: Oxford University Press, 1964.

AFTERWORD

Throughout this book there has been a recurrent theme which underlines the limitations of medical care in affecting health. This conclusion is not intended as a scathing criticism of the health care system. Rather, it is the result of a shift in perspective. If one looks at the health care system from the vantage point of the provider, one sees only the patients who present themselves for care. Some of these can be helped and some cannot. However, if one focuses on the community, the denominator becomes the entire population rather than only those who present themselves for care. Many in the community may never enter the system, perhaps because they do not give high priority to health care, perhaps because the obstacles placed in their way are too great. Of those who do get into the system, many are lost to follow-up after their initial entry, and the lack of effective outcomes is never appreciated by a system that may interpret failure to return for care as a sign of success.

Community medicine, then, provides a way whereby health professionals can keep their activities in context; that is, it provides a horizon upon which they can plot their own course on some relatively fixed points of reference. Because it does utilize this wide perspective, it often appears to be critical of many parts of the system. Such criticism should not be confused with antagonism, for it is born of the scientific method and of the rational interpretation of methodological observations.

It seems important that each health professional, whatever his discipline, develop a sense of context in which to better appreciate his own role. If that sense of context threatens to diminish one's self-image, the resulting threat to his professional ego may be justified on the ground that other forces may tend to magnify it out of proportion. Certainly the public has come to picture health care providers in a very positive way—whether we look at the increasing proportion of our gross national product being spent for health care, or the range of television heroes, or the amount of coverage given medical events in the press. This countervailing antidote may be perceived by some as a threat. It is certainly not intended as such. To the extent that a reasoned discussion threatens the dogmatic, community medicine may threaten some who hold steadfastly to their limited perceptions of the role of the health care system in today's society.

Community medicine then gives its practitioners a series of reference points for raising new questions and perhaps for challenging old answers. To its proponents it is an ever-changing, dynamic discipline, borrowing and synthesizing concepts and procedures from a variety of sources. To its detractors it sometimes appears ill-defined and uncertain, and often confusing. To its poets and philosophers it is "a star to every wandering bark, whose worth's unknown, although its height be taken."

Robert L. Kane

GLOSSARY

A

adequacy in the context of program evaluation, the degree to which a whole problem has been prevented or eliminated.

adjusted rate a single rate for the whole population based on projected rates for subgroups of that population.

age-adjustment the result of multiplying the age-specific rates serially by the number of individuals in the corresponding age band in a standardized population.

age-specific rate a rate in which population data are grouped according to age and rates calculated for each age group.

appropriateness the degree to which an objective is desirable.

artifactual association a false relationship due to bias, selection, or other faulty study techniques.

association the most general way of indicating that two variables are related. See also: **artifactual association, causal association, chance association**, and **secondary association.**

attack rate a special type of incidence rate (those persons who experienced the event, per unit population, per time interval of exposure), or of prevalence rate (persons having experienced an event as of termination of the time interval of exposure, per unit population).

secondary attack rate attack rate in those with known exposure to an infectious patient.

attributable risk the difference between two rates of a given condition; the rate in persons with a given characteristic minus the rate in persons without that characteristic (cf. **relative risk**). See also: **population attributable risk.**

B

bias any error in selection or classification that produces the invalid appearance of an association.

biochemical oxygen demand test (BOD) a test used for determining the relative oxygen requirements of municipal and industrial wastewaters.

C

case-control study an inquiry in which groups of individuals are selected in terms of whether they do (the cases) or do not (the controls) have the disease of which the etiology is to be studied; the groups are then compared with respect to the existing or past characteristics judged to be of possible relevance to the etiology of the disease.

case fatality rate a disease-specific measure of the frequency of death; the number of persons dying of a specific disease during a stated period divided by the total number of persons with the disease. See also: **rate.**

cause something that, if prevented, removed, or eliminated, will prevent the occurrence of the event in question, and/or, if permitted, introduced, or maintained, will be followed by the event in question.

necessary cause a condition that must exist if a given event is to occur or exist.

sufficient cause a condition whose existence is inevitably accompanied by a given event or the existence of a given thing.

causal association an inductively established relationship between two variables, one of which determines the other.

direct association a causal relationship without intermediary variables.

indirect association a causal relationship similar to the secondary association except that an arbitrary alteration of the independent variable does not produce a change in the dependent variable.

multifactorial association a causal relationship characterized by complex interaction of variables.

chance association a non-causal association which can be ruled out effectively by biostatistical tests of significance.

cluster analysis a commonly used method of detecting the presence of disease outbreaks by looking for aggregations in time and/or place.

cohort study a study in which a group is chosen for the presence of a specific characteristic or independent variable and followed over time for the appearance of a particular dependent variable (condition).

cohort effect a change in mortality or morbidity rates over time related to changing susceptibility of succeeding cohorts or to changes in the environment. See also: **secular trend.**

confounding an association between two variables that occurs because there exists a third variable that itself determines one of the two and is therefore associated with the other.

cost-benefit analysis a measure of the relationship between the cost of a project, in terms of resources, to its efficiency in accomplishing program objectives.

cost-effectiveness analysis a measure of the effects for the costs invested, when the costs and benefits cannot be measured in the same terms, e.g., dollars.

coverage the extent to which statistical measures are applied to each instance of the phenomenon of interest.

cross-sectional study an epidemiologic study in which the measurements of cause and effect are made at the same time.

crude rate a rate adjusted for only time or unit factors; a frequency measure of disease, or characteristic, expressed per unit of population in which the factor is observed. See also: **rate.**

D

dependent variable the condition or characteristic that is assumed to be preceded by or associated with the independent variable.

double blind technique a method that eliminates much of the conscious or unconscious bias of both subject and investigator by keeping them unaware of who is getting what specific treatment. Classically, this involves the use of the look-alike placebo in intervention studies.

E

ecologic fallacy an erroneous association between the characteristic of a group and a condition of that group when in fact the characteristic and condition do not necessarily coexist in any one individual within that group.

effectiveness a measure of the actual accomplishment of a program compared with the amount intended or planned, which may be less than total eradication or prevention. The effectiveness of a prophylactic measure is the percentage of cases expected in a population that are prevented by the measure.

efficiency a measure of the cost in resources necessary to accomplish the program's objectives, or the ratio between an output (net attainment of program objectives) and an input (program resources expended).

excess fertility the delivery of more children by a woman than she, her husband, or her family desires. **National excess fertility** is the birth of more children than the nation can feed, house, clothe, and educate in the ways consistent with accepted cultural values. The **excess level of fertility** is that number of births greater than the presumed ideal number of births.

experimental study an investigative technique that tests a cause-effect hypothesis by the deliberate application or withholding of the independent variable and observation of the effects on the dependent variable.

F

false positives cases wrongly diagnosed as having the disease characteristic/condition.

G

general fertility ratio (GFR) the number of births in a population during a specified time period divided by the number of females in the childbearing age group.

H

hypothesis a proposition set up for examination which purports to explain a given set of conditions; an assumption or theory to be tested.

I

incidence the number of *new* cases during a period of time (cf. **prevalence**).

independent variable a characteristic or condition under study that is assumed to precede or influence the appearance of another (altered) characteristic or condition.

interval scale an ordered list of mutually exclusive and collectively exhaustive categories with a systematic assignment of intervals but without a meaningful absolute reference point (cf. **nominal scale, ordinal scale, probability scale, ratio scale**).

L

longitudinal study an epidemiologic study in which the observations of cause and effect are made at two different points in time. Most cohort studies are longitudinal.

M

matching a study technique for neutralizing confounding variables. It matches each individual exposed with an unexposed individual who is identical with respect to all confounding factors.

Medicaid (Title 19) the program under federal law that provides payments for medical care services to recipients of categorical public assistance. This program is administered by the individual states, which in turn receive matching federal funds to support it.

Medicare (Title 18) an amendment to the Social Security Act, which provides a federal health insurance program to persons over 65 years of age and those younger with chronic disabilities. This program is funded and administered federally.

misclassification an error in assignment of variables to appropriate classes; a form of bias.

morbidity ratio a ratio of the sick/well in a given area; expressed in terms of population, usually 100,000. See also: **ratio.**

mortality rate (death rate) a measure of the frequency of death for a specified period of time, usually a year, in relation to the total population. See also: **rate.**

N

nominal scale an unordered list of mutually exclusive and collectively exhaustive categories (cf. **interval scale, ordinal scale, probability scale, ratio scale**).

O

observational study the non-experimental, non-interventional technique that may be used in case-control, cohort, and cross-sectional studies.

ordinal scale a list of mutually exclusive and collectively exhaustive categories amenable to and arranged in some logical order or rank, but without any systematically assigned intervals (cf. **interval scale, nominal scale, probability scale, ratio scale**).

P

person-years a way of simultaneously combining time and the number of units observed. Five persons for one year each and one person for five years are both equal to five person-years.

population attributable risk an estimate of the impact that a specific exposure may have on the total population with respect to a particular outcome and thus an estimate of the amount by which a particular disease might be reduced if the exposure were removed. See also: **attributable risk.**

population pyramid an age- and sex-specific prevalence histogram.

preciseness the extent to which a measurement technique discriminates between differences in magnitude.

presumptive evaluation an assessment of the process by which an effect is achieved based on data concerning the resources and activities of a program rather than its objectives.

prevalence the number of persons with a given condition in a population during a specified time (cf. **incidence**). Prevalence = Incidence × Duration.

period prevalence prevalence over a specified period of time.

point prevalence prevalence at one point in time.

prevention the avoidance of a disease and/or its morbid consequences.

primary prevention the actual prevention of a disease from occurring.

secondary prevention detection and early action taken to minimize the ramifications of the disease.

tertiary prevention that which we often call clinical medicine, i.e., treatment and the prevention of complications.

rehabilitation prevention only to the extent that it may discourage the development of sequelae that lead to further deterioration following the arrest of a disease process.

probability scale an ordered list of mutually exclusive and collectively exhaustive categories, with systematic assignment of intervals including a meaningful absolute reference point, but with the scale altered to reflect not only the relationship of each value to a reference point, but of the distribution of all values to a standard theoretical distribution (cf. **interval scale, nominal scale, ordinal scale, ratio scale**).

Professional Activity Survey—Medical Audit Program (PAS—MAP) an automated data reporting system that supplies information about hospital activities and diagnoses.

prospective study a study planned to observe events that have not yet occurred (cf. **retrospective study**). See also: **cohort study.**

R

randomization a method of selecting subjects that is unaffected by any characteristic of those subjects; the operation of chance is essential in achieving randomization.

rate a specifically defined subset of ratios, wherein the numerator is contained by the denominator. See also: **adjusted rate, age-specific rate, attack rate, case fatality rate, crude rate, mortality rate, specific rate.**

ratio a comparison of two sets, neither of which is wholly contained within the other (cf. **rate**). A ratio can be expressed as A/B while a rate can be expressed as A/(A + B). See also: **fertility ratio, morbidity ratio.**

ratio scale an ordered list of mutually exclusive and collectively exhaustive categories, with systematically assigned intervals having a meaningful absolute reference point. The actual quantity to which the ratio of "1 to 10" on the scale refers is the same as the actual quantity to which "40 to 400" on the scale refers (cf. **interval scale, nominal scale, ordinal scale, probability scale**).

relative risk (risk ratio) a ratio of the incidence of cases among those exposed to the risk or causal factor to the incidence among those not exposed (cf. **attributable risk**).

reliability the reproducibility of a result, i.e., how closely a second go-around would yield the same answer.

retrospective study a study that deals with persons who have already developed the condition and examines the record for the characteristic; often called the case-control study (cf. **prospective study**).

S

scope (generalizability) those conditions of time and space under which the statement holds true.

secondary association an apparent relationship between two unrelated variables because of mutual relation with a third factor.

secular trend (cohort effect) a change in mortality or morbidity rates over time related to changing susceptibility of succeeding cohorts or to changes in the environment.

selection the method for obtaining a population for study; usually used with the negative connotation of obtaining an unrepresentative group from a population.

sensitivity (of a predictor or a screening test) the proportion of true cases correctly identified. Sensitivity = True Positives ÷ (True Positives + False Negatives).

specific rate a rate for a segment of the population, selected by age, race, sex, or other characteristic.

specificity (of a predictor or a screening test) the percentage of healthy persons (true noncases) correctly assessed by a negative report as healthy. Specificity = True Negatives ÷ (True Negatives + False Positives).

stochastic predictive based on probabilities.

stratification a method of controlling for confounding variables by separating study subjects into layers or groups based on those variables. **prognostic stratification** separates patients into groups on the basis of severity with respect to effect upon outcome.

surveillance the process of gathering routine data for the purpose of identifying and responding to outbreaks.

T

threshold limit values (TLVs) safe exposure limits expressed as time-weighted, airborne concentrations that are set to protect nearly all workers who may be exposed eight hours a day, forty hours a week, and presumably for a working lifetime.

V

validity the degree to which the data actually assess the phenomenon of interest; the extent to which a situation as observed reflects the "true" situation, or the situation as evaluated by other criteria that are thought to reflect the true situation accurately.

INDEX